Statistical Methods for Quality of Life Studies

Statistical Methods for Quality of Life Studies

Design, Measurements and Analysis

Edited by

Mounir Mesbah
Université de Bretagne-Sud,
France

Bernard F. Cole
Dartmouth College,
U.S.A.

and

Mei-Ling Ting Lee
Harvard University,
U.S.A.

KLUWER ACADEMIC PUBLISHERS
DORDRECHT / BOSTON / LONDON

A C.I.P. Catalogue record for this book is available from the Library of Congress.

ISBN 1-4020-0142-8

Published by Kluwer Academic Publishers,
P.O. Box 17, 3300 AA Dordrecht, The Netherlands.

Sold and distributed in North, Central and South America
by Kluwer Academic Publishers,
101 Philip Drive, Norwell, MA 02061, U.S.A.

In all other countries, sold and distributed
by Kluwer Academic Publishers,
P.O. Box 322, 3300 AH Dordrecht, The Netherlands.

Printed on acid-free paper

Printed in the Netherlands.

Contents

Acknowledgements

The workshop and this volume would not have been possible without the hard work of many people. We thank Patrice Kermorvant, Jean-François Petiot, Jean Marie Tricot and Ion Grama for their help in organizing the workshop. We thank the University of Bretagne-Sud and The Regional Council of Bretagne for their financial support. We also thank the Association of French Speaking Epidemiologists, the French Group of Biometric Society and the Biopharmacy Group of the French Statistical Society for their support and cooperation. We are grateful to the authors and the many anonymous reviewers for their efforts in preparing the manuscripts in this volume. Finally, we thank André Gall, the mayor of the city of Arradon, as well as the city hall staff for their kind hospitality and for allowing our use of the conference center for the workshop. And last but not least, we thank the many people at the University of Bretagne-Sud who helped to organize the conference and ensure its success.

Preface

On October 16 and 17, 2000, we hosted an international workshop entitled "Statistical Design, Measurement, and Analysis of Health Related Quality of Life." The workshop was held in the beautiful city of Arradon, South Brittany, France with the main goal of fostering an interdisciplinary forum for discussion of theoretical and applied statistical issues arising in studies of health-related quality of life (HRQoL). Included were biostatisticians, psychometricians and public health professionals (e.g., physicians, sociologists, psychologists) active in the study of HRQoL.

In assembling this volume, we invited each conference participant to contribute a paper based on his or her presentation and the ensuing and very interesting discussions that took place in Arradon. All papers were peer-reviewed, by anonymous reviewers, and revised before final editing and acceptance. Although this process was quite time-consuming, we believe that it greatly improved the volume as a whole, making this book a valuable contribution to the field of HRQoL research.

The volume presents a broad spectrum of papers presented at the Workshop, and thus illustrates the range of current research related to the theory, methods and applications of HRQoL, as well as the interdisciplinary nature of this work. Following an introduction written by Sir David Cox, it includes 27 articles organized into the following chapters.

Chapter 1: Measurement, Scale Development and Study Design

Chapter 2: Analysis and Interpretation of Multiple Endpoints

Chapter 3: Item Response Theory and Rasch Models

Chapter 4: Joint Analysis of Quality of Life and Survival

Chapter 5: Quality-Adjusted Survival Analysis and Related Methods

Chapter 6: Methods for Informatively Missing Longitudinal Quality-of-Life Data

Chapter 1 covers many important issues related to developing a quality-of-life study, including the development and validation of tools for measuring HRQoL as well as study design considerations to ensure that, ultimately, the results from a HRQoL study will provide a useful interpretation. Chapter 2 describes methods for handling multiple endpoints that arise in nearly all HRQoL studies because of the inherent multi-dimensional nature of quality of life. Chapter 3 focuses on item response theory and the distilling of responses on many individual items (e.g., questions on a questionnaire) into useful scales. Included in this chapter is the important Rasch model for item response. Chapter 4 presents methods for combining survival data and HRQoL data in a joint analysis. These methods are especially useful in studies of fatal diseases, where survival time is a critical endpoint and the HRQoL information must be interpreted in light of a patient's time of death. Chapter 5 describes techniques for evaluating survival time after adjustment for the quality of life experienced. These methods are useful for comparing interventions that differ in their impact on both quality of life and survival time. Finally, Chapter 6 presents a variety of methods for handling the important problem of missing data in quality-of-life studies, particularly the case where the missingness is related to the actual, unobserved quality of life at the time of the planned assessment.

While each paper in this book is an individual advancement in the field of HRQoL study, we believe that the full value of this volume exceeds the sum of its individual parts. In large part, owing to the valuable discussions in Arradon, this volume represents enhanced connections between biostatistics, psychometry and economics, with contributions from methodologists, clinicians and health scientists in academia, industry and regulatory agencies. Nevertheless, we cannot claim to exhaust, or come anywhere near exhausting, the creative ideas for new and useful methods. In particular, additional attention can easily be paid to the following (which of course is only a partial list): Bayesian analysis and subjective probability considerations, decision theoretic perspectives, optimal design for quality-of-life measurement in the longitudinal context with occurrence of death, and the responsiveness of a quality-of-life instrument under the item response modeling theory.

We sincerely hope that this volume will serve as a valuable reference for current HRQoL researchers as well as encourage new researchers to work in this important area.

Mounir Mesbah, Bernard F. Cole and Mei-Ling Ting Lee, editors

April, 2002

Presenting Authors

The following authors of papers in this volume presented talks at the workshop, "Statistical Design, Measurement, and Analysis of Health Related Quality of Life," held October 16 and 17, 2000 in Arradon, South Brittany, France.

Lucile Awad
Aventis
Department of Biostatistics, Tri N 13
20, rue Raymond Aron
92 165, Antony Cedex
France
Tel: +33 1 55 71 41 47
E-mail: lucile.awad@aventis.com

Serge Briançon
Ecole de Santé Publique
9 avenue de la Forêt de Haye
BP 184
F 54505 Vandoeuvre les Nancy Cedex
France
Tel: +33 (0) 3 83 59 25 89
Fax: +33 (0) 3 83 59 26 90
E-mail: briancon@sante-pub.u-nancy.fr

David Cella
Institute for Health Services Research and Policy Studies
Center on Outcomes, Research and Education
Northwestern University
1000 Central Street, Suite 101
Evanston, Illinois 60201
USA
Tel: +1 (847) 570-1730
Fax: +1 (847) 570-1735
E-mail: d-cella@nwu.edu

Michel Chavance
Inserm U472
Hôpital Paul Brousse
94 807 Villejuif Cedex
France
Tel: +33 1 45 59 50 63
Fax: +33 1 45 59 51 69
E-mail: chavance@vjf.inserm.fr

Arin Judith Chwalow
INSERM Unité 341
Service de Diabétologie, Hôtel-Dieu
1, Place du Parvis Notre Dame
75181 Paris Cedex 04
France
Tel: +33 1 42 34 84 02
Fax: +33 1 56 24 84 29
E-mail: judith.chwalow@htd.ap-hop-paris.fr

Bernard F. Cole
Dartmouth-Hitchcock Medical Center
7927 Rubin Building
Lebanon, New Hampshire 03756
USA
Tel: +1 (603) 650-7247
Fax: +1 (603) 650-6485
E-mail: bernard.cole@dartmouth.edu

David R. Cox
Nuffield College
New Road
Oxford OX1 1NF
United Kingdom
Tel: +44 1865 278 690
Fax: +44 1865 278 621
E-mail: david.cox@nuf.ox.ac.uk

Dominique Dubois
Janssen Resaerch Foundation
Turnhoutseweg 30
B-2340 Beerse
Belgium
Tel: +32 14 60 3003
Fax: +32 14 60 54 25
E-mail: ddubois@janbe.jnj.com

Jean-François Dupuy
Laboratoire Sabres
IUP de Vannes-Tohannic
rue Yves Mainguy
56 000 Vannes
France
Tel: +33 (0) 2 97 68 32 43
Fax: +33 (0) 2 97 68 32 26
E-mail: jean-francois.dupuy@univ-ubs.fr

Diane Fairclough
AMC Cancer Research Center
1600 Pierce Street
Denver, Colorado 80214
USA
Tel: +1 (303) 239-3406
Fax: +1 (303) 239-3394
E-mail: fairclough@amc.org

Francis Guillemin
Ecole de Santé Publique
9 avenue de la Forêt de Haye
BP 184
F 54505 Vandoeuvre les Nancy Cedex
France
Tel: +33 (0) 3 83 85 21 63
Fax: + 33 (0) 3 83 59 26 90
E-mail: francis.guillemin@sante-pub.u-nancy.fr

Clare Gnecco
U.S. Food and Drug Administration
1401 Rockville Pike
HFM-215
Rockville MD 20852
USA
E-mail: gnecco@cber.fda.gov

Agnes Hamon
Unité de Biostatistique
Pavillon Pillore
Hôpital Charles Nicolle
Chu de Rouen
1 rue de Germont
76031 Rouen Cedex
France
Tel: +33 (0) 2 32 88 83 86
Fax: + 33 (0) 2 32 88 64 29
E-mail: hamon.agnes@chu-rouen.fr

Natacha Heutte
Université de Paris V
Laboratoire de Statistique Médicale
45 rue des Saints Pères
75006 Paris
France
Tel: +33 (0) 1 42 86 33 57
E-mail: heutte@biomedicale.univ-paris5.fr

Andrew Kramar
CRLC Val D'Aurelle
Unité de Biostatistique
rue des Apothicaires
Parc Euro Médecine
34 298 Montpellier Cedex 5
France
Tel: +33 (0) 4 67 61 31 61
Fax: + 33 (0) 4 67 61 37 18
E-mail: akramar@valdorel.fnclcc.fr

Svend Kreiner
University of Copenhagen
Deptartment of Biostatistics
PANUM
Blegdamsvej 3
DK-2200 Copenhagen N
Denmark
Tel: +45 35 32 75 97
Fax: +45 35 32 79 07
E-mail: s.kreiner@biostat.ku.dk

Catherine Le Galès
INSERM U357
Hôpital de Bicêtre/Pavillon de la Force
78 rue du Général Leclerc
94275 Le Kremlin-Bicêtre Cedex
France
Tel: +33 (0) 1 49 59 19 70
Fax: +33 (0) 1 46 71 32 70
E-mail: legales@kb.inserm.fr

Peter Lachenbruch
U.S. Food and Drug Administration
1401 Rockville Pike
HFM-215
Rockville, Maryland 20852
USA
Tel: +1 (301) 827-6055
Fax: +1 (301) 827-3529
E-mail: lachenbruch@a1.cber.fda.gov

Mei-Ling Ting Lee
Department of Medicine
Channing Laboratory
181 Longwood Avenue
Boston, Massachusetts 02115-5804
USA
Tel: +1 (617) 525-2732
Fax: +1 (617) 731-1541
E-mail: stmei@channing.harvard.edu

Ivo W. Molenaar
Rijkuniversteit Groningen
Vakgroep Statistiek en Meettheorie
Grote Kruisstraat 2/I
9712 TS Groningen
Netherlands
Tel: +31 50-3636185
Fax: +31 50-3636304
E-mail: w.molenaar@ppsw.rug.nl

Geert Molenberghs
Limburg Universitair Centrum
Department of Biostatistics
B-3590 Diepenbeek
Belgium
Tel: +32 11 26 82 38
Fax: +32 11 26 82 99
E-mail: gmolenb@luc.ac.be

Geoff Norman
Clinical Epidemiology and Biostatistics
Health Sciences Centre, Room 2C14
McMaster University
1200 Main Street W
Hamilton, Ontario L8N 3Z5
Canada
Tel: +1 (905) 525-9140 x22119
Fax: +1 (905) 577-0017
E-mail: norman@mcmaster.ca

Dennis A. Revicki
MEDTAP International
7101 Wisconsin Avenue, Suite 600
Bethesda, Maryland 20814
USA
Tel: +1 (301) 664-7261
Fax: +1 (301) 654-9864
E-mail: revicki@medtap.com

Pranab K. Sen
Department of Biostatistics
University of North Carolina
Chapel Hill, North Carolina 27599-7400
USA
Tel: +1 (919) 966-7274
Fax: +1 (919) 966-3804
E-mail: pksen@bios.unc.edu

Pascale Tuber-Bitter
Inserm U472
Hôpital Paul Brousse
94 807 Villejuif Cedex
France
Tel: + 33 (0) 1 45 59 52 62
Fax: + 33 (0) 1 45 59 51 69
E-mail: tubert@vjf.inserm.fr

Hans C. van Houwelingen
Leiden University
Department Medische Statistiek
PO 9604 Leiden
2300 RC Leiden
Netherlands
Phone: +31 71 527 68 26
E-mail: jcvanhouwelingen@lumc.nl

Samuel Wieand
NSABP Biostatistics Center
230 McKee Place, Suite 403
Pittsburgh, Pennsylvania 15213
USA
Tel: +1 (412) 383-2243
Fax: +1 (412) 383-1387
E-mail: wieand@nsabp.pitt.edu

Janet Wittes
Statistics Collaborative, Inc.
1710 Rhode Island Avenue, NW; Suite 200
Washington, DC 20036
USA
Tel: +1 (202) 429-9267
Fax: +1 (202) 429-9268
E-mail: janet@statcollab.com

Margaret C. Wu
6 Spruce Tree Court
Bethesda, MD 20814
Tel: +1 (301) 564-6699
Fax: +1 (301) 564-9666
E-mail: mcjwu@aol.com

Introduction

David R. Cox

INTRODUCTION

DAVID R. COX

Nuffield College

Professor Mounir Mesbah and his colleagues are to be warmly congratulated first on organizing in Arradon a most stimulating and enjoyable meeting and then, with remarkably few missing values, compiling and editing the papers into this comprehensive volume.

There is a temptation in these introductory remarks to try and comment on every paper. I have managed to resist this temptation. All the papers, however, merit careful discussion, as indeed occurred at Arradon. I shall instead concentrate on a few themes chosen if not at random certainly somewhat arbitrarily.

The great majority of the papers argue or implicitly accept that health-related quality of life is a multidimensional concept and that this multidimensionality is to be preserved in analysis and interpretation. Of course, in particular applications special aspects will be of concern, for example in patients undergoing hip surgery the issue of pain will predominate, although even then the analysis may require more than one dimension. See, in particular, the paper of S. Briançon et al. A different view is, of course, taken in health economic studies of resource allocation and in the overall assessment of the impact of health care, where reduction to units such as the QALY (quality-adjusted life year) or the DALY (disability-adjusted life year) is commonly made. The paper of C. Le Gallès discusses the application of multi-attribute utility theory to the construction of a single preference-based index. This is a very important if extremely difficult field, with implications for resource allocation far beyond the health fields. In particular, it seems desirable that if different groups of respondents have radically different and indeed conflicting disinterested priorities decisions taken should if possible respect the interests of various groups.

More broadly, dimension-reduction is a recurring theme in the analysis and interpretation of empirical data on complex phenomena. The extensive economic literature on index-numbers is rarely considered in the statistical world, by and large for good reason. P.K. Sen's contribution brings out parallels with the literature on poverty indices in welfare economics. A serious problem is that difficult but unavoidable choices of the relative weight to put on different features cannot really be bypassed by formalistic specifications of structure.

The broader implication is the need to distinguish distinct purposes for the use of these instruments. The helpful statement by C. Gnecco and P. Lachenbruch that the Food and Drug Administration's (USA) attitude to these issues inevitably and correctly involves some element of rigidity. It is to be hoped that this rigidity does not carry over into other areas of application. J. Wittes's very thoughtful paper

M. Mesbah et al. (eds.), Statistical Methods for Quality of Life Studies, 3–5.

addresses difficult issues of translating the results of instruments into clinically meaningful information. The possible role of such instruments in monitoring the progress of and adjusting the therapies of individual patients does not seem to have been addressed either in this volume or very much elsewhere.

The clear formal connection between the analysis of quality of life instruments and psychometric studies more generally is the theme of several papers. S. Kreiner and K.B. Christensen's important paper relates the Rasch model to the currently very popular topic of Markov graphs as incisive representations of independencies among a set of variables. It leads on to a constructive and critical approach to the isolation of discrepant items. I.W. Molenaar emphasizes a nonparametric development. A. Hamon and M. Mesbah discuss the connections between classical measurement theory and the Rasch model, including the role of Cronbach's alpha as a general measure of reliability. A general issue in all these discussions is that, especially in dimensions with a relatively small number of items, the individual items are likely to be of intrinsic interest. This contrasts with educational testing where individual items are unlikely to be of concern. If the individual items are essentially unlikely to be interpreted on their own there are, of course, powerful reasons for making the instruments simple by keeping the number of items per dimension small.

Continuous rating scales, typically 10 cm lines, seem to be out of favour, although one or two papers mention them in passing. One possible advantage of them is that even if the final analysis is say on a 5 or even 3 point scale the division points can be chosen in the light of the data and yet at least some element of inter-study comparability can be preserved.

Quite a number of the papers were more technical statistically. Not surprisingly some dealt with missing values in this context and with the issue of informative "drop-outs." Some of these papers follow a longish line of argument stemming originally from the econometric literature. This is to postulate a model for the observed responses and explanatory variables supplemented by an assumed dependence on missing future responses. When marginalized over these latter variables the induced model is of different form than the original model. That is, a lack of fit of the original model is induced. Essentially if the appropriate lack of fit is observed it is interpreted as informative drop-out. The difficulty with this argument is that it depends crucially on the adequacy of the originating model. Therefore, there should be strong external evidence for that adequacy, or a sensitivity analysis should be performed to judge the dependence on other types of failure, for example distortions of distributional form. The contrasting pattern mixture models described and illustrated by G. Molenberghs *et al.* are appealing mathematically but seem somewhat contrived unless there are indeed two "natural" groups of patients, non droppers out and droppers out.

Another technically very interesting theme, well represented in the book, is the combination of quality of life and survival data. Here the most natural approach for many purposes is to describe first the distribution of survival time and its dependence on explanatory variables and then to discuss the conditional distribution of quality of life trajectory conditional on survival time, for example separately within different treatment arms. It is known that the tempting possibility of using the Kaplan-Meier method directly to assess a monotone development in a single measure of quality of life is biased, essentially because censoring uninformative in time is in general informative on the artificially induced time scale.

Finally, as in so many areas of work the construction of suitable measuring devices is crucial to the securing of accurate and repeatable conclusions and these design issues are discussed in a valuable group of papers. I conclude by repeating congratulations to all those involved in the organization of the meeting in Arradon and this book.

Chapter 1

Measurement, Scale Development and Study Design

REGULATORY ASPECTS OF QUALITY OF LIFE

CLARE GNECCO AND PETER A. LACHENBRUCH

U. S. Food and Drug Administration, Center for Biologics Evaluation and Research

We discuss some issues in using quality of life endpoints in studies that will lead to an application to license a product or add an indication to an already licensed product. Studies of this sort should be double blinded, randomized and use validated questionnaires. The duration of the study should be appropriate for the indication. Missing values can be a serious problem and plans for handling them should be included. Sensitivity analyses are important in this context. An example of a sensitivity analysis shows how substitutions for missing values can offer insight into the effect of these missing values. An alternative model is given to analyze data of this sort. Other analytic methods are discussed in the second part of the paper. The views and opinions expressed in this paper are those of the authors and do not necessarily represent those of the Food and Drug Administration.

1. Introduction

Health related quality of life (HRQOL) studies can provide supporting evidence to a regulatory agency for a labeling indication for a pharmaceutical product. The product may be a synthesized drug, a biological therapeutic product, or a device. The issues largely revolve around issues of experimental design, instrument design, and analysis. In this paper, we discuss issues in using quality of life endpoints in the regulatory setting. It may be noted that the U.S. Food and Drug Administration (FDA) does not consider pharmacoeconomic issues in licensing, and we will not consider them in this paper. However, we note that these are often widely discussed in utilization reviews and by the manufacturers.

HRQOL is an ill-defined term. The World Health Organization defines health as "a state of complete physical, mental and social well-being, and not merely the absence of disease." Thus, HRQOL will measure these three (or four) components. HRQOL may be broadly measured as a response to one or more questionnaires. Validation of the questionnaire is a complex issue that is discussed in other contributions to this volume and in many other sources in the psychometric literature. The questionnaires may be related to general health or a specific health issue. Some examples of questionnaires are listed below.

ADL	Activities of Daily Living general health questionnaire
ESSI	A seven item questionnaire on social support
EORTC QLQ-30	A 30 item questionnaire for cancer clinical trials
FACT-An	A 13 item subscale of the FACT (for cancer trials) for anemia
HAQ	Health Assessment Questionnaire – used in arthritis studies
PAR-Q	A questionnaire relating to readiness for physical activities

M. Mesbah et al. (eds.), Statistical Methods for Quality of Life Studies, 9–19.

SAQ	The Seattle Angina Questionnaire (20 questions)
SDS	A symptom distress scale (18 questions)
SF-36	The RAND Corporation 36 item questionnaire on general health

Many dimensions of quality of life can be measured. These may include general health, physical functioning (can the subject accomplish basic activities?), social function (support networks), mental health (depression, anxiety, etc.). The questionnaires should be validated within the context they will be used. For example, a scale that has been shown "valid" for patients with cardiovascular disease may not be appropriate for cancer patients. Investigators may not know this unless an attempt is made to study the questionnaire in the oncology setting. A series of anecdotes cannot serve as a measure of QOL, although such a series can serve as the basis for selecting or developing an instrument.

2. Measurement Issues

2.1 Design

Because responses to questionnaires are usually subjective, there is a substantial potential for a biased response if the subject is aware of his or her treatment. To minimize this bias, studies should be conducted in a double-blinded manner. In some cases, side effects or laboratory results can unblind the investigator or patient. In addition, differing dose schedules make blinding difficult (e.g., in a cancer trial that evaluates two different chemotherapy cycle lengths). If unblinding is a concern, the questionnaire may be administered by a study assistant who remains masked to the treatment. Alternatively, the questionnaire may be self-administered or computer-administered. This can remove the effect of possible investigator cues to the subject, but cannot remove bias due to known and predictable side effects that unblind the patient. Comparator groups are important in this context. If the standard of care has similar side effects, this can reduce the potential for bias. Informed consent documents are required to disclose known side effects, making it easier for patients to determine their treatment. Note that comparator groups can be standard of care, active controls, or placebos if their use is deemed ethical. Most often, a "no treatment" arm is not used because of the ethical concerns. Thus, an active control or a standard of care arm is used.

If HRQOL is a secondary endpoint, the sample size of the study will have been driven by the primary endpoint, presumably without adjustment for multiple testing associated with the HRQOL comparisons. In the conservative sense, if all of the type I error rate (α) is concentrated on the primary endpoint, then the HRQOL comparisons are considered exploratory. Alternatively, the primary endpoint can be viewed as a gatekeeper and comparisons of HRQOL can be done only if a significant treatment effect is observed in terms of the primary endpoint. This controls the α level of the study. If there are many secondary endpoints (e.g., many subscales of the HRQOL instrument), adjustment for testing of multiple endpoints should be done.

2.2 Interpretation

The regulatory agency will want to understand the meaning of the HRQOL response and interpret it in the context of the disease. For this reason, any HRQOL instrument should be described and submitted to the regulatory agency. The scoring system needs to be understood by the regulatory group. Submitting the instrument's scoring manual can be helpful to the regulatory agency. References from peer-reviewed publications can discuss the validation of the instrument. If pertinent, additional studies in a relevant patient population may be submitted so that a meaningful assessment of the instrument's performance in that group can be done.

2.3 Reliability and Validity

Reliability and validation issues continually arise in HRQOL studies. It is well known that the validity of an instrument depends on many factors including the method of administration, culture, language, and type of disease. For example, a measure of neurologic function, which consists of listing as many words as possible that begin with a given letter, depends on the subject's native language. Similarly, questions relating to social support in the elderly might be answered differently by individuals having access to universal health care versus those that do not. If a measure has not been used in a disease population before, it will be important to establish the measure's reliability and validity before using it in a phase III study. Thus, a depression questionnaire appropriate in a normal population may not be appropriate in a population with rheumatoid arthritis (RA). One study (Berkanovic and Hurwicz, 1990, Hurwicz and Berkanovic, 1993) found that twice as many RA patients scored in the depressed range than did normal subjects. Is this evidence of clinical depression in these patients or a realistic assessment of their life condition? If one of the major questions of interest is to show that a new treatment has a positive effect on depression, then evidence of depression should be an eligibility criterion. In addition, a comparator group becomes essential since the depression scale may be elevated in the population. The goal of the study may be to demonstrate a change in the depression scale, or it may be to show that fewer patients in the treated group are depressed following therapy as compared to the control group. These may be quite distinct outcomes. A scale that gives results about general health may not encompass responses related to social support or mental health.

Many HRQOL scales are proprietary, and their scoring algorithms are not available to the public. This may be problematic if the agency wishes to examine them. The FDA must maintain confidentiality of all submissions, so if the proprietor of the HRQOL scale wishes to submit the scoring algorithm directly to the agency, it is possible to maintain the proprietary nature of the scale.

A HRQOL instrument must be valid in the population being studied. Validity is usually established in a separate study conducted prior to the phase III study and in the appropriate patient population. One cannot validate the instrument in the same clinical trial that is being submitted for approval, as such a strategy has many pitfalls, including false positive error inflation, lack of replicability, and lack of extendibility to a more heterogeneous patient group where the treatment would be applied. One suggestion has been to validate the instrument in a run-in phase of the clinical trial. This approach might create the problem of conducting much of the study and then discovering the instrument was not valid. We recommend that a validation study be conducted prior to the clinical trial that would lead to an HRQOL claim. We take as the definition of validity that the

HRQOL scale measures what it is purported to measure. Various measures of validity may be considered. First, a proposed measure of HRQOL may be compared to a gold standard instrument. For example, a long-form version of a widely used scale can be compared to a short-form version that takes less time to complete. Comparing these scales would constitute *criterion validity*. Secondly, the HRQOL measure may need to reflect a range of responses in the disease being studied. For example, in rheumatoid arthritis, a measure that looked only at the time needed to walk 25 feet might not reflect joint pain or a global evaluation by the physician. An instrument has *content validity* if the range of responses reflects the range of disease burden. Thirdly, clinicians working in a particular disease area generally have an idea of how subjects with the disease should respond to the questions. This correspondence is called *construct validity*.

Scientists wish the HRQOL scale to be responsive to changes in the disease. These changes may be due to evolution of the disease, a response to treatment or familiarity with the instrument. Several measurement approaches have been proposed. Let D be the difference of population means, σ be the standard deviation of the measure at baseline, σ_D be the standard deviation of the difference in means, and σ_S be the standard deviation among "stable" subjects (those subjects in the control group who show little difference between baseline and final measurements). The *effect size* is defined as D/σ, the difference of population means divided by the baseline standard deviation. This is often used to estimate sample size requirements. The *standardized response mean* is D/σ_D, the difference in means divided by the standard deviation of the mean difference. Finally, the *responsiveness statistic* is D/σ_S, the mean difference divided by its standard deviation among stable subjects. There is an extensive focus on these topics in the psychometric literature. In the regulatory context, it is usually necessary to define a *clinically important difference* (i.e., one that is likely to have a meaningful impact on the patient) and a *minimally important difference*. An effect size is convenient in determining sample size requirements, but may have limited relevance to a clinically important difference. Additionally, since repeated measures analyses are often applied that involve assumptions about the covariance matrix, the sample size estimation is rarely as simple as a *t*-test computation for a specific effect size.

The HRQOL measure must also be reliable. Reliability refers to the ability to measure the HRQOL trait repeatedly and consistently. *Test-retest reliability* implies that if the test is repeated the outcomes will be similar. There are pitfalls here, of course. The time period between the two tests must be sufficiently long so that question recall does not affect responses. Similarly, the time difference cannot be so long to allow actual changes in HRQOL (e.g., disease progression or cure) to affect responses. These considerations hold whether the questionnaire is self-administered or given by an interviewer. A second reliability question relates to *internal consistency* of the questions. This is a function of the number of items and their correlation. Cronbach's α is an intraclass correlation that is widely used in this context. A third reliability measure is *inter-rater* reliability, the ability of two raters to agree on the HRQOL score. See Staquet, Hays and Fayers (1998) for more details in this area. This may not be appropriate for patient reported outcomes since there cannot be multiple raters.

HRQOL measurements should be taken over time to allow a longitudinal evaluation. The pattern of HRQOL scores may be a linear, quadratic, a threshold model, or something more complex. The timing of measurements should be precise – that is, if measurements are to be taken every two weeks, gaps of 5 and 6 weeks will make it difficult to interpret the measurements for that individual. In chronic diseases, it is important that the study be able to reflect a durable effect on HRQOL. Thus, if the disease leads to mortality within one year, a short-term response (e.g., 1–3 months) may be acceptable. If the disease has a long-term survival (e.g., breast cancer, diabetes), there is a need to show a longer-term benefit (e.g., 6–24 months). Finally, there are potential bias and measurement error problems if the pre-specified HRQOL assessment time points are not adhered to rigorously. Overly liberal time windows are to be avoided.

Many drug development clinical trials are multi-national, and this might cause problems when standards vary across cultures and languages, etc. A natural way to address this issue would be to consider the country as a stratum and compare effects across strata. In particular, it would be important to show a consistent effect over the strata. A single large stratum that dominates the treatment effect might be due to some cultural specificity of the questionnaire.

Missing values plague all studies. It is important to recognize that in HRQOL studies, death is not a missing value. It corresponds to a poor outcome. However, it may not correspond to the worst possible HRQOL since there may be dire disease states worse than death (e.g., constant agonizing pain without the ability to communicate needs). In some scales, a score of 0 may be assumed for death. However, other scales do not have a clearly defined minimum value. In such cases a decision should be made prospectively about the score that will be assigned for death and for dropouts due to other reasons. When the data are collected over time, a missing time point is more serious than a single missing item. Appropriate rules can be constructed for the latter. For the former (the missed visit), plans for several sensitivity analyses are appropriate. Imputation methods can be outlined in the study protocol. The most serious missing values arise from study dropouts, where all observations following dropout are missing. If possible, the subjects should be encouraged to obtain evaluations on schedule to reduce the number of missing values as much as possible. In addition, efforts should be made to obtain evaluations for a period after dropout. Such information is an important component in structuring sensitivity analyses.

The outcome of the clinical trial is used to determine whether a product will be approved (or a new indication listed on the label of an existing product). Thus, it is crucial to pre-specify what the endpoint will be. If a subscale is to be used, it must be specified before the study is unblinded, preferably well before that time. It is not acceptable to examine the data and then select an outcome variable. If several scales are co-primary endpoints, plans to adjust for false positive error inflation due to multiplicity (multiple endpoints) need to be specified in the protocol.

It is important to ensure that the trial sponsor and the FDA have agreed on the design of the study, sample size, outcome measures, and analysis. The FDA strongly encourages trial sponsors to discuss the trial with them, either by telephone or in person. The sponsor should submit plans for studies as an investigative new drug (IND) application at least 30 days in advance of the meeting so that FDA staff can review it and react to it. It is in everyone's interest to have trials that are designed and conducted to meet their stated objectives.

3. Statistical Analytic Issues

Features that make the analysis of HRQOL endpoints more challenging to analyze than other longitudinal measures are: complex correlation structures, temporal patterns induced by repeated evaluations, greater subjectivity of these measurements, multidimensionality, and greater potential for informative dropout. When evaluating a HRQOL claim for product approval, the same level of rigor pertains as for other efficacy endpoints. Thus, many statistical analysis issues need to be addressed. The majority of these are important in the regulatory setting. We discuss six important issues below.

3.1 Intent-to-Treat Analysis

The standard for efficacy analysis is that all randomized patients be included in the statistical analysis and that patients be grouped according to their originally-randomized treatment without regard to the treatment actually administered. We believe this standard applies equally in the HRQOL setting.

3.2 False Positive Error Inflation

This can occur due to multiplicity of endpoints and/or when multiple statistical tests are performed. HRQOL questionnaires usually contain many individual questions (in excess of 30 in many cases), and these are usually grouped into sets of related questions or domains (five or six domains are common). Thus, it is essential to pre-specify a small number of important HRQOL questions to avoid multiplicity problems. The definition of "important" is driven by the clinical issues that the drug or product is attempting to address. The primary HRQOL endpoints are specified by the pharmaceutical company in their protocol. Adjustment for multiplicity is required. As it is difficult or impossible to impose many of these adjustments *post hoc*, appropriate endpoint multiplicity adjustment should be pre-specified in the protocol. Another source of false positive error inflation is multiple comparisons of post-baseline values to baseline. In addition to lack of independence of these tests, such a strategy results in false positive error inflation.

3.3 Univariate Versus Multivariate Analytic Approaches

Univariate techniques are attractive since they are straightforward to implement and yield results that are not difficult to interpret. Such approaches include: comparison of baseline score to a pre-specified post-baseline value, endpoint analysis (comparison of baseline to the last recorded value), utility score Q-TWiST (Quality Adjusted Time without Symptoms or Toxicity), and summary measures (patient slopes, area under the curve). There are limitations to these techniques. They do not enable one to adequately assess the missing data mechanism (informative or not). Endpoint analysis yields unbiased results only if the missing data follow a non-informative mechanism. These methods do not provide an assessment of HRQOL over time. For example, time to event analyses (i.e., time to a pre-specified deterioration in HRQOL) may not capture important temporal patterns (e.g., gradual versus abrupt decline). Summary measures should be used cautiously because statistical testing can be sensitive to the measure chosen. In addition, they can be subject to bias if follow-up duration differs by treatment group and if the missing data mechanism is informative. Sensitivity analyses are useful to address these limitations. In Q-TWiST analysis, utility scores are assigned to various health states (e.g., toxicity, relapse of disease, or death) and a competing-risks time-to-event analysis is employed. It is important to have sufficient follow-up before undertaking these analyses because the outcomes may not be relevant to HRQOL in the disease context. With short follow-up time, many subjects will be censored. This leads to large variances of the time to event distributions. There is an element of subjectivity in choosing the utility weights. Sensitivity analysis is needed to demonstrate relative insensitivity to the choice of weights. Multivariate approaches, such as MANOVA of the subscales of the HRQOL instrument, require complete data (or assume a missing at random mechanism) and somewhat restrictive assumptions (e.g., normally-distributed data). MANOVA is known to be sensitive to non-normal data and outliers, and to have a low breakdown point (i.e., the proportion of outliers that affect the analysis is small).

3.4 Missing Data Imputation

Complete case analysis or missing data imputation methods, such as last observation carried forward (LOCF), are often used to obtain a "complete" data set. Imputation assumes that missing values are a random sample of all cases. LOCF assumes the patient's last-observed score remains constant for subsequently missing observations. An in depth investigation of the type of missing data mechanism at work with appropriate sensitivity analyses should be undertaken. The LOCF assumption is untenable in most cases, as it leads to underestimation of the variability of the data, and consequent inflation of the false positive error rate. Other simple imputation techniques include worst outcome and worst case approaches. In the worst outcome method, a missing observation in a treatment group is replaced by the worst outcome in that treatment group. The worst-case method is most conservative since a missing value in the treatment group is replaced by the worst overall value and a missing value in the control group is replaced by the most favorable value. These methods are biased, but are useful for sensitivity analyses. Another more sophisticated, computer-intensive technique is multiple imputation, which uses observations from patients with complete data to predict values for patients with missing data. One defines classes of data based on other variables (e.g., initial value, and clinically relevant covariables). A set of "close" observations with complete data (perhaps 10 or 20 cases) is identified. A value to impute is randomly selected and this is done several times generating a data set at each cycle (five is common). A parameter (e.g., a mean) is estimated for each data set. These estimates are combined, and we compute the variability due to the imputation and due to the data. The key assumption is that the data are missing completely at random within each stratum. Again, this is not a testable assumption, and sensitivity analyses are essential with this methodology. No matter what imputation technique is used, it must be emphasized that death is not a missing value; it needs to be scored appropriately. From a regulatory standpoint, informative missingness is a major problem because if hypothesis tests are marginally significant, missing values can change conclusions substantially. Informative missingness may arise from the prior values of the dependent variable (e.g., the patient experienced no improvement on therapy and the treatment is changed). It may also arise from a value that cannot be measured (e.g., pulmonary function may not be measurable at later stages of lung disease). In structuring a statistical analysis plan for a pivotal study in a regulatory submission, sponsors should plan for sensitivity analyses for the methods employed. Such strategies explore methods to examine the degree to which the missing value methods affect analytic results (e.g., a change in directionality is a serious concern). A reviewer of this paper commented that LOCF could be appropriate in situations where patients might be switched to alternative medication because of lack of efficacy with the randomized treatment. In this case, the last observation would be the "best" one. Unfortunately, this does not account for trends in the data, nor does it address the reduction of variability of the outcome associated with LOCF. We view a level of 5% missing as unlikely to affect the analysis greatly, while 20% raises questions and concerns regarding adequacy of study conduct.

3.5 Longitudinal Approach

Perhaps with the exception of short-term studies, a longitudinal analysis generally should be an essential component of the statistical evaluation of the HRQOL measures. Longitudinal analyses are needed to characterize temporal patterns, investigate the effects of dropouts, study the influence of baseline covariates on time trends, and place univariate comparisons in context. One approach makes use of growth curve analysis in the context of a pattern mixture model (Little, 1993, 1995) to study missing data mechanisms. These mixed effects models are useful in this setting because the evaluations are often not performed at the specified times and invariably there are missing observations. The growth curve analysis fits polynomial growth curves to each HRQOL component using time as the predictor. Then one examines the mean HRQOL response in the subgroups that did or did not drop out within a time frame constituting minimum adequate treatment. A prospective definition of dropout classes is obtained from clinical input. Sensitivity analyses are needed to assess the robustness of the cut-point chosen. Thus, two strata or homogeneity classes for a modified pattern mixture model are obtained. If the time trend for dropouts is different from that for completers, that provides evidence that the missingness mechanism is informative. In such a case, the investigator cannot ignore the missingness mechanism and cannot use all of the data to estimate time trends. Completers and dropouts need to be modeled separately. If the two trends are not different, then this suggests the missingness mechanism is noninformative. In that case, we can use all of the data in estimation. Other longitudinal approaches often used include selection models and general estimating equations (GEE; Zeger, Liang and Albert, 1988). Selection models posit a statistical model for the missing data mechanism. An example is the Schluchter (1992) two-stage mixed effects model. Again, sensitivity analyses are crucial for these models since they are based on untestable assumptions. The GEE approach (also requiring the non-informative missingness assumption) provides a robust estimate of the variance-covariance structure of the data. This method can be used in sensitivity analyses for the growth curve/modified pattern mixture strategy previously described.

3.6 Robustness Concerns

Stating major hypotheses and analytic approaches prospectively is essential in the regulatory setting. Robustness of results is also an important concern. Thus, well-considered sensitivity analyses need to be undertaken to examine the sensitivity of analytic findings to the missing data imputation algorithm chosen and the modeling approach undertaken. Substantial changes in significance or directionality are the major concern.

4. A Sensitivity Study

DeMetri, *et al.* (1998) studied the quality of life of patients with a variety of cancers using the FACT-An scale and estimated the change from baseline following administration of erythropoeitin. They obtained baseline measurements of HRQOL from

2,289 patients with various cancers. They note that about 35% did not have a final measurement due to death (223), progressive disease (136), loss to follow-up (129), and adverse events (35), among other reasons. There were 1,484 patients with both baseline and follow-up. The authors report a p-value for the difference in HRQOL scores of 0.001, based on a paired *t*-test. If the reason for a missing final observation were unrelated to outcome, this statistical-testing approach would be appropriate. However, death, progressive disease and adverse events suggest that the missing final observation is dependent on actual HRQOL. Let us consider how we might perform a sensitivity analysis in this context.

Let the proportion of patients who have complete observations be π. Suppose that observations among patients with complete data and patients with incomplete data are normally distributed with respective means μ_{complete} and $\mu_{\text{incomplete}}$ and variances $\sigma^2_{\text{complete}}$ and $\sigma^2_{\text{incomplete}}$. Then the overall mean and variance are respectively given by

$$\mu = \pi\mu_{\text{complete}} + (1 - \pi)\mu_{\text{incomplete}}$$

$$\sigma = \pi\sigma^2_{\text{complete}} + (1 - \pi)\sigma^2_{\text{incomplete}} + \pi(1 - \pi)(\mu_{\text{complete}} - \mu_{\text{incomplete}})^2.$$

Using these results, we computed the paired t statistic for various values of $\mu_{\text{incomplete}}$ while holding all other parameters equal to their respective estimates based on the data. We found that for $\mu_{\text{incomplete}} = 113$, the baseline mean for the entire sample, the p-value for the paired *t*-test is below 0.05; however for $\mu_{\text{incomplete}} \leq 110$, the p-value is increased to above 0.075. Thus, only if the dropouts have scores that are not much below baseline, is significance maintained. The highly significant outcome ignoring the dropouts is sensitive to the assumption of no difference among dropouts and completers. In this case, the paired *t*-test was affected by the mean difference being reduced and by the variance being increased.

Generally, analyses should account for all subjects in a study since dropouts and protocol violations usually are a non-random subset of the group being studied. We could not attempt a multiple imputation process because we did not have the patient-level data.

5. An Alternative Model

Lachenbruch (2000) studied a two-part model that compared the proportion of patients who dropped out using a binomial test and the difference in means using a *t*-test. This can be extended to using a Wilcoxon rank-sum test. This leads to a two degree of freedom χ^2 test of the form $B^2 + Z^2$, where B is the test statistic for the binomial test, and Z is the test statistic for the comparison of means. In this example, suppose we wish to test the combined null hypothesis H_0: $\pi = 0.6$ and $\mu_d = 0$. Then the statistic is $\chi^2 = 5.396^2 + 3.29^2 = 39.94$, which has a p-value less than 0.001. In this case, we would note that the treatment seems to improve those who complete, but that we have a higher than hypothesized proportion of dropouts.

We can easily generalize this to multiple reasons for not completing the study. Suppose we wished to consider death, medical reasons not including death and other reasons for non-response. Each such category adds a degree of freedom to the overall χ^2. Suppose the combined null hypothesis is H_0: $\pi_{\text{death}} = 0.1$, $\pi_{\text{medical}} = 0.19$, $\pi_{\text{other}} = 0.06$ and $\mu_d = 0$. In this case, $\chi^2 = 0.152 + 1.334 + 1.497 + 10.824 = 13.81$ which has a p-value of 0.008. The χ^2 due to the dropouts has a p-value of 0.394. Note the null hypotheses values were arbitrarily selected. For a sample size of 2,289, small changes in the null hypothesis values can lead to large changes in the χ^2.

6. Conclusions

Recently, the FDA has proposed the term Patient Reported Outcomes as an alternative to HRQOL because it is a term descriptive of the outcome being studied. Whether this term gains acceptance remains to be seen. Below we summarize our main concerns in this article. The ordering of these points is not intended to imply any value judgement (nor has this scale been validated or found reliable).

- There should be an *a priori* plan for analyzing the study, including explicit criteria for "success."
- Studies should be randomized and double-blind to remove or reduce effects of treatment knowledge on the response.
- The HRQOL scale should be validated in the population/study group to which it is being applied. Both reliability and validity measures will be needed.
- Measurements should be timed to reflect the disease context.
- Missing values must be proactively minimized, and plans should be in place to evaluate the sensitivity of the results to missing observations.
- Address multiplicity issues in the analysis plan.
- Talk to the regulatory agency before committing to a clinical trial to ensure it will be acceptable for product approval. In particular, discuss plans for any claims that will be made for the product.

ACKNOWLEDGEMENTS

We thank the three referees for helpful comments and suggestions. Our colleagues at the FDA have also provided us with useful insights.

REFERENCES

Berkanovic, E. and Hurwicz, M.L. (1990). Rheumatoid arthritis and comorbidity. *Journal of Rheumatology* **17**, 888–892.

DeMetri, G.D., Kris, M., Wade, J., Degos, L. and Cella, D. (1998). Quality-of-life benefit in chemotherapy patients treated with epoetin alpha is independent of disease response or tumor type: results from a prospective community oncology study. *Journal of Clinical Oncology* **16**, 3412–3425.

Hurwicz, M.L. and Berkanovic, E. (1993). The stress process in rheumatoid arthritis. *Journal of Rheumatology* **20**, 1836–1844.

Lachenbruch, P.A. (2000). Comparisons of two-part models with competitors. *Statistics in Medicine* **20**, 1215–1234.

Little, R.J.A. (1993). Pattern mixture models for multivariate incomplete data. *Journal of the American Statistical Association* **88**, 125–134.

Little, R.J.A. (1995). Modeling the drop-out mechanism in repeated-measures studies. *Journal of the American Statistical Association* **90**, 1112–1121.

Schluchter, M.D. (1992). Methods for the analysis of informatively censored longitudinal data. *Statistics in Medicine* **11**, 1861–1870.

Staquet, M.J., Hays, R.D. and Fayers, P.M., eds. (1998). *Quality of Life Assessment in Clinical Trials: Methods and Practice*. Oxford: Oxford University Press.

Zeger, S.L., Liang, K.Y. and Albert, P.S. (1988). Models for longitudinal data: a generalized estimating equations approach. *Biometrics* **44**, 1049–1060.

BIASES IN THE RETROSPECTIVE CALCULATION OF RELIABILITY AND RESPONSIVENESS FROM LONGITUDINAL STUDIES

GEOFF NORMAN, PAUL STRATFORD AND GLENN REGEHR

McMaster University and University of Toronto, Canada

We critically examine the common practice in quality of life assessment of identifying improved, unchanged and worsened subsamples retrospectively using some form of global rating, and then calculating test-retest reliability coefficients from the unchanged subsample and responsiveness coefficients from the changed subsample. We use data derived from Monte Carlo simulations to examine the relation between measures of reliability and responsiveness derived from retrospective studies using an unchanged subsample and coefficients based on prospective studies with known treatment effect sizes. We also use actual data from longitudinal studies to examine the fit between simulated and published data. Our results show that calculation of reliability from an unchanged subsample leads to an inflation of the computed coefficient from a typical range of 0.6–0.8 up to 0.85–0.95. We similarly demonstrate that responsiveness coefficients based on the changed subsamples overestimate the responsiveness of the instrument, so that even in situations where there is no overall change, the methods lead to an acceptably large responsiveness coefficient. Based on these results, we conclude that retrospective methods of calculating reliability and responsiveness coefficients based on unchanged samples lead to upwardly biased estimates, and should be discontinued.

1. Introduction

A number of authors have pointed out that reliability (or reproducibility) and responsiveness are fundamental measurement characteristics for quality of life measures. Wright and Feinstein [1, p. 1206] put it strongly: "The demand for reproducibility is a *sine qua non* of any method of measurement." Similarly, Kirshner and Guyatt [2] argue convincingly that, since the goal of therapy was to effect change in health status, some assessment of the ability of an instrument to be responsive to clinically important treatment effects is an important prerequisite for the use of such instruments in clinical trials.

Reliability has been a standard for educational and psychological testing for about five decades. The basic expression for reliability, the intraclass correlation, was devised over seven decades ago. The reliability coefficient is based on the fundamental idea that any observation of an individual can be separated in two components: the true score for that individual, and the error associated with the particular observation. Each individual has only one true score which is stable across observations and thus is fairly accurately estimated by averaging a very large number of observed scores. Given this assumption of stability over time in the true score, any variation in the observed score, whether resulting from measurement error or random change in the underlying characteristic will, by definition, be interpreted as arising from error of measurement and will therefore end up in the error term of the equation.

The reliability coefficient follows from this equation, and is a measure of the signal to

M. Mesbah et al. (eds.), Statistical Methods for Quality of Life Studies, 21–31.

noise ratio in the measurement instrument. That is, how much of the difference in individuals' scores is a function of real differences on the dimension of interest (the true score) and how much is a function of error in the measurement process (the error score). The reliability coefficient, the so called *intraclass correlation*, expresses these two components as a ratio, whose numerator is the variance due to true differences among patients and whose denominator is the sum of true variance between patients and error variance—the total variance in the scores. This leads to the familiar expression:

$$\text{Reliability} = \frac{\sigma^2_{\text{True}}}{\sigma^2_{\text{Total}}} = \frac{\sigma^2_{\text{True}}}{\sigma^2_{\text{True}} + \sigma^2_{\text{Err}}}$$

By contrast, the notion of responsiveness has a short history. It was originally based on a simple construct: the assessment of the ability of an instrument to be responsive to clinically important treatment effects. Kirshner and Guyatt [2] recognized that the conventional assessment of reliability was a measure of the extent to which an instrument could detect stable differences between subjects, and thus had no direct bearing on the assessment of responsiveness.

A number of measures of responsiveness based on the measurement of change from therapeutic interventions have been proposed. These include a simple paired *t*-test on difference scores [3], (which has the undesirable property that it is related to sample size), a ratio of the mean change in a treatment group to the standard deviation of the initial score [4] and intraclass correlations [5]. All can be viewed as variants on an effect size (mean change/standard deviation of change). We will call this class of coefficients, based on an overall mean change of a group, responsiveness-treatment (RT) coefficients. The specific version of the RT coefficient used in the present paper is defined as:

$$\text{RT} = \frac{\Delta_{\text{Pre-post}}}{\sigma_{\text{Pre-post}}}$$

where $\Delta_{\text{Pre-post}}$ is the mean change score, based on a comparison of individual scores before and after treatment (where "treatment" is interpreted generally, and may include simply the passage of time), and $\sigma_{\text{Pre-post}}$ is the standard deviation of the change scores. All of these methods are a direct assessment of the overall responsiveness of a cohort of patients, since they explicitly involve the mean change.

2. The Retrospective Approach

Although the computation of responsiveness and reliability using these methods is straightforward, the general approach has some limitations. With respect to responsiveness, the magnitude of the coefficients are dependent on the actual change induced by the treatment, and consequently cannot be viewed as a property of the instrument itself. Because of the dependence on the size of the treatment effect, studies of responsiveness generally proceed by administering a battery of instruments to patients who have undergone some treatment, then comparing the relative responsiveness of the various instruments under conditions of a common overall treatment effect.

In order to conduct such a study one must have some confidence *a priori* that the treatment is efficacious, and so is faced with the prospect of trying to conduct a trial of a treatment with known efficacy, simply to determine a property of a new measurement instrument. Some investigators [6,7,8] have abandoned this strategy and instead have opted to estimate responsiveness retrospectively, and independently of any particular intervention, by identifying those patients who have, and have not, changed over time to a clinically important extent and then examining their change scores on various measures.

In the retrospective approach, "true" change is assessed by comparison with some other measure, usually by having the patient or a clinician assess the amount of change retrospectively, using a global scale (GS) to measure change such as a 15 point scale ranging from –7 = "much worse" to +7 = "much better." Below one cutpoint, patients are said to have a clinically important worsening of their condition; above a second cutpoint, patients are assumed to have undergone a clinically important improvement; between the two there is no clinically important change. Generally the cutpoint is based on verbal anchors; for example, those whose scores are greater than +1 or less than –1, where +/–1 is "almost the same," +/–2 is "a little better" or "a little worse," etc. This cutpoint is referred to as the minimally important difference (MID) [9]. One then determines the mean change on the HRQL instrument of those who have improved and worsened. If these are approximately the same, then the sign of the worsened group is reversed and the two means added together. Finally this mean change is divided by the standard deviation of the group who has stayed the same [6].

The idea of assessing clinically important change independent of any experimentally induced treatment effect has considerable appeal. One need only follow a group of patients for some period of time, identify who have changed by some clinically meaningful amount, and then examine the amount of change on the HRQL measure in those who "truly" have changed (that is, those who have reported a clinically important change on a retrospective global scale) standardized to the variability in scores among those who have not changed. We will call coefficients of this form responsiveness- retrospective (RR) coefficients. In this paper, we will formally define these coefficients by the following formula:

$$RR = \frac{\Delta_{\text{Improved}}}{\sigma_{\text{Unchanged}}}$$

where Δ_{Improved} is the mean change in the improved group, and $\sigma_{\text{Unchanged}}$ is the standard deviation of the unchanged group.

Having adopted the position that one can assess responsiveness by identifying those patients who have improved or changed, and compute a responsiveness coefficient based on the mean change in the changed group, it would then be illogical to include the same changed patients in a calculation of reliability. Some patients clearly get better over time, from response to therapy, spontaneous remission or natural healing, whereas others are clearly worse as a result of progression of the disease. It makes no sense to compute a reliability coefficient which presumes the hypothesis that all patients are stable over time when clearly they are not. Both methods are in common use; computing responsiveness based on changed subsamples [6,7,8] and computing reliability based on unchanged subsamples [9–13]. However, we will show that, although this practice may appear clinically reasonable, on close inspection, it is logically flawed. In addition, we will demonstrate that calculation of reliability from unchanged subsamples and responsiveness from changed samples results in estimates which are systematically biased upward by as much as 50% in comparison with coefficients computed in the usual way from the whole sample.

2.1 Problems with Retrospective Approaches

Despite its logic and appeal, the retrospective method has two distinct problems. First, we have already discussed elsewhere the dangers and difficulties associated with the use of a single global rating of change as a gold standard measure to which the health-related quality of life (HRQL) measure is compared [14]. We will not repeat the discussion other than to say that identifying a good independent measure is fraught with difficulties and will not be as easy as it might seem. Certainly a global rating based on a single response is unlikely to stand as a reasonable gold standard for no other reason that, all things being equal, reliability and responsiveness are directly (although not linearly) related to the number of items on the scale, so it seems highly unlikely that a single global scale could provide a better measurement than the detailed, multi-item HRQL. Indeed, if it could, there seems little point to go through the laborious exercise of developing the new measure.

However, a second, more fundamental problem leads us to question the use of any approach to separate "true" change in subjects from measurement error. Retrospective approaches to assessment of change will be heavily influenced by the present state [15] so that it is likely that patients will be highly vulnerable to the influence of transient changes in their recent state. Including patients in the responsiveness calculation and eliminating patients from the reliability study because they claim, retrospectively, to have changed, amounts to eliminating disease fluctuation from the error estimate, and thereby inflating the measure of reliability as well as creating a responsiveness coefficient derived from what may amount to nothing more than transient improvements in disease.

In the extreme case, we can envision a situation where (a) the overall treatment effect is zero, but there is, naturally a distribution of changes around zero, so that many patients report small changes, positive or negative, and a few report large changes, which would be viewed, in isolation, as clinically significant, and (b) the nature of the changes are such that patients who report improvements in one time period report worsening in the next, with no resultant net change, either overall or individually. Under these circumstances, it would appear that all changes amount to error in estimates of treatment effects. Yet a calculation of reliability based on the unchanged sample and responsiveness based on the changed sample could yield credible estimates. As we shall see, although this scenario is hypothetical, there are indications that it is not an unrealistic model of real data.

3. Responsiveness Computed Retrospectively from Changed Subsamples Compared to Responsveness Based on Treatments

3.1 Methods

In a previous paper [14], we used Monte Carlo simulations to determine the relation between RT and RR coefficients. In order that it would not depend on observed data, we conducted a series of simulations of the process using computer-generated data. We began with 1,000 pairs of observations that represented the change scores for 1,000 individuals on both a global scale and on an HRQL instrument. Both sets of change scores were drawn from normally distributed populations, each with a standard deviation of 1.0.

We systematically varied three parameters in the simulations. First, we varied the correlation between the GS and the HRQL from 0.0 to 0.8 in steps of 0.2. Second, we varied the mean of both change score distributions from 0.0 to 1.0 in steps of 0.2 (the means of both distributions were changed concurrently so that, regardless of the correlation, the means of the GS and HRQL distributions were always identical). Finally, we varied the MID on the GS from 0.2 to 1.0 in steps of 0.2. The simulations were conducted using a spreadsheet program; further details are given in the paper. Because the standard deviation of the HRQL was set at 1.0, the mean change score (the effect size) was also the RT coefficient for each simulation.

For each of the 150 resulting parameter combinations, we simulated the retrospective calculation of the RR coefficient by using the MID on the GS to divide the 1,000 simulated subjects into worse, unchanged, and improved groups. We then calculated the mean and standard deviation on the HRQL measure for the unchanged and improved groups (as defined by the GS). Finally, we computed the RR coefficient as the mean change of the Improved group divided by the standard deviation of the unchanged group. Finally, we plotted observed data derived from a number of studies that reported sufficient information to compute both RR and RT coefficients.

3.2 Results

A first observation is that the relationship between RT and RR, while positive is relatively small. The major determinant of the value of RR is the correlation with the GS. The choice of the MID has a relatively smaller effect, generating families of curves for each value of the correlation.

Figure 1 shows the calculated curves for correlations with the GS of 0.0, 0.4, 0.6, and 0.8; for values of the RT coefficient (effect size) of 0 to 1 in steps of 0.2, and for MID's of 0.2, 0.5, and 0.8 and the observed data.

More detailed inspection reveals a number of other important relationships:

1. The lower limit of the RR occurs when the correlation with the GS equals zero. At this minimum, the RR and RT coefficients are identical.
2. As the correlation with the GS increases, so does the RR relative to the RT coefficient, reflecting the extent to which the use of the GS selects individuals at the extreme of the distribution. The result is that RR coefficients can be as high as 1.5 even in the absence of a treatment effect. In the extreme case where the correlation equals 1 (not shown), the distributions of changed and unchanged no longer overlap, and RR coefficients as high as 20 may be observed.
3. The selection of the MID has a small positive relation to the size of the RR, because a higher MID results in the selection of more extreme changed groups, and a higher mean change score.
4. The experimental data are consistent with the theoretical relationships.

The effect of these three parameters in combination is that the direct relationship between the RT and RR coefficients is virtually impossible to predict. For example, an RR coefficient of 1.5 can result from an effect size (RT) of zero (with $r = 0.8$ and MID about 0.7) or an RT of one (with $r = 0.6$ and MID about 0.2).

Figure 1. Relation between responsiveness computed retrospectively from an improved subsample (vertical axis, RR) and responsiveness computed prospectively from the entire sample expressed as an effect size (RT). The legend on the right side indicates the correlation between the HRQL and the global scale (GS). Within each value of r, the top solid line corresponds to an MID of 0.8, the middle dotted line to an MID of 0.5, and the lower dashed line to an MID of 0.2. Also on the figure are experimental points derived from several studies.

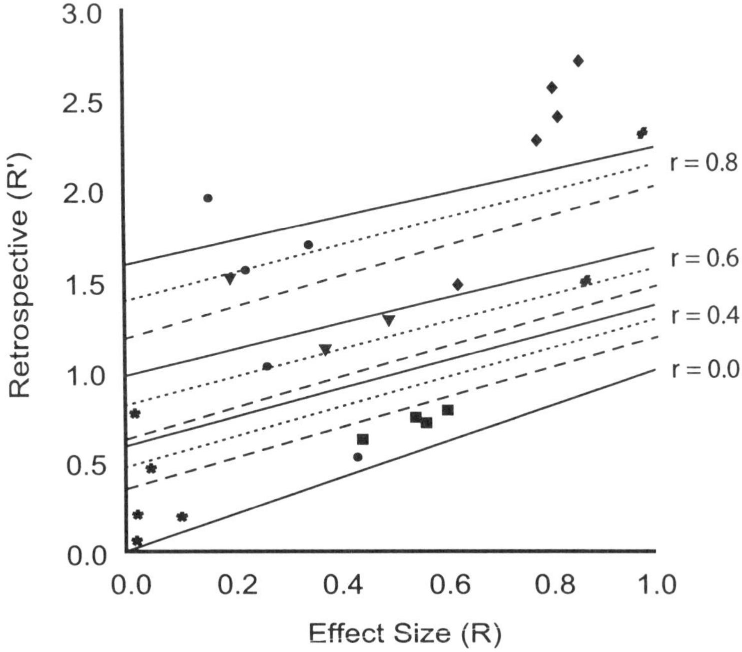

3.3 Discussion

While the simulation theoretically would make it possible to move from one coefficient to the other given knowledge of the MCID and the correlation with GS, likely this would result in considerable uncertainty, as the individual estimates would have fairly large associated errors. The precise relationship between the RT and RR coefficients is nearly impossible to determine because of the influence of other variables. Furthermore, the experimental data, while consistent with the simulated curves, shows a similar uncertain relationship between RT and RR coefficients.

4. Reliability Computed from Stable Samples and Retrospectively from Unchanged Subsamples

4.1 Methods

The simulation in the previous section also provided the information needed to examine the relation between reliability coefficients computed from the whole sample and from an unchanged subsample. We used the same data sets to compute the subject and error variance from the entire sample and the unchanged subsample (left over after we identified the subsample with significant change). Again, we computed a family of curves corresponding to differing values of the MID and the correlation with the gold standard. These are shown, with observational data described later, in Figure 2.

The interpretations parallel the interpretation of the responsiveness simulations. When the correlation between GS and HRQL approach zero, there is no bias in the computed reliability. However, as the correlation rises, the error variance in the unchanged group is reduced and the unchanged group reliability rises relative to the reliability from the whole sample. Similarly, the dependence on the MID is minimal until the correlation exceeds 0.8, at which point increasing the MID removes the tails and increases the retrospective reliability.

In order to explore the fit of the curves, we located raw data from a study conducted by Elizabeth Juniper of pediatric asthma [16] that involved 52 patients and a complex observational schema, where patients were examined at weeks 1, 2, 5 and 8 of the total 9-week follow up period. In addition, a global assessment of change was made in two ways: (1) retrospectively by patients for weeks 2 to 5 and 6 to 8, using a conventional –7 to + 7 scale, and (2) retrospectively by the investigator using all the data from both quality of life and

Figure 2. Relation between reliability computed retrospectively from an unchanged subsample (vertical axis) and reliability computed from the whole sample for different correlations with the global scale (GS) from 0.2 to 1.0. For R = 0.2 to 0.8, there is no visible effect of the choice of MID; for R = 1.0, values of the MID of 0.2 and 0.5 are shown on the figure. Also shown are experimental points derived from Juniper (16)

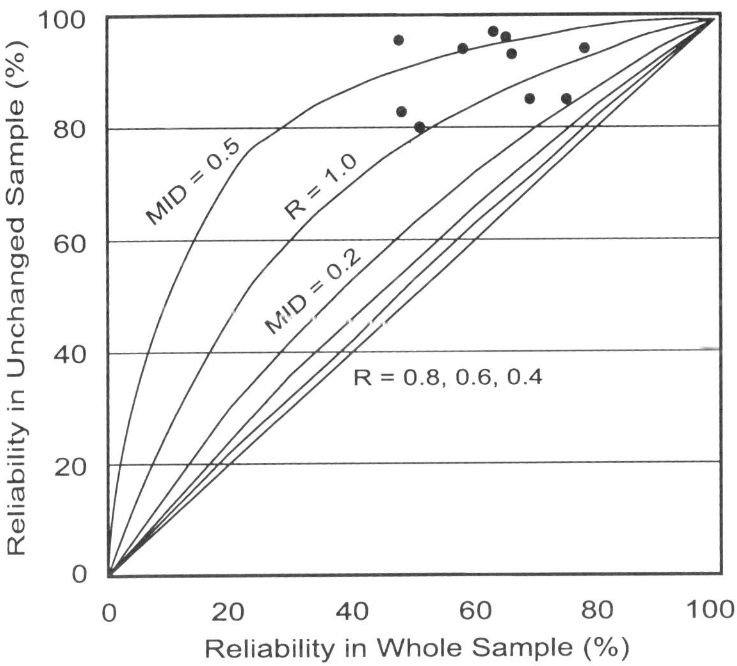

physiological measures for two time intervals: week 2 to week 5 and week 6 to week 8, using a three point scale (–1,0,1). In the paper, they report reliability coefficients for the unchanged patients, roughly half the total, aggregating data from both the first and second time period. Reliability was reported for the total score and four subscales. In our reanalysis we computed intraclass correlation coefficients for all patients and patients who were judged to have not changed by self-report (global scores of –1 to +1) and by investigator judgment (score = 0) for each time period separately, resulting in a subsample of 22 and 26 in the first time period and 23 and 27 in the second period.

The results are shown on the figure. It is apparent that the observed values fall in a range where considerable bias is present, resulting in an inflation of the reliability coefficient from relatively low values averaging about 0.62, to very high values averaging 0.84 using the patient-identified sample and 0.90 using the investigator-derived sample. We also compared our calculations with those reported in the paper, from the same data base, but using a different method of selection where both time periods were analysed together, and patients contributed to the stable group in any time period where there was no reported change. These coefficients averaged 0.90.

Generally, reliability coefficients lower than 0.6 are viewed as unsatisfactory, whereas coefficients greater than 0.8 or 0.9 are accepted as high. Thus, the identification of samples of unchanged patients retrospectively, whether by self-report or by clinician judgment using all available data, results in a substantial and clinically important upward bias. Further, it is apparent that the availability of prospectively gathered data is no safeguard, since, if anything, retrospective clinician judgment resulted in larger coefficients than those based on self-report.

5. Evidence that Changes in HRQL Scores Result from Fluctuations, not Trends

The second point we want to make is that the observed changes, however compelling they may be to the clinician, amount to nothing much more than transient fluctuations in the disease. The counter view is that individuals who report that they have improved over a single time period really are on their way to a slow and steady recovery, and conversely those who report a worsening state are really on a progressively downhill course. If this is so, then we may well regard that the reported changes in those cohorts are far more important and enduring than transient fluctuations. Indeed, this was the basis for the original formulation of responsiveness as a separate measurement property [2].

It is self-evident that a simple pre-post design with only two observations does not permit separation of fluctuations from monotonic trends. However the Juniper data, as we indicated, encompassed a total of four observations. We reanalysed these data two ways. First we examined the reliability coefficients computed for the entire sample over three time periods: one week (week 1 to week 2); three weeks (week 2 to week 5 and week 6 to week 8) and eight weeks (week 1 to week 9). Since measurement error, as isolated in the retrospective calculations is small, we can consider the relative impact of trends and fluctuations. If the changes in individuals are based on trends over relatively long times, we would expect the reliability coefficients to begin close to one and drop monotonically with greater time separation. Conversely, if the changes result from fluctuations with short periodicity, we would expect that the reliability coefficients would begin relatively low and remain relatively constant over the successive time periods. The results are shown in Table 1.

The intraclass correlation coefficients for a one week, three week and eight week delay are all moderately low and show a small negative change with increasing time interval, averaging 0.74, 0.58 and 0.48 for the three time periods. Thus, while there may be a small effect of trend in HRQL arising over the 8 week period, much of the contribution to error variance appears to be occurring with periodicity of less than one week, and must be due to fluctuations in HRQL.

If the changes result from trends, a patient who was improving in the first 3-week period (week 2 to week 5) would continue to improve over the second (week 6 to week 9); conversely one who was deteriorating in the first period would also deteriorate in the second. Thus the change scores in the two periods would be positively correlated. Examining the correlations of the two change scores (between week 2 and week 5 and between week 6 and week 8), in fact all the correlations were negative and ranged between –0.38 and –0.57 on the various subscales (with no overall difference in HRQL over the time periods). That is, an improvement in the first time period was associated with a deterioration in the second and vice versa, suggesting that the identified changes simply represent fluctuations in disease, not monotonic and permanent changes in individual patients.

Table 1. Reliability computed from the whole sample in the pediatric asthma study over successive time periods

Scale	Time period		
	1 week (weeks 1 to 2)	3 weeks (weeks 2 to 5 and 6 to 8)	7 weeks (weeks 1 to 8)
Overall	0.81	0.61	0.53
Activities	0.63	0.58	0.44
Symptoms	0.85	0.66	0.55
Emotional	0.74	0.50	0.45

6. Relation between Reliability and Responsiveness

Although some early writings [2,17] attempted to make the case that reliability and responsiveness are unrelated, this is not the case. While each employs a different measure as signal (in the one case, variance due to differences among individuals; in the other, the average change over time), both involve the same error term [5]. Thus any factor such as disease fluctuations which reduces the reliability coefficient will also suppress the responsiveness coefficient.

The original motivation for using retrospective methods to identify stable and changed subgroups was to compute responsiveness on a subgroup of patients who had improved (or improved and worsened). The arguments advanced above with respect to the calculation of reliability apply equally well to the measurement of responsiveness. To the extent that individual patient's HRQL fluctuates over time, the researcher will be unable to detect overall effects of treatment as well as identify stable differences among patients.

In the first analysis we showed that restricting the calculation of responsiveness to only those patients who have "truly" changed, by self-report, results in an upward bias in the responsiveness coefficient, typically by a factor of two or three in comparison to a coefficient computed by examining overall change resulting from a treatment. In the second analysis we showed that this retrospective approach similarly results in an upward bias in the calculation of reliability. The retrospective identification of changed and unchanged subgroups combined with the strategy of restricting calculation of change to only those who changed, and restricting calculation of stability to those who remained stable, amounts to proving a tautology and results in inflated estimation of both coefficients.

7. Conclusions

This paper demonstrates that the common approach to calculation of reliability retrospectively from a sub-sample who have been selected because they did not change over time and calculating responsiveness retrospectively from a subsample who report that they have changed results in an upward bias in the estimates. Calculations showed that the bias is not trivial, and amounts to a proportionate increase of the reliability coefficient by as much as 50% over one computed from the total sample and a larger increase in the responsiveness coefficient.

While we believe that the use of global self-ratings of change is poor practice for a number of reasons, it is evident that the bias cannot be solely due to this methodology. Our conclusion is that using methods based on retrospective selection of unchanged subsamples, whether by a global self-rating or clinician judgment, is ill-advised, and should be discouraged.

Instead, reliability must be computed prospectively. This can be based either on sampling of a cohort who would be unlikely to show trends in HRQL over the duration of the study, or selection prospectively of a subgroup who would judged by clinicians to remain stable [18]. Similarly, responsiveness should be computed according to the original formulation by examining the relative changes in different instruments resulting from a treatment of known efficacy.

ACKNOWLEGEMENTS

Portions of this article were taken from Norman, G.R., Regehr, G. and Stratford, P.W. (1997). Bias in the retrospective calculation of responsiveness to change: the lesson of Cronbach. *Journal of Clinical Epidemiology* **50**, 869–879. Permission of the editors is acknowledged.

REFERENCES

1. Wright J.G. and Feinstein, A.R. (1992). A comparative contrast of clinimetric and psychometric methods for constructing indices and rating scales. *Journal of Clinical Epidemiology* **45**, 1201–1218.
2. Kirshner, B. and Guyatt, G.H. (1985). A methodological framework for assessing health status indices. *Journal of Chronic Diseases* **38**, 27–36.
3. Liang, M.H., Cullen, K.E. and Schwartz, J.A. (1985). Comparative measurement efficiency and sensitivity of five health status instruments for arthritis research. *Arthritis Rheumatism* **28**, 542–547.
4. Kazis, L.E. and Anderson, J.J. (1989). Effect size for interpreting changes in health status. *Medical Care* **27**, S178–S189.
5. Norman, G.R. (1989). Issues in the use of changes scores in randomized trials. *Journal of Clinical Epidemiology* **42**, 1097–1105.
6. Jaeschke, R., Singer, J. and Guyatt, G.H. (1989). Measurement of health status: ascertaining the minimum clinically important difference. *Controlled Clinical Trials* **10**,

407–415.

7. Guyatt, G.H., Deyo, R.A., Charlson, M., Levine, M.N. and Mitchell, A. (1989). Responsiveness and validity in health status measurement: a clarification. *Journal of Clinical Epidemiology* **42**, 403–408.
8. Deyo, R.A. and Centor, R.M. (1986). Assessing responsiveness of functional scales to clinical change: an analogy to diagnostic test performance. *Journal of Chronic Diseases* **39**, 897–906.
9. Juniper, E.F., Guyatt, G.H., Feeny, D.H., Ferrie, P.J., Griffith, L.E. and Townsend, M. (1996). Measuring quality of life in children with asthma. *Quality of Life Research* **5**, 35–46.
10. Abello-Banfi, M., Cardiel, M.H., Ruiz-Mercado, R. and Alarcon-Segov, D. (1994). Quality of life in rheumatoid arthritis: validation of a Spanish version of Arthritis Impact Measurement Scales. *Journal of Rheumatology* **21**, 1250–55.
11. Ruta, D.A., Garratt, A.M., Leng, M., Russell, I.T. and MacDonald, L.M. (1994). A new approach to the measurement of quality of life: the patient generated index. *Medical Care* **32**, 1109–1126.
12. Ruta, D.A., Garratt, A.M., Wardlaw, D. and Russell, I.T. (1994). Developing a valid and reliable measure of health outcomes for patients with low back pain. *Spine* **19**; 1887–1896.
13. Rowe, B.H. and Oxman, A.D. (1993). Performance of an asthma quality of life questionnaire in an outpatient setting. *American Review of Respiratory Diseases* **148**, 675–682.
14. Norman, G.R., Regehr, G. and Stratford, P.W. (1997). Bias in the retrospective calculation of responsiveness to change: the lesson of Cronbach. *Journal of Clinical Epidemiology* **50**, 869–879.
15. Ross, M. (1989). Relation of implicit theories to the construction of personal histories. *Psychological Review* **96**, 341–347.
16. Juniper, E.F., Guyatt, G.H., Feeny, D.H., Ferrie, P.J., Griffith, L.E. and Townsend, M. (1996). Measuring quality of life in children with asthma. *Quality of Life Research* **5**, 35–46.
17. Guyatt, G.H., Walter, S.D. and Norman, G.R. (1987). Measuring change over time: assessing their usefulness of evaluative instruments. *Journal of Chronic Diseases* **40**, 171–178.
18. Francis, D.J., Fletcher, J.M., Stuebing, K.K., Davidson, K.C. and Thompson, N.M. (1991). Analysis of change: modelling individual growth. *Journal of Consultant in Clinical Psychology* **59**, 27–37.

APPLICATION OF THE MULTIATTRIBUTE UTILITY THEORY TO THE DEVELOPMENT OF A PREFERENCE-BASED HEALTH-RELATED QUALITY OF LIFE INSTRUMENT

CATHERINE LE GALÈS

Centre of Health Economics and Administration Research, INSERM U537

The Health Utilities Index is a generic multiattribute preference-based system for assessing health-related quality of life and is widely used in economic evaluations in North America and in international multicentre studies. As the HUI3 consists of 8 attributes deliberately selected to be structurally independent and specifies 5 or 6 levels by attribute, the explicit approach of the multiattribute utility theory (MAUT) provides an efficient framework to determine the utility scores of the 972,000 health states of this system. After reviewing the theoretical foundations used to model the multiattribute utility function, this article describes the protocol for revealing individual preferences and the analysis of a study carried out on a French population in June 1999. Results obtained at the person-mean level will be presented and discussed. This research illustrates the contribution of the MAUT to develop a weighting function for a health-related quality of life instrument. The analysis showed the importance of accounting for an individual's risk attitude when modelling preferences for health states.

1. Introduction

Over the past two decades, particular attention has been focused by many health economists on the measurement of health effects associated with conditions or interventions. As a result, new measurement strategies are now available to assess health-related quality of life (HRQL). Some of these strategies, such as the Health Utilities Index (Furlong *et al.*, 1998; Torrance, 1976; Torrance *et al.*, 1996), the Quality of Well Being scale (Kaplan, Bush and Berry, 1978) or the EuroQol scale (Dolan *et al.*, 1995; Dolan and Sutton, 1997) are generic preference-based health classification systems and capture, directly or indirectly, a person's value for health states. Among these instruments, the HUI is the unique preference-based system for which the weighting by preferences is based explicitly on the economic theory of rational choices (von Neumann and Morgenstern, 1947). According to the expected utility theory, when facing a choice between options, a rational individual will choose the best one according to the preferences he or she has for the consequences of the options. There are two types of preferences. Values are preferences measured in situations of certainty. That is, no probabilities pertain to the decision into which the measurement is applied. If this is not the case, measured preferences are called utilities and the rational person will choose the option with the higher expected preference (utility).

M. Mesbah et al. (eds.), Statistical Methods for Quality of Life Studies, 33–50.

The Health Utilities Index (HUI) is composed of two complementary elements: a multiattribute classification system which is used to describe health states and a weighting function used to value the health states. The classification is based on a multidimensional conception of health. It allows us to describe an individual's or a population's health status at a given moment and over a period of time. Based on Fanshel and Bush (1970) and then, Cadman and Goldsmith (1986), different versions of the HUI were developed.[1] In its most recent version (HUI3), it includes 8 dimensions (vision, hearing, elocution, ambulation, dexterity, emotion, cognition, and pain), each of which has 5 or 6 levels.[2] A health state is thus a vector of 8 elements; the first shows the pertinent level in the first dimension (vision) for the individual whose health state is being described; the second gives the level in the second dimension (hearing), so that 972,000 health states are possible. Because the health states are multidimensional, the multiattribute utility theory (MAUT) put forward by Keeney and Raiffa (1976), an extension of the expected utility theory when the consequences are complex, allows one to construct the weighting function of the multidimensional classification whilst supposing that each dimension of the HUI classification is an argument (or attribute) of the weighting function. Thus, the weighting function is called the aggregate multiattribute utility (MAU) function associated with the health states built upon the basis of preferences found in a sample of persons belonging to the general population. After reviewing the theoretical foundations used to model the MAU function, this paper describes the protocol for revealing individual preferences and the analyses of data obtained from a French population in June 1999.[3]

2. Methods

2.1 Theoretical and Methodological Foundations

The MAUT allows us to deal with the multidimensional nature of the health state without having to adopt a holistic approach (Fischer, 1979) which would involve directly revealing individual preferences for all health states in the HUI3 classification. Within this framework, the MAU function linked with a health state is characterised by several arguments which respectively correspond to the specific level of each of the dimensions of the health state.

The specificity of the MAUT is, on the basis of the axiomatic theory of expected

[1] For a complete presentation of the HUI classification system development, see Feeny, Torrance and Furlong (1996).

[2] As the original HUI3 classification was developed in English, the first step of the development of the instrument was to culturally adapt the classification and to validate it in different populations of patients in France (Costet *et al.*, 1998; Le Galès *et al.*, 1999). More precisely, the HUI2 and 3 classifications were both culturally and psychometrically validated in French adult and paediatric populations. The French weighting function was only constructed for HUI3. For a presentation of the French HUI2 or 3 classifications, see Le Galès *et al.* (1997). The 15Q questionnaire that allows mapping the answers whether in the HUI 2 or the HUI 3 classifications is available upon request to the author.

[3] The psychometric properties of the original classification, developed in English, were already adapted and validated for different populations of patients in France (Costet *et al.*, 1998; Le Galès *et al.*, 1999).

utility, to establish additional hypotheses that allow us to express a MAU function as a mathematical combination of utility functions defined for each dimension (conditional single-attribute utility functions).

The fundamental hypothesis of the MAUT is the first-order utility independence hypothesis (Farquhar, 1977; Fischer, 1979; Fishburn, 1965; Keeney, 1971, 1974; Keeney and Raiffa, 1976). This hypothesis states that an attribute X_i (or a sub-group of attributes) is deemed to be independent in terms of the utility of its complementary group if the order of preference for the lotteries, whose health states only differ in terms of the level of attribute X_i, is identical if we modify the attribute levels of the complementary group. If this hypothesis is verified for each of the eight attributes, the MAU function is said to be multilinear (equation 1). This strengthened, or completed hypothesis leads to multiplicative (equation 2) or additive forms (equation 3):

$$\begin{aligned} u(\mathbf{E}) &= \sum_{i=1}^{8} k_i u_i(x_i) + \sum_{i=1}^{8}\sum_{j>i} k_{ij} u_i(x_i) u_j(x_j) + \cdots + \\ & \sum_{i=1}^{8}\sum_{j>i}\sum_{\ell>j} k_{ij\ell} u_i(x_i) u_j(x_j) u_\ell(x_\ell) + \cdots + k_{12\cdots 8} u_1(x_1) \cdots u_8(x_8) \quad (1) \end{aligned}$$

$$u(\mathbf{E}) = \frac{1}{k}\left[\prod_{i=1}^{8}(1 + kk_i u_i) - 1\right] \quad \text{with} \quad k = \prod_{i=1}^{8}(1 + kk_i) - 1 \qquad (2)$$

$$u(\mathbf{E}) = \sum_{i=1}^{8} k_i u_i(x_i) \quad \text{with} \quad \sum_{i=1}^{8} k_i = 1, \qquad (3)$$

where: the MAU function $u(\mathbf{E})$ is defined on the basis of the health states $\mathbf{E}$ characterised by 8 attributes ($i = 1, \ldots, 8$), and is normalised on $[0, 1]$ so that $u(\mathbf{E}^\star) = u(x_1^\star, \ldots, x_8^\star) = 1$ and $u(\mathbf{x}^\circ) = u(x_1^\circ, \ldots, x_8^\circ) = 0$, where $x_i^\star$ represents the best level of attribute i and x_i° represents the worst level; the conditional single-attribute utility functions $u_i(x_i)$, defined for each attribute X_i are also normalised on $[0, 1]$, such that $u_i(x_i^\star) = 1$ and $u_i(x_i^\circ) = 0$; the k_i are scalar constants, such that $k_i = u(x_1^\circ, \ldots, x_{i-1}^\circ, x_i^\star, x_{i+1}^\circ, \ldots, x_8^\circ)$, which respectively correspond to corner state utilities, the respective weightings of the conditional single-attribute utilities. A corner state associated with a particular attribute is such that all the attributes are characterised by their lowest levels, with the exception of the attribute concerned, which is characterised by its highest level; the parameters $k_{i\ell}, k_{i\ell m}, \ldots, k_{12\cdots 8}$ are second- through eigth-order interactions.

The modelling which we selected to construct the MAU function for the French HUI classification was based on a twin choice: on the one hand, that of a MAU function of a multiplicative type; on the other hand, adherence to the mode of construction qualified as an explicitly decomposed approach.

The choice of a multiplicative type stems from a compromise between a form which best represents the characteristics of the preferences—empirically revealed—and the need for the empirical protocol for revealing individual preferences to be feasible from the interviewees' point of view. Unlike the additive form, the multiplicative composition also has the advantage that it takes into account the interactions between preferences on the different dimensions of a health state. However, unlike a multilinear composition, the dimensions must all be preference complements, or all be preference substitutes. Furthermore, a protocol for revealing preferences, which is based upon a multiplicative type allows us to evaluate an additive utility function, as the two types have most of their parameters in common.

Producing the information to assess a MAU function requires making a choice between two main designs: the statistically inferred modeling or the explicitly decomposed approach. The first requires fewer subjective multiattribute judgments than the holistic approach, in addition, to a statistically inferred technique such as functional measurement method, analysis of variance or multiple regression (Anderson, 1970; Fischer, 1979). Although a few studies have successfully used this approach, its practicability remains to be seen, and it is prudent to limit the number of attributes (Fischer, 1979; Llewellyn-Thomas *et al.*, 1984). The general class of the explicitly decomposed approach constitutes the standard MAU method. It asks the respondents to evaluate each level of a particular attribute, assuming all other attributes are held constant and, then, to provide scaling constants by assessing utilities of selected multiattribute states (Farquhar, 1977; Fishburn, 1965; Keeney and Raiffa, 1976). Finally, the explicitly decomposed approach is particularly suitable when the MAU function is defined on the basis of numerous attributes. Given the large number of attributes (8) and levels (5 or 6 per attribute) in the HUI3 classification, we therefore opted for this approach.

2.2 Adapting the Explicitly Decomposed Approach

Using the explicitly decomposed approach to construct a multiplicative utility function for health states involves revealing the preferences, under uncertainty, for the different levels of each attribute in the HUI3 classification and for the multidimensional health corner states. However, both for reasons of the specificity of the notion of health state, and for feasibility, and following Furlong *et al.* (1998) we modified the specification for health corner states. Rather than using corner states as they are defined by the MAU theory, we chose corner states of type $(x_1^\circ, \ldots, x_{i-1}^\circ, x_i^\star, x_{i+1}^\circ, \ldots, x_8^\circ)$. This new specification involves changing the referent for weighting the single-attribute functions, and constructing, to begin with, the multiplicative disutility function for health states:

$$du(\mathbf{E}) = 1 - u(\mathbf{E}) = \frac{1}{c}\left[\prod_{i=1}^{8}(1 + cc_i du_i) - 1\right] \tag{4}$$

where

$$c = \prod_{i=1}^{8}(1 + cc_i) - 1, \quad c_i = (x_1^\circ, \ldots, x_{i-1}^\circ, x_i^\star, x_{i+1}^\circ, \ldots, x_8^\circ). \tag{5}$$

The parameters c_i correspond to the corner state disutilities, c is the parameter expressed as a function of these disutilities, and du_i is the single-attribute disutility function defined for the i-th attribute.

2.3 The Mode of Construction of the Aggregate Function

The objective of the research was to build the aggregate utility function for the HUI health states on the basis of aggregated individual preferences. This explicitly required interpersonal comparison of utilities and defining a consistent aggregation rule. Two modes of construction can be distinguished. The first is to construct the MAU function for each interviewee on the basis of its elicited preferences. Then, the aggregate MAU function is modeled as a composition of these individual MAU functions. Excluding a dictatorial composition which makes one particular individual MAU function the aggregate one, the simplest modeling is linear. This modeling gives a weight to each individual MAU function. If all weights are equal, the aggregate MAU function is the mean of the individual ones. The second mode of construction requires modeling a fictional individual which aggregates all the interviewees. In such a mode, the aggregate MAU function is the MAU of this fictional individual. By consequence, this mode makes impossible to calculate confidence intervals for the function parameters (Le Galès *et al.*, forthcoming 1). This last mode of construction will be applied here, with the aggregated fictional individual's preferences being the mean of the interviewees' elicited preferences (person-mean).

3. The Study of Revelation of Preferences in the French Population

3.1 Protocol for Eliciting Health State Preferences

To obtain the parameters of the multiplicative disutility function, one needs to use methods for revealing individual preferences in a risk universe which are suitable for the sphere of health. Given the specificity of our field of application, the standard gamble (SG) seemed to be the most pertinent. However, exclusive use of this method would have made the process long and repetitive for the interviewees, so we also used a method for revealing preferences within a certain universe[4] (the visual analog scale [VAS] method) to obtain values.[5] These methods were applied to each interviewee by setting the value of the best possible state, or perfect health (PH), of the HUI3 *a priori* at 100, and leaving a choice between two states, worst possible state or (PITS) or death, for 0. PH is the best possible health state of the HUI3 classification as all attributes are at their best level of capacity. PITS it the most deteriorated HUI3 health state, as it is the one with all attributes being at their worst level of capacity.

The VAS method was used to reveal each of HUI3's uniattribute value functions (that is 28 uniattribute health states consisting of all intermediate levels of capacity for all eight attributes) and the values of 12 multiattribute health states.[6] These 12

[4]A choice between two options is in a certain universe if the consequences of these options are certain. If not, the decisional context is uncertain or probabilistic.

[5]Following Keeney and Raiffa (1976), a value qualifies any preference revealed within a certitude decisional context (i.e., using VAS technique for example), and a utility qualifies any preference revealed within a risk or uncertain one (i.e., SG for example).

[6]In our protocol, interviewees used a support called the "preference thermometer" and positioned the states of health described on cards along a scale graded from 0 to 100 in such a way that the greater the satisfaction with the state, the closer the position to the top of the scale should be, with the difference in grade between two states reflecting the difference in the level of satisfaction

multiattribute states were the 8 corner states, the state which had not been chosen as equalling 0 (PITS or death), and 3 multidimensional states:

MA(2,1,1,1,1,1,1,3)—Able to see well enough to read ordinary newsprint and recognize a friend on the other side of the street, but with glasses or contact lenses; able to hear what is said in a group conversation with at least 3 other people, without a hearing aid; able to be understood completely when speaking with strangers or people who know me well; able to walk around the neighborhood without difficulty, and without walking equipment; full use of 2 hands and 10 fingers; happy and interested in life; able to remember most things, think clearly and solve day to day problems; moderate pain that prevents a few activities.

MB(2,1,1,3,1,2,1,3)—Able to see well enough to read ordinary newsprint and recognize a friend on the other side of the street, but with glasses or contact lenses; able to hear what is said in a group conversation with at least 3 other people, without a hearing aid; able to be understood completely when speaking with strangers or people who know me well; able to walk around the neighborhood with walking equipment, but without the help of another person; full use of 2 hands and 10 fingers; somewhat unhappy; able to remember most things, think clearly and solve day to day problems; moderate pain that prevents a few activities.

VI(5,1,1,3,1,1,3,1)—Unable to read ordinary newsprint and unable to recognize a friend on the other side of the street, even with glasses or contact lenses; able to hear what is said in a group conversation with at least 3 other people, without a hearing aid; able to be understood completely when speaking with strangers or people who know me well; able to walk around the neighborhood with walking equipment, but without the help of another person; full use of 2 hands and 10 fingers; happy and interested in life; somewhat forgetful, but able to think or solve day to day problems; free of pain and discomfort.

The latter 3 states had been defined by supposing that they would relate to relatively distinct values which were likely to be spread along the entire scale. Furthermore, MA and MB are the states used in the Canadian protocol (Furlong *et al.*, 1998). They are thus important with regard to any comparison between the Canadian and French weightings. The utilities of 5 among the 12 multidimensional states were revealed using the SG method.[7] These data enable one to establish the function for transforming the values into utilities using the theoretical framework developed by Dyer and Sarin (1982) as we anticipate that the value of a given health state can be different from its utility.

felt.

[7]The SG was presented on a support which resembled a board game and on which there were two propositions. In the first, the interviewee was with certainty in the described health state; in the second, he/she was either in the best possible state with a certain probability, or in the state he/she considered to be the worst possible state with complementary probability. Different probability values were proposed in an iterative manner until the interviewee stated him/herself to feel indifferently towards both propositions.

3.2 Characteristics of the Sample

The study took place in June 1999 and included 365 persons from the general French population, aged between 20 and 65, and not suffering from any chronic or incapacitating illness. As our survey was the first one to be conducted on the French population, there were no scientific and rigorous data to calculate the required sample size. So the choice of 365 was determined in discussion with the Canadian developers on the basis of the precision of the MAUF they previously achieved. The sample was created using the quota method under five criteria. These criteria were selected for two reasons. Following the current recommendations (Gold *et al.*, 1996), the first reason was to define a sample as representative as possible of the French general population. The second reason was to be able to investigate the variability of the revealed preferences according to major socio-demographic characteristics. So, the splits by geographical zone, by size of village or town where the interviewee lives and by socio-professional category are representative of the French population. On the other hand, the splits by sex and age are balanced.

The recruitment procedure was based on a random selection of individuals from each of the main geographical zones, using the telephone directory. If during the telephone call, the contacted individual met all the inclusion criteria and accepted to participate, the interview was organized at home. The rate of acceptance was 25%, similar to what one would expect with this type of population survey design in France. After agreeing to take part in the study, the interviewees all saw the interview through to the finish. For conducting the interviews, 30 interviewers were specifically trained in the field of preference revelation by our research team. They used specifications which included both instructions for managing the interviews and the instructions to be read out to the interviewees. To minimise the bias created by what the interviewers said during the process of revealing preferences, the specifications had to be followed to the letter. Furthermore, each interviewer only carried out a limited number of interviews (maximum of 15).

The socio-demographic characteristics of the sample are shown in Table 1. To familiarise the interviewees with the HUI3 classification, the interviews began with a description of the interviewee's own health state over the previous 7 days, using the HUI3 classification. The notion of chronicity of a health state was then introduced, with the interviewee being asked to estimate how many years he or she had left to live, either by referring to the life expectancy of French people of the same age and sex, or by referring to personal or family history. During the remainder of the interview, every time the preference for a health state was elicited, the interviewee had to imagine that it was a question of his or her own health state and that it would remain unchanged for the rest of his or her life. The interview ended with the interviewee answering personal socio-demographic questions.

4. Results

4.1. Choice of Preference Anchoring

Of the 355 individuals for whom the anchoring was clearly identified, 93% put the PITS at the lower end of the multiattribute scale, the remaining 7% chose death.

Table 1. Socio-demographic characteristics of the sample

Characteristic	Group	Number	(Percent)
Gender	Female	184	(50)
	Male	181	(50)
Age (years)	20 to 30	97	(27)
	31 to 40	89	(24)
	41 to 50	94	(26)
	51 to 65	85	(23)
Marital status	Married	246	(68)
	Single	87	(24)
	Divorced	21	(6)
	Widowed	9	(2)
Employment status	Active	246	(67)
	Inactive	63	(17)
	Sick leave	5	(1)
	Unemployed	14	(4)
	Other	37	(10)
Religious practice	None	213	(58)
	Casual	111	(30)
	Regular	41	(11)
Education level	Primary education	41	(11)
	Vocational training certificate	73	(20)
	G.C.S.E	24	(7)
	Prof./Tech. education	40	(11)
	High school diploma	51	(14)
	University degree	134	(37)
Number of children	0	105	(29)
	1	57	(16)
	2	124	(34)
	3	50	(14)
	4 or more	28	(8)
Income (FF)	Under 3,000	17	(5)
	3,001 to 6,000	45	(13)
	6,001 to 12,000	120	(34)
	12,001 to 20,000	112	(31)
	More than 20,000	64	(18)

Table 2. Uniattribute values observed for the capacity levels of attributes with VAS

Attribute		N	Mean	SD	Median
Vision	5	341	15.3	16.8	10
	4	341	35.2	22.0	32
	3	341	50.3	23.6	50
	2	341	85.9	15.0	90
Hearing	5	341	22.8	19.8	20
	4	341	35.0	21.9	33
	3	341	56.6	24.9	60
	2	341	64.9	25.4	70
Elocution	4	341	29.2	23.1	22
	3	340	47.8	27.1	50
	2	341	65.5	25.2	70
Ambulation	5	341	12.1	14.9	10
	4	341	23.9	18.7	20
	3	341	45.2	23.4	50
	2	341	68.3	23.9	75
Dexterity	5	341	14.4	15.8	10
	4	341	27.2	19.5	25
	3	341	42.2	23.4	45
	2	341	63.4	25.1	70
Emotion	4	341	12.0	15.1	10
	3	341	30.9	22.2	30
	2	341	75.7	22.6	82
Cognition	5	341	17.8	17.2	10
	4	341	37.1	22.0	37
	3	341	56.8	24.1	60
Pain	4	341	18.8	15.6	15
	3	341	52.1	22.9	55
	2	341	76.1	21.8	85

This choice was not linked to the different socio-demographic characteristics of the respondents, nor to the health state of the interviewee. Due to the low number of individuals who chose death as the lower grading, the following analysis is focused on individuals who chose PITS as the lower grading (341 persons). Results concerning the 24 individuals who chose death at the bottom of the scale are presented elsewhere (Le Galès *et al.*, 2000).

4.2. Observed Values and Utilities in the PITS-PH Scale

Tables 2 and 3 show the values and utilities directly observed within the PITS-PH sub-sample. For each attribute, the mean value for the different levels of capacity is coherent with their logical order. We see high variability in the scores (standard deviations of between 14.9 and 27.1). Death is the consequence with the lowest score (10.4), with variability lower than that of the other states (standard deviation = 15.6). The MA and MB states are coherently ordered. No particular order was envisaged for the other states.

For all evaluated states (including death), the mean utility is higher than the mean value. The order of scores for value and utility is the same. The variability of utilities is higher than that for values (standard deviations of between 25.2 and 32.1). The test for the explicative character of the available socio-demographic variables (age, sex, socio-professional category, income level and religious practice) does not allow us to determine any predictive factors for the values and utilities attributed to the multidimensional states. We also looked for an interviewer's influence on the collected data but found none.

4.3 Aggregation of Individual Data and Definition of Person-Mean

The aggregated fictional individual (person-mean) was calculated after excluding individuals having put both PITS and death at 0 and in separately considering the uniattribute and multiattribute sections. Regarding the uniattribute preferences, there are two sorts of reason for exclusion: first of all, systematic scoring of 0 or 100 for all of the intermediary capacity levels for a given attribute and over at least 3 attributes (7 individuals were excluded for this reason); secondly, the non-respect of the logical order for certain capacity levels over several attributes (1 excluded).[8] At the end of the day, the number of individuals excluded for the calculation of aggregated individuals is relatively low (8 excluded). Regarding multiattribute preferences, the responses of certain individuals could not be retained due to an error which occurred at the time of the interview (change of anchoring for the VAS and SG methods). Furthermore, because the MA and MB states are ordered (in as much as MB corresponds to MA, but with two attributes that are lower),[9] the MB state should not have a higher score than the MA, either for value or for utility.

[8]The intermediate levels of the HUI3 attributes are not necessarily ordinal but for some attributes non-logical rankings could be identified (e.g., valuing level 4 of the pain attribute [moderate to severe pain that prevents some activities] higher than level 3 [moderate pain that prevents a few activities]. Only such cases of inversion were considered for exclusion.

[9]For these two attributes (ambulation and emotion) the logical order for capacity levels is from full capacity (level 1) to total incapacity (level 6 or 5).

Table 3. Observed scores for multidimensional health states (for value and for utility)

Attribute	N	Mean	SD	Median
Multiattribute values (VAS method)				
Vision*	341	23.1	22.8	15
Hearing*	341	42.6	26.0	40
Elocution*	340	38.8	24.8	40
Ambulation*	340	31.2	22.8	30
Dexterity*	341	36.4	24.6	34
Emotion*	341	18.2	24.2	5
Cognition*	341	30.1	28.4	20
Pain*	341	24.2	24.2	15
MA	341	76.7	21.4	85
MB	339	56.3	25.8	64
VI	341	36.3	25.1	34
Death	331	10.4	15.6	5
Multiattribute values (SG method)				
Elocution*	340	64.2	32.1	75
MA	341	80.0	25.2	92
MB	341	71.0	26.9	75
VI	341	56.3	31.8	60
Death	340	37.8	31.7	35

*Corner state of the attribute

Individuals who reversed MA or MB for value (20 subjects) or utility (34 subjects) were therefore excluded. The surveyed people who were excluded did not belong to any particular age, income or qualifications group. Finally, the calculation of the person-mean integrated data from 275 individuals (PITS-PH scale).

4.4. Function for Transforming Values into Utilities

To find a transformation of the value function into a utility function, we analysed the type of relationship between the values and the utilities attributed by the respondents during the survey to the health states MA, MB, VI, CEL and death in as much as they expressed their preferences for these states both in a certain universe (by VAS) and in a risk universe (by SG). After verifying, for these health states, the coherency of the ordering of the certain preferences with that obtained in a risk universe, the following adjustment models for the relationship between values and utilities were tested (Buron, 1999):

Adjustment A (linear): $u_e[v(\mathbf{E})] = v(\mathbf{E})$

Adjustment B (exponential): $u_e[v(\mathbf{E})] = \dfrac{e^{-\alpha v(\mathbf{E})-1}}{e^{-\alpha}-1}$, $\alpha \neq 0$

Adjustment C (logarithmic): $u_e[v(\mathbf{E})] = \dfrac{\ln[1+\alpha v(\mathbf{E})]}{\ln(1+\alpha)}$

Adjustment D (log-power): $u_e[v(\mathbf{E})] = \dfrac{[1+\beta v(\mathbf{E})]^{\ln(1+\alpha)/\ln(1+\beta)}-1}{\alpha}$,
$\alpha = k,\ \beta = w$

Adjustment E (power): $u_e[v(\mathbf{E})] = v(E)^{\alpha}$, $\alpha > 0$

The first four models tested correspond to the theoretical relationships between utility and value functions established by Dyer and Sarin (1979). Certain studies have shown the pertinence of the fifth model when analysis covers health states (Llewellyn-Thomas *et al.*, 1984; Mehrez and Gafni, 1987; O'Connor *et al.*, 1987; Torrance, 1976; Read *et al.*, 1984). Indeed, in many studies, the power function has provided a good adjustment of the relationship between value and utility (Torrance, 1976; Torrance *et al.*, 1996; Wolfson *et al.*, 1982).

The decision on which of the five models was the best adjustment model was made in two stages. First, the α parameter (and β in the case of adjustment D) was estimated for each model by minimizing the root mean square error (RMSE; Dyer *et al.*, 1973; Fishburn and Kochenberger, 1979). The RMSE is the root of the mean squared error given by

$$\frac{1}{N}\sum_{n=1}^{N}\left(u_e[v(E_n)] - u(E_n)\right)^2,$$

where $N = 5$ states (MA, MB, CEL, VI and death). Use of the RMSE criterion enables us to measure and judge how close the adjustment for each estimated model $u_e[v(\mathbf{E})]$ was to the observed data $u(\mathbf{E})$. Once the α (and β) estimator with the lowest RMSE has been obtained for each adjustment model, the various models were compared on the basis of their respective RMSE's. The model with the lowest RMSE was then considered to be the model which best adjusted the relationship between values and utilities. In order to judge how close each adjustment model was to reality, we defined an *ad hoc* rule: a model was considered to be acceptable when its RMSE was no greater than 0.055. There are very few articles that test the relational form between utilities and values, and to which we could refer in order to establish the RMSE threshold. We used the work by Keller (1985) to set the threshold. The test of the different relational forms between utilities and values on the basis of the RMSE criterion highlights the superiority of the power model (Table 4).

This observation corroborates the results of the above-mentioned studies when preference revelation relates to health states. The linear model is the model with the highest RMSE values. Given the hypothesis underlying the linear model,[10] this

[10]The linear relational form between values and utilities expresses neutrality with regard to "relative" risk. This means that a decision-maker's choices in a risk universe are only determined by the differences in preferences for certain states of health, and that the risk inherent in the decisional situation does not influence his/her choice.

suggests that the individuals in our sample are not neutral with regard to "relative" risk. This is confirmed when we examine the sign of the attitude measurement regarding "relative" risk in the case of the best adjustment model (the power model): $v(\mathbf{E})r_v[v(\mathbf{E})] = 1 - \alpha = 1 - 0.47$. Indeed, because the value of the α parameter is lower than 1, we can conclude that the interviewees are expressing, on average, an aversion to "relative" risk. This is easily seen by computing first and second derivatives of $e(\mathbf{E}) = v(\mathbf{E})^\alpha$ with respect to $v(\mathbf{E})$.

Table 4. Best adjustment model for the relationship between values and utilities ($N = 275$). For model D, the log-power model, convergence was not obtained

Model	RMSE	α
A (linear)	0.218	–
B (exponential)	0.091	2.16
C (logarithmic)	0.067	9.68
E (power)	0.044	0.47

Table 5. Person-mean MAU function on a PITS(6,6,5,6,6,5,6,5) PH(1,1,1,1,1,1,1,1) scale. Shown are the resulting disutility and utility functions.

Attribute	x_1	x_2	x_3	x_4	x_5	x_6
Disutility function						
Vision	0.00	0.07	0.28	0.39	0.59	1.00
Hearing	0.00	0.18	0.23	0.39	0.50	1.00
Elocution	0.00	0.18	0.29	0.44	1.00	
Ambulation	0.00	0.16	0.31	0.49	0.63	1.00
Dexterity	0.00	0.19	0.33	0.46	0.60	1.00
Emotion	0.00	0.12	0.42	0.63	1.00	
Cognition	0.00	0.14	0.23	0.37	0.56	1.00
Pain	0.00	0.12	0.26	0.55	1.00	
Utility function						
Vision	1.00	0.96	0.86	0.80	0.70	0.49
Hearing	1.00	0.94	0.92	0.87	0.83	0.66
Elocution	1.00	0.93	0.89	0.84	0.64	
Ambulation	1.00	0.93	0.87	0.79	0.73	0.57
Dexterity	1.00	0.93	0.87	0.82	0.77	0.61
Emotion	1.00	0.93	0.77	0.65	0.45	
Cognition	1.00	0.94	0.90	0.84	0.76	0.56
Pain	1.00	0.94	0.87	0.73	0.51	

4.5 Person-Mean Multiattribute Utility Function

Having chosen the best adjustment model relating values and utilities, the uniattribute values were converted into uniattribute disutilities ($du(x_i) = 1 - v(x_i)^{0.47}$).

The c_i parameters of the equation (4) were calculated from the values (directly measured) of the corner states, which had been converted into utilities and then transformed into disutilities ($c_i = 1 - v(x_1^\star, \ldots, x_{i-1}^\star, x_i^\circ, x_{i+1}^\star, \ldots, x_8^\star)^{0.47}$). Finally, parameter c was obtained by solving equation (5) and the formula for calculating the disutility and utility of each state in the HUI3 classification was established (Table 5) for the person-mean. The parameter values are $c = 0.990$, $c_1 = 0.5118$, $c_2 = 0.3408$, $c_3 = 0.3659$, $c_4 = 0.4316$, $c_5 = 0.3909$, $c_6 = 0.5546$, $c_7 = 0.4415$, $c_8 = 0.4952$. The multiattribute disutility function was on a scale from 0 (PITS) to 1 (PH), and the form of the disutility function was

$$du(\mathbf{E}) = \frac{1}{c}\left[\prod_{i=1}^{8}(1 + cc_i du_i) - 1\right].$$

The disutility of the health state $\mathbf{E}$ was calculated as $u(\mathbf{E}) = 1 - du(\mathbf{E})$ or using the following scoring formula: $u(\mathbf{E}) = 1.01a_1a_2a_3a_4a_5a_6a_7a_8 - 0.01$, where the a parameters are given by the utility values shown in Table 5.

Although the utilities of the corner states cannot be interpreted using the MAU theory as being the relative weights of the attributes, they do enable us to distinguish the emotion and vision attributes which have the lowest corner state utilities: 0.46 and 0.49 respectively. Overall, the deviations between attributes remain limited: the lowest corner utility stands at 0.46, with the highest being 0.66 for the hearing attribute. It is possible to calculate the utility of the MA, MB, VI and CEL states whose utilities were directly measured. Only, the death utility, which is not a classified state, cannot be calculated by this formula. Therefore, the related level of utility is that which was directly measured during the study.

A comparison of these calculated utilities with the observed ones provides a primary indicator of the validity of the constructed person-mean function (Table 6). The slight absolute differences obtained between observed and calculated utilities and the low RMSE scores lead us towards a favourable conclusion.

Similarly, the results obtained in terms of the differences between calculated and observed utilities and RMSE values through modelling the MAU function of additive type do not call the choice of a multiplicative model into question.

Table 6. Calculated and observed utilities for the states MA, MB, VI and CEL for the multiplicative and additive models at the person-mean level (PITS-PH scale). RMSE is 0.0288 for the multiplictative model and 0.0710 for the additive model.

	Multiplicative model			Additive model		
State	U_{obs}	U_{calc}	Diff.	U_{obs}	U_{calc}	Diff.
MA	0.8387	0.8384	0.0003	0.8387	0.8338	0.0049
MB	0.7127	0.6771	0.0356	0.7127	0.6329	0.0798
VI	0.5758	0.5426	0.0332	0.5758	0.4626	0.1132
ECS	0.6649	0.6340	0.0309	0.6649	0.6340	0.0309

5. Conclusion

To the best of our knowledge, this is the first survey on individual preferences for health states using VAS and SG methods carried out in France. In accordance with the economic welfare theory, the interviewed population came from the general French population. A recent review of the literature on the existence of differences in preferences between patients and other raters (Ardine de Wits, Busschbach and de Charro, 2000) reports growing evidence that patients assign in general higher values than other raters. So, as it is the case for the other existing weighting functions based on this type of population preference survey, the French HUI3 function does not necessarily reflect the preferences of ill persons.

The limited number of questionnaires excluded at the various different stages of building the multiattribute utility function demonstrates that such surveys are viable instruments for gathering original and high-quality information on the values and judgements held by individuals with regard to health. Reasons of exclusion were inconsistencies of individuals' answers with the expected utility theory. This is not surprising as a great deal of empirical research indicate that individual preferences do not always conform to this modelling of rationality. Nevertheless, because of the low number of exclusions and its limited impact of the function, these empirical results are not convincing enough to abandon expected utility theory in the domain of preference-weighted health index. To examine the impact of exclusions on calculated utilities, we recalculated the MAUF taking into account all the collected data of our survey. The differences were important for the health states which utilities were less than 0.50 and have only a very small impact on the weighting function (Le Galès *et al.*, 2002).

The analogies of our protocol with that chosen to construct the HUI3 multiattribute utility function in Canada allow us to make an international comparison of our results. A rough preliminary comparison of the two functions suggests that the results are relatively similar as far as the form and the parameters of the MAU functions are concerned. If these results were confirm there will be of particular importance for the overall international development strategy of HrQL instruments based on the economic theory.

In conclusion, the practical consequences of our work must be highlighted. The development of the French HUI preference-based system is now achieved and from now it is possible to perform economic evaluation studies in France which combine length and quality of life in accordance with the international recommendations (Gold *et al.*, 1996).

ACKNOWLEDGEMENTS

This research was mainly financed by the Programme Hospitalier de Recherche Clinique (Direction des Hôpitaux) during 1995 and 1996 offers to tender. Special thanks to Nathalie Costet, Catherine Buron, Samuel Aballéa and Sophia Rosman.

REFERENCES

Anderson, N. (1970). Functional measurement and psychophysical judgment, *Psychological Review* **77**, 153–170.

Ardine de Wits, G., Busschbach, J. and de Charro, F. (2000). Sensitivity and perspective in the valuation of health status: whose values count? *Health Economics* **9**, 109–126.

Buron, C. (1999). *Utilities and Preferences under Risk and Uncertainty: An Application of Multiattribute Utility Theory to Health Economics* (French). Doctoral thesis. Université Panthéon-Assas (Paris II).

Cadman, D. and Goldsmith, C. (1986). Construction of social value or utility-based health indices: the usefulness of factorial experimental design plans. *Journal of Chronic Disease* **39**, 643–651.

Costet, N., Le Galès, C., Buron, C. Kinkor, F., Mesbah, M., Chwalow, J. and Slama, G. (1998). French cross-cultural adaptation of the Health Utilities Indexes Mark 2 (HUI2) and 3 (HUI3) classification systems. Clinical and Economic Working Groups. *Quality of Life Research* **7**, 245–256.

Dolan, P., Gudex, C., Kind, P. and Williams, A. (1995). A social tariff for EuroQol: results from a UK general population survey. Discussion Paper 138, Center for Health Economics, University of York, York.

Dolan, P. and Sutton, M. (1997). Mapping visual analogue scale health state valuations onto standard gamble and time trade-off values. *Social Science and Medicine* **44**, 1519–1530.

Dyer, J.S., Farrell, W. and Bradley, P. (1973). Utility functions for test performance. *Management Sciences* **20**, 507–519.

Dyer, J.S. and Sarin, R.A. (1979). Measurable multiattribute value functions. *Operations Research* **24**, 220–243.

Dyer, J.S. and Sarin, R.K. (1982). Relative risk aversion. *Management Sciences* **28**, 875–886.

Fanshell, S. and Bush, J.W. (1970). A health status index and its application to health services outcomes. *Operations Research* **18**, 1021–1066.

Farquhar, P.H. (1977). A survey of multi-attribute utility theory and application. *TIMS Studies in the Management Sciences* **6**, 59–89.

Feeny, D.H., Torrance, G.W. and Furlong W.J. (1996). Health Utilities Index. In: Spilker, B. (ed.), *Quality of Life and Pharmacoeconomics in Clinical Trials, 2nd Edition.* Philadelphia: Lippincott-Raven.

Fischer, G.W. (1979). Utility models for multiple objective decisions: do they accurately represent human preferences? *Decision Sciences* **10**, 451–479.

Fishburn, P.C. (1965). Independence in utility theory with whole product sets. *Operations Research* **13**, 28–45.

Fishburn, P.C. and Kochenberger G. (1979). Two-piece Von Neumann-Morgenstern utility functions. *Decision Sciences* **10**, 503–518.

Furlong, W., Feeny D., Torrance G.W., Goldsmith, C.H., DePauw, S., Zhu, Z., Denton, M. and Boyle, M. (1998). Multiplicative multi-attribute utility function for the Health Utilities Index Mark 3 (HUI3) system: a technical report. Working paper series 98-11, CHEPA, McMaster University.

Gold, M.R., Siegel, J.E., Russel, L.B. and Weinstein, M.C., Eds. (1996). *Cost-Effectiveness in Health and Medicine.* New York: Oxford University Press.

Kaplan, R.M., Bush, J.W. and Berry, C.C. (1978). The reliability, stability and generalisability of a health status index. *Proceedings of the Social Statistics Section of the American Statistical Association*, 704–709.

Keeney, R.L. (1971). Utility independence and preferences for multiattributed consequences. *Operations Research* **19**, 875–893.

Keeney, R.L. (1974). Multiplicative utility functions. *Operations Research*, **22**, 22–34.

Keeney, R.L. and Raiffa, H. (1976). *Decision with multiple objectives.* New York: Wiley.

Keller, L.R. (1985). An empirical investigation of relative risk aversion. *IEEE Transactions on Systems, Man and Cybernetics* **15**, 475–482.

Le Galès, C., Costet, N., Gentet, J.C., Kalifa, C., Frappaz, D., Edan, C., Sariban, E., Plantaz, D. and Doz, F. (1999). Cross-cultural adaptation of a health status classification system in children with cancer. First results of the French adaptation of the Health Utilities Index Marks 2 and 3. *International Journal of Cancer - Supplement* **12**, 112–118.

Le Galès, C., Costet, N., Buron, C. et le groupe HUI (1997). Methodology of the trans-cultural adaptation of a preference-weighted health status classification system (French). *Journal d'Economie Médicale* **15**, 529–548.

Le Galès, C., Costet, N., Buron, C. and Slama, G. (2000). Development of a preference-weighted health index (French). Working paper, CHEAR, INSERM U537, Le Kremlin-Bicêtre.

Le Galès, C., Buron, C., Costet, N., Rosman, S. and Slama, G. (forthcoming 1). Development of a preference-weighted health status classification system in France (French). *Economie et Prévision.*

Le Galès, C., Buron, C., Costet, N., Rosman, S. and Slama, G. (2002). Development of a preference-weighted health status classification system in France: the Health Utilities Index 3. *Journal of Health Care and Management Science* **5**, 41–51.

Llewellyn-Thomas, H., Sutherland, H.J., Tibshirani, R., Ciampi, A., Till, J.E. and Boyd, N.F. (1984). Describing health states. Methodologic issues in obtaining values for health states. *Medical Care* **22**, 543–552.

Mehrez, A. and Gafni, A. (1987). An Empirical evaluation of two assessment methods for utility measurement for life years. *Socio-Economic Planification Science* **21**, 371–375.

O'Connor, A.M., Boyd, N.F., Warde, P., Stolbach, L. and Till, J.E. (1987). Eliciting preferences for alternative drug therapies in oncology: influence of treatment outcome description, elicitation technique and treatment experience on preferences. *Journal of Chronic Diseases* **40**, 811–818.

Read, J.L., Quinn, R.J., Berwick, D.M., Fineberg, H.V. and Weinstein, M.C. (1984). Preferences for health outcomes. Comparison of assessment methods. *Medical Decision Making* **4**, 315–329.

Torrance, G.W. (1976). Social preferences for health states: an empirical evaluation of three measurement techniques. *Socio-Economic Planification Science* **10**,

129–136.

Torrance, G.W., Feeny, D., Furlong, W., Barr, R.D., Zhang, Y. and Wang, Q. (1996). Multiattribute utility function for a comprehensive health status classification system. Health Utilities Index Mark 2. *Medical Care* **34**, 702–722.

Von Neumann, J. and Morgenstern, O. (1947). *Theory of games and economic behaviour, 2nd Edition.* Princeton: Princeton University Press.

Wolfson, A.D., Sinclair, A.J., Bombardier, C. and McGeer, A. (1982). Preference measurements for functional status in stroke patients: interrater and intertechnique comparaisons. In: Kane, R.L. and Kane, R.A. (eds.), *Values and Long Term Care.* Lexington: Lexington Books.

STRATEGY AND METHODOLOGY FOR CHOICE OF ITEMS IN PSYCHOMETRIC MEASUREMENT: DESIGNING A QUALITY OF LIFE INSTRUMENT FOR HIP AND KNEE OSTEOARTHRITIS

FRANCIS GUILLEMIN,[1] JOEL COSTE,[2] NATHALIE RETEL-RUDE,[3] ELISABETH SPITZ,[4] MICHÈLE BAUMANN,[1] CYRILLE TARQUINIO,[4] CATHERINE LUTTENBACHER,[3] JACQUES POUCHOT[5] AND THE FRENCH QUALITY OF LIFE IN RHEUMATOLOGY GROUP

[1]*University of Nancy,* [2]*Hôpital Cochin-Paris,* [3]*Université de Besançon,* [4]*Université de Metz,* [5]*Hôpital Louis Mourier-Paris*

The construction of composite health status or quality of life (QoL) measurement scales includes various steps, and aims to generate items with meaningful content. Standard scale construction has three stages: a qualitative stage, designed to achieve coverage of all potentially affected areas, a quantitative stage designed to test instrument scaling properties, and a stage of item selection to address feasibility and acceptability of the scale. The objectives of this paper are to investigate the relative contribution of several methods of item development and choice, to highlight the need for structuring the conceptual reflection on building an instrument, and to propose guidelines for structuring a quality of life questionnaire. As a model, we present a protocol for developing a QoL instrument for lower limbs osteoarthritis (OA). OA is a chronic disease with prevalence increasing with age. It may produce potentially severe ability limitations and social participation restrictions according to the ICIDH-2 classification. However, no real OA quality of life questionnaire has been yet developed. This study was conducted with 3 working hypotheses: (1) a generic questionnaire, the SF-36, is relevant to target consequences of lower limbs OA on patients QoL; (2) a condition specific questionnaire for lower limbs OA can be built as the combination of the SF-36 and a disease specific module; and (3) various item generation methods may each contribute relevant statements and words. These methods include cognitive interview of patients, individual or focus group interviews of patients, individual or focus group interviews of health professionals, followed by various methods of content analysis. Accordingly, the study will comprise five pathways aimed at generating items. A total of 128 OA patients and 32 health professionals will be interviewed. A trained team of sociologists will perform a semantic theme content analysis of tape-recorded and transcribed interviews. The next step consists of running content analysis completed by hierarchical cluster analysis. This will be used to identify relevant QoL dimensions. The second task will be to review the data analysis to identify verbatims pertaining to each dimension. Further analyses will identify the respective contribution of each method employed to generate items. The primary stages of composite scale construction include concepts specification and content descriptions. We expect to better document the relative contribution of each approach within each stage. We hope to contribute to future methodological guidelines to generate quality of life questionnaires.

1. Composite Measurement Scales Construction

The construction of composite health status measurement scales (CMS) includes various steps, and their validation requires empirical study involving multiple researchers and many patients (including those required for cross-validation or application studies).

M. Mesbah et al. (eds.), Statistical Methods for Quality of Life Studies, 51–61.

Clinicians, methodologists and statisticians should be aware of the rationale for the use of a particular instrument, as well as the different facets of the construct and choices made during its construction.

The first step in the construction of a scale is to establish content validity. Content validity, as defined by the American Psychological Association [1,2], is the property of a measurement method to measure what it is intended to measure. This depends primarily on the adequacy and exhaustiveness with which a specified domain is sampled. Much effort has been put in developing methods to (1) select components, group items, cover a construct, and aggregate different items on different dimensions, (2) model, define and choose between candidate items, and (3) address scaling properties of items and answering modalities [3,4]. Although much work has been performed in this area, with a focus on the metric properties of such scales, item construction methodology is somewhat neglected. The current biomedical literature remains scarce regarding the very first step of this process, item and scale generation. Very few studies are presenting a structured protocol for the way items are generated and assembled into dimensions to form a scale. Little is known on the respective contribution of various methods developed in qualitative research to elicit patients' opinions and perceptions about their conditions. The development of a new scale gives the opportunity to create a protocol by exploring the contribution of several methods.

Quality of life (QoL) is multifaceted. Previous reviews have identified poor content description and specification [5,6]. The content validity should generally rely on critical definition and specification of the concept, constructs and facets explored. Unfortunately, such work is rarely reported in the literature [7–9].

Several works [10,11] have been done recently to document the respective merit of item selection through a clinimetric approach in which experts (clinicians, sometimes with patients) are proposing items informally or through structured group processes and are making decisions, and a psychometric approach, which relies on statistical analysis of data collected according to psychometric standards [2]. These statistical analyses are performed after items have been generated, formulated and administered to a sample of subjects. Further research regarding the scaling properties of answering modalities has been recently boosted by the development of new statistical models particularly suited for ordinal scales and based on item response theory (IRT). These models include Rasch models, logistic models for binary or rating scales, partial credit models, nominal response models for polytomous scales, and factor analysis [12].

Generating items involves making explicit, relevant items or questions targeting a specific concept. The goal is to make the item's meaning fit the targeted population in the desired objective of measurement. Little methodology has been formalised for this initial stage (i.e., building the items themselves). Several issues are considered separately and have been mainly developed by health psychologists well aware of problems with metric or item bias [13,14].

The current standard for scale construction consists of three stages:

1. A qualitative stage including (in no particular order) literature review, items bank, and patient or expert opinion. The aim of this stage is to cover all potentially affected areas with a particular focus of the definition for disease-specific instruments. Combinations of these approaches have been reported to generate pools of items [15]. Standardised focus groups have proved useful in providing condition-specific items [16].

2. A quantitative stage designed to test instrument-scaling properties and optimise measurement by minimizing expenses, preparing acceptable scaling properties, and making the measurement efficient.

3. A stage of item selection to address feasibility and acceptability of the CMS.

Scale validation is the classical examination of the product issued from scale construction with regard to standard metric properties. We will not address this in this paper.

The objective of item generation is to develop a scale with meaningful content before it is used in further statistical modelling (metric scaling, validity testing, or data analysis). Current literature on CMS scales understates these stages, leaving one to assume that items have been adequately generated and chosen. Methods regarding the respective contribution of each of these qualitative stages are poorly reported. Combinations of various methods have already proved useful in the field of subjective CMS scales [17,18].

2. Objectives

The objectives of this research are to:

1. Investigate the relative contribution of several methods of item development and selection.

2. Highlight the need for structuring the conceptual reflection for building an instrument.

3. Propose guidelines for structuring a quality of life questionnaire, with an application to designing a QoL scale for lower limbs osteoarthritis (OA).

The framework for addressing these objectives consists of two parts. The first is dimension identification based on concept dimension specification. Here we use a general framework embracing the WHO definition of health, the ICIDH-2 framework for defining a handicap [19] and the standard WHOQOL definition of quality of life [20], combined with patients' expression of feelings. Because we are in a subjective measurement paradigm, we will weight highly the latter source. Second, item generation and formulation will be possible when dimensions have been identified. We will use a patient-structured elicitation approach.

2.1 Hip and Knee Osteoarthritis

Osteoarthritis of the lower limbs is a chronic disease with prevalence increasing with age. Hip osteoarthritis is slightly more frequent in males, while knee osteoarthritis is predominantly affecting females. It may produce potentially severe physical and social limitations according to the ICIDH-2 classification (Figure 1). Current medical treatment is not highly effective, with many patients remaining symptomatic. Surgical treatment, particularly total hip or knee replacement, where indicated, is costly but helpful to restore function and relieve pain. Quality of life in patients with lower limbs OA has been explored using generic instruments such as the Nottingham Health Profile [21] or the SF-

36. Limitations in the responsiveness of the SF-36 have been documented [22]. Generic and condition specific questionnaires have been frequently advocated to be administered jointly in chronic OA patients [23, 24].

No real OA-specific quality of life questionnaire has yet been developed. Although disability instruments like the WOMAC [25] are available, they are restricted to exploration of mobility in daily life. A quality-of-life questionnaire for lower limbs OA should reflect patients' expectations, account for their needs in daily life, address invisible or poorly recognised aspects of their condition, and give attention to emotional reaction and social participation.

Figure 1. Current understanding of interactions between the dimensions of ICIDH-2

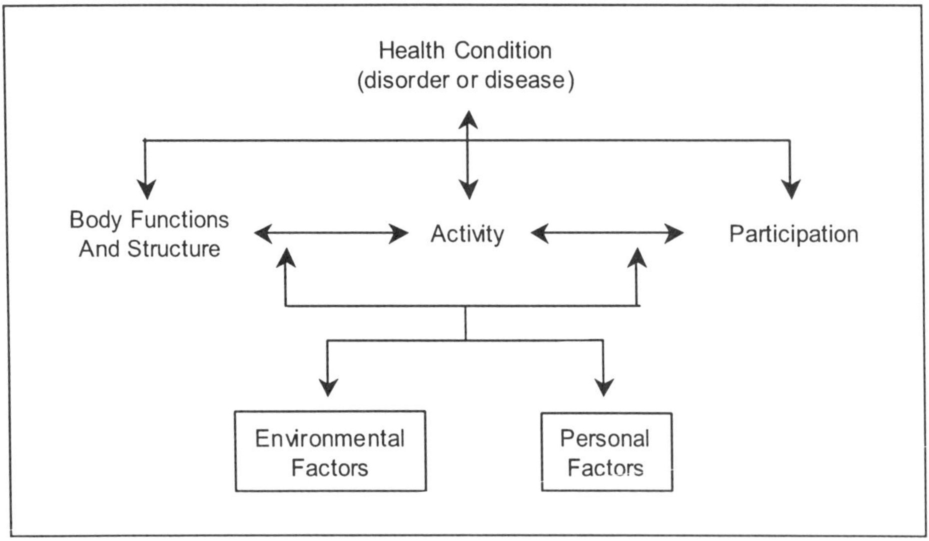

2.2 The SF-36 and Its Modules

The content of the SF-36 questionnaire has been analysed by quality of life experts and found unsatisfactory in the OA setting. Being generic in nature, items are too general and do not focus on specific lower limb OA problems. Nevertheless, the SF-36 has been suggested as a tool for measuring responsiveness in clinical trials. As such, it is likely to miss disease-specific aspects such as self-consciousness of joint deformations, having fear of needing a wheelchair, suffering pain when cold or in humidity, or avoiding certain activities because of OA.

The modular approach to quality-of-life assessment is interesting. Generic instruments address overall health or quality of life, while specific instruments focus on the impact of a particular disease on a patient's QoL. Several instruments use generic dimensions tailored to a specific condition by adding insight into a particular aspect and adapting the framing of questions.

The addition of modules to the SF-36 has proved successful for kidney disease (KD-QOL) [26,27] and multiple sclerosis (MS-54) [28]. Such approaches are not unique and have been developed with the EORTC QLQC-30 [29] or the FACT [30] instruments. Our objective is to test the possibility of developing an SF-36 module for lower limbs OA.

2.3 Working Hypothesis 1

A generic questionnaire, the SF-36, can target the impact of lower limbs OA on patients' QoL. Acceptance of this hypothesis will require further work to document whether it is sufficiently comprehensive to target this condition. If so, the process can end there. If not, a new instrument will be needed.

2.4 Working Hypothesis 2

A condition-specific questionnaire for lower limbs OA can be built by combining the SF-36 with a disease-specific module. Thus, dimension testing of patients' expressions will identify additional specific dimensions. Acceptance of this hypothesis will lead to the addition of a module to the SF 36. Rejection of this hypothesis will lead us to build a new instrument.

2.5 Working Hypothesis 3

We hypothesise that various generation methods may each contribute relevant statements and words useful in the construction of relevant items. Acceptance of this hypothesis will lead to use a variety of methods to generate items. These methods include cognitive interviews, individual or focus group interviews with patients, and individual or focus group interviews with health professionals. These will be followed by various methods of content analysis. Rejection of this hypothesis will lead to select only items suggested in common by each method.

3. Study design

The study will consist of five paths aimed at generating wordings, speech and verbatims to develop an interview guide (Figure 2).

Path 1: Patients will be interviewed using the cognitive interview technique which has four components: recall emotional and environmental context, recall as many details as possible, recall situations in different orders, and adopt various perspectives of narration [31].

Path 2: Spontaneous wordings and speeches will be collected from traditional patient/health professional interactions.

Path 3: Focus groups of patients will be interviewed. These interviews will be guided by previously identified quality-of-life issues.

Path 4. Health professionals will be individually interviewed as experts.

Path 5. Health professionals will be interviewed in focus group.

The material obtained from all five paths will be examined by a number of field experts first to consider whether the SF-36 will be adequate, and second to analyse and to extract the verbatims.

OA patients will be sampled using a quota method in a balanced design according to 4 stratification factors: gender, age, type of OA (hip versus knee), and medical/surgical stage. The sample size will be a minimum of 8 persons per focus group (which is considered an optimal number [32]), and 16 persons per individual sample at each stage to balance 2 subjects in each cell of the design. The cognitive interview sample will be double in size (32 patients), because it is a new field of application of this method.

Figure 2. Design of the study in five paths to generate words, speeches and verbatims to construct an OA-specific SF-36 module, or an independent OA-specific questionnaire

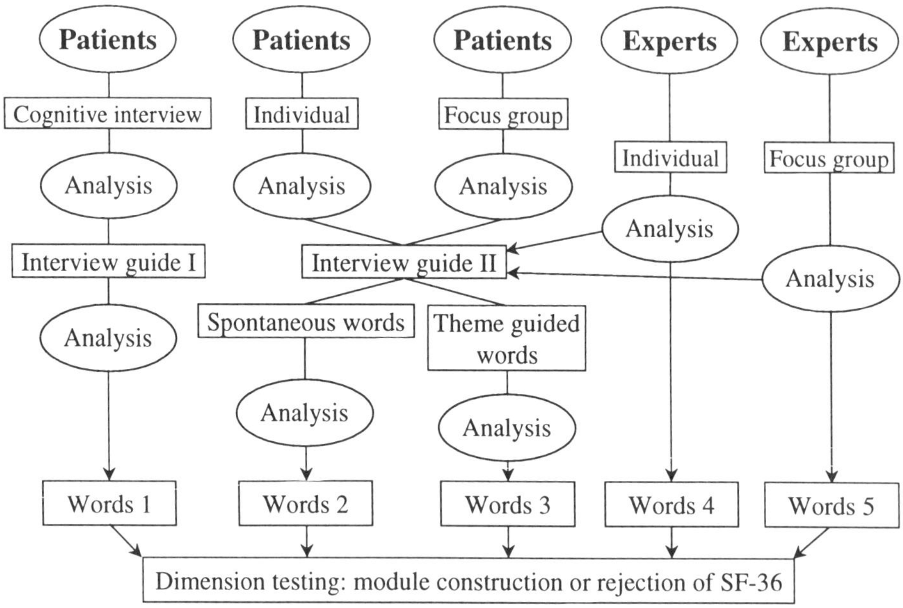

4. Analysis

The analysis will deal with five different types of wordings, speeches and verbatims, each issued from a separate structured source. A trained team of sociologists will operate a semantic theme content analysis of tape-recorded and transcribed interviews. The pre-specified conceptual framework (health status perception and quality of life) will be used as a benchmark to decide what level of association will be useful for defining themes. The description of concepts will be a priority over item formulation at this stage. The next step will be to run content analysis completed by hierarchical cluster analysis. This will identify frequently associated words or subgroups, groups, families, or superfamilies of associations, further grouped into clusters.

Once themes are identified, the second task will be to identify verbatims pertaining to each dimension. This will be done by performing a second look at the data analysis with emphasis on the list of words, speeches and verbatims grouped under each cluster previously selected. Relevant items will be constructed based on consensus.

At the end of these analyses, a judgmental approach to item selection will be conducted with experts involving interacting group, consensus group, nominal group techniques or the Delphi technique [33]. Both dimension identification and item or verbatim listings will be provided to an expert group composed of health psychologists, medical sociologists, rheumatologists, rehabilitation specialists, orthopedists, linguists, methologists, epidemiologists, osteoarthritis patients, self-help group members, and consumer representatives. It is expected that the expert group will select a manageable number of items.

In addition, separate analyses will be conducted to evaluate each of the following:

1. The effect that the number of patients selected has on the number and relevance of items generated, and the degree of their association and clustering at the dimensional level.
2. The contribution of the new cognitive interview technique as compared to the usual semi-structured interview.
3. The respective contributions of experts, health professionals and patients by the usual semi-structured interviews. It is assumed that each group contributes differently [11].
4. The contributions of focus groups versus individual interview of experts. One may assume that individuals contribute more intimate items and focus group contribute more comprehensive items.
5. The contribution of spontaneous versus theme-guided interview of patients.

Finally, item formulation will be in accordance with response modality choices. Items will be formulated according to the verbatim, frequency and severity. If the SF-36 is the retained model, it will also govern the choice.

4.1 Limitations

This study does not use a crossed design since the research focuses only on the steps in standard scale construction. The representativeness of our sample has been questioned: quota was the best sampling method to elicit possible items, although it is not representative of the epidemiology of the disease. Furthermore, the sample involves a rather high number of subjects which is unusual in such a study.

The basis of triangulation methods is the multiple employment of several techniques to investigate the same phenomenon. The goal is to strengthen the validity of the overall findings through congruence and/or complementarity of the results from each method [34,35]. The essence of the triangulation logic is that the methods represent independent assessments of the same phenomena and contain offsetting biases and measurement errors [36]. It has successfully been applied to questionnaire validity testing [16]. It has been recommended for use with data sources, investigators contribution, theory perspectives and methodological approaches [37], recognising that it may be limited by the impossibility to make a case for the validity, since each method can be flawed [38]. We will apply it for the first time to questionnaire development.

Such research does not preclude the usual validity testing of a questionnaire, which requires extensive investigation involving many patients. It addresses only the content of the instrument, and it is a contribution for standardisation of method and publication of scale generation process guidelines.

4. 2 Further Stage: Item Selection

After the stage of item generation, item selection will be conducted to ensure easy acceptability and feasibility of the questionnaire administration. A method developed by the French Quality of Life in Rheumatology Group, which combines psychometric and clinimetric information, will be used [39]. It requires carefully organised analysis of content by experts (patients and professionals), and secondary information on psychometric properties, reliability over sensitivity to change. It has been successfully used in rheumatoid arthritis [40].

5. Conclusion

The primary stages of composite scale construction include concept specification and content descriptions that can rely on several strategies. We will analyse, but not test statistically, the contribution of each strategy. Although this protocol represents a large amount of work, it is expected to provide a number of benefits:

1. Development of a quality of life instrument for lower limb OA.
2. Identification of the contributions of various methods and viewpoints (patients, experts) in eliciting statements for item generation.
3. Exploration of the cognitive interview in this field.
4. Investigation of the stability of items produced by several teams using the same qualitative methods.

We will make recommendations regarding the contribution of open or semi-structured interview as well as patient and expert usefulness.

We expect to better document the relative contribution of each approach within each stage, the relative importance of statistical selection and of content analysis, and the complementarity of informal and formal experts (patients) contributions. We hope to contribute to future methodological guidelines to generate quality of life questionnaires.

REFERENCES

1. American Psychological Association (Ed.) (1985). *Standards for Educational and Psychological Tests.* Washington DC: American Psychological Association.
2. American Psychological Association (Ed.) (1974). *Standards for Educational and Psychological Tests.* Washington DC: American Psychological Association.
3. Juniper, E.F., Guyatt, G.H., Streiner, D.L. and King, D.R. (1997). Clinical impact versus factor analysis for quality of life questionnaire construction. *Journal of Clinical Epidemiology* **50**, 233–238.
4. Guyatt, G.H., Feeny, D.H. and Patrick, D.L. (1993). Measuring health-related quality of life. *Annals of Internal Medicine* **118**, 622–629.
5. Gill, T.M. and Feinstein, A.R. (1994). A critical appraisal of the quality of quality-of-life measurements. *Journal of the American Medical Association* **272**, 619–626.
6. Leplège, A., Ecosse, E., Verdier, A., Perneger, T.V., Gandek, B. and Ware, J.E. (1998). Translating functional health and well-being: international quality of life

assessment (IQOLA) project studies of the SF-36 health survey. *Journal of Clinical Epidemiology* **51**, 1013–1023.

7. Wechsler D. (1974). *Manual for the Wechsler Intelligence Scale for Children-Revised.* New York: Psychological Corp.
8. Dazord, A., Gerin, P. and Boissel, J.P. (1994). Subjective quality of life assessment in therapeutic trials: presentation of a new instrument in France (SQLP: subjective quality of life profile) and first results. In: Orley, J. and Kuyken, W., (eds.), *Quality of Life Assessment: International Perspectives.* Berlin: Springer-Verlag.
9. Coste, J., Fermanian, J. and Venot, A. (1995). Methodological and statistical problems in the construction of composite measurement scales: a survey of six medical and epidemiological journals. *Statistics in Medicine* **14**, 331–45.
10. Marx, R.G., Bombardier, C., Hogg-Johnson, S. and Wright, J.G. (1999). Clinimetric and psychometric strategies for development of a health measurement scale. *Journal of Clinical Epidemiology* **52**, 105–111.
11. Lomas, J., Pickard, L. and Mohide, A. (1987). Patient versus clinician item generation for quality of life measures. The case of language-disabled adults. *Medical Care* **25**, 764–769.
12. Cella, D. and Chang, C.H. (2000). A discussion of item response theory and its applications in health status assessment. *Medical Care* **38** (supplement II), II-66–II-72.
13. Nunnally, J.C. (1978). *Psychometric Theory.* New York: McGraw-Hill.
14. Streiner, D.L. and Norman, G.R. (1989). *Health Measurement Scales. A Practical Guide to their Development and Use.* Oxford: Oxford University Press.
15. Frost, N.A., Sparrow, J.M., Durant, J.S., Donovan, J.L., Peters, T.J., Brookes, S.T. (1998). Development of a questionnaire for measurement of vision-related quality of life. *Ophthalmic Epidemiology* **5**, 185–210.
16. Mangione, C.M., Berry, S., Spritzer, K., Janz, N.K., Klein, R., Owsley, C. and Lee, P.P. (1998). Identifying the content area for the 51-item National Eye Institute Visual Function Questionnaire: results from focus groups with visually impaired persons. *Archives of Ophthalmology* **116**, 227–233.
17. Etter, J.F. and Perneger, T.V. (1997). Validating a satisfaction questionnaire using multiple approaches: a case study. *Social Science & Medicine* **45**, 879–885.
18. Anderson, J.S. and Ferrans, C.E. (1997). The quality of life of persons with chronic fatigue syndrome. *Journal of Nervous and Mental Disorders* **185**, 359–367.
19. ICIDH-2. (1999). *International Classification of Functioning and Disability.* BETA-2 DRAFT short version – July 1999. Geneva: WHO
20. The WHOQOL Group. (1995). The world health organization quality of life assessment (WHOQOL): position paper from the world health organization. *Social Sciences & Medicines* **41**, 1403-1409.
21. Wiklund, I., Romanus, B. and Hunt, S.M. (1988). Self-assessed disability in patients with arthrosis of the hip joint. Reliability of the Swedish version of the Nottingham Health Profile. *International Disability Studies* 10, 159–163.
22. McGuigan, F., Hozack, W.J., Moriarty, L., Eng, K. and Rothman, R.H. (1995). Predicting quality-of-life outcomes following total joint arthroplasty. Limitations of the SF-36 Health Status Questionnaire. *Journal of Arthroplasty* **10**, 742–747.
23. Bombardier, C., Melfi, C.A., Paul, J., Green, R., Hawker, G., Wright, J. and Coyte, P. (1995). Comparison of a generic and a disease-specific measure of pain and

physical function after knee replacement surgery. *Medical Care* **33** (supplement 4), AS131–144.
24. Melfi, C., Holleman, E., Arthur, D. and Katz B. (1995). Selecting a patient characteristics index for the prediction of medical outcomes using administrative claims data. *Journal of Clinical Epidemiology* 48, 917–926.
25. Bellamy, N., Buchanan, W.W., Goldsmith, C.H., Campbell, J. and Stitt, L.W. (1988). Validation study of WOMAC: a health status instrument for measuring clinically important patient relevant outcomes to antirheumatic drug therapy in patients with osteoarthritis of the hip or knee. *Journal of Rheumatology* **15**, 1833–1840.
26. Hays, R.D., Kallich, J.D., Mapes, D.L., Coons, S.J. and Carter, W.B. (1994). Development of the Kidney Disease Quality of Life (KDQOL^{TM}) Instrument. *Quality of Life Research* **3**, 329–338.
27. Wu, A.W., Fink, N.E., Cagney, K.A., Bass, E.B., Rubin, H.R., Meyer, K.B., Sadler, J.H. and Powe, N.R. (2001). Developing a health-related quality-of-life measure for end-stage renal disease: the CHOICE health experience questionnaire. *American Journal of Kidney Disease* **37**, 11–21.
28. Vickrey, B.G., Hays, R.D., Harooni, R., Myers, L.W. and Ellison, G.W. (1995). A health-related quality of life measure for multiple sclerosis. *Quality of Life Research* **4**, 187–206.
29. Aaronson, N.K., Ahmedzai, S., Bergman, B., Bullinger, M., Cull, A., Duez, N.J., Filiberti, A., Flechtner, H., Fleishman, S.B. and de Haes, J.C. S Kaasa, M Klee, Osoba, D., Razavi, D., Rofe, P.B., Schraub, S., Sneeuw, K., Sullivan, M. and Takeda, F. (1993). The European Organization for Research and Treatment of Cancer QLQ-C30: a quality-of-life instrument for use in international clinical trials in oncology. *Journal of National Cancer Institute* **85**, 365–376.
30. McQuellon, R.P., Russell, G.B., Cella, D.F., Craven, B.L., Brady, M., Bonomi, A. and Hurd, D.D. (1997). Quality of life measurement in bone narrow transplantation: development of the Functional Assessment of Cancer Therapy-Bone Marrow Transplant (FACT-BMT) scale. *Bone Marrow Transplant* **19**, 357–368.
31. Geiselman, R.E., Fisher, R.P., McKinnon, D.P. and Holland, H.L. (1986). Enhancement eyewitness memory with the cognitive interview. *American Journal of Psychology* **99**, 385–401.
32. Krueger, R.A. (1988). *Focus Groups: A Practical Guide for Applied Research.* Newsbury park, CA, Sage
33. Gustafson, D.H., Fryback, D.G., Rose, J.H., Yick, V., Prokop, C.T., Detmer, D.E. and Moore, J. (1986). A decision theoretic methodology for severity index development. *Medical Decision Making* **6**, 27–35.
34. Greene, J. and McClintock, C. (1985). Triangulation in evaluation, design and analysis issues. *Evaluation Review* **9**, 523–545.
35. Maggs-Rapport, F. (2000). Combining methodological approaches in research: ethnography and interpretive phenomenology. *Journal of Advanced Nursing* **31**, 219–225.
36. Campbell, D.T. and Fiske, D.W. (1959). Convergent and discriminant validation by the multitrait-multimethod matrix. *Psychological Bulletin* **56**, 81–106.
37. Denzin, N.F. and Lincoln, Y.S. (1994). *Handbook of Qualitative Research.* London: Sage.

38. Silverman, D. (1993). *Interpreting Qualitative Data Methods for Analysing Talk, Text and Interaction*. London: Sage.
39. Coste, J., Guillemin, F., Pouchot, J. and Fermanian, J. (1997). Methodological approaches to shortening composite measurement scales. *Journal of Clinical Epidemiology* **50**, 247–252.
40. Guillemin, F., Coste, J., Pouchot, J., Ghezail, M., Bregeon, C., Sany, J. and the French Quality of Life in Rheumatology Group. (1997). The AIMS-2-SF. A short form of the Arthritis Impact Measurement Scales 2. *Arthritis and Rheumatism* **40**, 1267–1274.

CONCEPTION, DEVELOPMENT AND VALIDATION OF INSTRUMENTS FOR QUALITY OF LIFE ASSESSMENT: AN OVERVIEW

ARIN JUDITH CHWALOW[1] AND ADEKUNLE B. ADESINA[2]

[1]*Institut National de la Santé et de la Recherche Médicale,*[2] *Bernadir Consult*

Health related quality of life should be considered a therapeutic objective in the conduct of clinical trials, epidemiological studies and economic evaluations. The development of a new scale or instrument is a long and difficult process, requiring both qualitative and quantitative perspectives. The methodology necessary for the elaboration of a new instrument or the evaluation of the quality of an existing one is often assumed or ignored. Therefore, when indices are required to measure subjective dimensions of well-being in populations, the use of existing standardized measures, already cross-culturally validated, is usually recommended. This chapter will discuss precise psychometric elements to be considered in the decision to develop or to use an existing scale. The principles discussed here, serve as general guidelines for those planning to assess health related quality of life in research and practice settings.

1. Introduction

Traditionally, biomedical or clinical outcomes have been the main foci of attention in the care of the chronically ill. Efforts are now being made to measure other outcomes that are not only of direct interest to patients but that actually derive from their own reported experiences. Conventional measures of clinical outcomes include survival, signs and symptoms of disease, markers of disease control, complications, and disability. While these are valid indices of severity and/or success of treatment, there now seems to be a growing consensus among researchers, clinicians, policy-makers and payers on measuring outcomes in terms of the perceptions of the patients who are having to live with illness on a daily basis. In public health, optimal assessment of quality of life (QoL) allows the integration of a long-term perspective of the prevention of disease and complications and the short-term perspective of possible QoL impacts of preventive treatment regimens. Until recently, integration of survival and QoL was not always incorporated into outcome measures when evaluating the effectiveness of health care interventions.

2. Conceptual Issues

The definition of QoL has evolved along different lines since the introduction of the term into principles of health care about ten years ago. The exact meaning of quality of life has also been a subject of debate in various quarters. However, there is a general agreement on the spectrum of domains encompassed by the concept of QoL: mental, physical and social well-being. In its broadest sense, quality of life, as defined by the World Health Organization, refers to "individuals' perceptions of their position in life in the context of

M. Mesbah et al. (eds.), Statistical Methods for Quality of Life Studies, 63–70.

their culture and the value systems in which they live, and in relation to their goals, expectations, standards and concerns. It is a broad ranging concept affected in a complex way by the persons' physical health, psychological state, level of independence, social relationships, personal beliefs, and their relationship to the salient features of their environment" (Brazier, Jones and Kind, 1993).

Health-related quality of life (HRQoL) is a more restricted term defined as "the value assigned to duration of life as modified by the impairments, functional states, perceptions, and social opportunities that are influenced by disease, injury, treatment, or policy" (Patrick and Erickson, 1993). HRQoL covers domains of general well-being, psychological and social functioning and symptom status. These include, among others, areas of physical health, sleep, sex life, stress, school/work life and specific as well as non-specific symptoms.

Functional status may be considered as a separate outcome as this is a relatively objective dimension of QoL. Indeed, HRQoL includes subjective dimensions such as health perceptions and satisfaction with health. For instance, the type of treatment regimen may determine patients' compliance and HRQoL depending on their socio-demographic characteristics. Information on the QoL of patients may be an indicator of how well they are coping with the stress of living with illness, and this information should be used to help determine treatment needs, which may result in increased costs for health care (Torrance *et al.*, 1995).

Our review of the literature on HRQoL revealed that, in contrast to established generic scales such as the Sickness Impact Profile (SIP; Bergner, 1993), the Nottingham Health Profile (NHP; Hunt, McEwen and McKenna, 1986) and the Medical Outcome Study 36 item Short Form (SF-36; Ware and Sherbourne, 1992; Ware *et al.*, 1993), many condition-specific instruments in current use have been designed without clear statements of their conceptual basis and how this lack of a conceptual basis affected their final development and format. Also, there are psychological scales that address issues such as health beliefs, locus of control and knowledge. Though related to patient well-being, these are not, strictly speaking, adequately comprehensive measures of the concept that may be referred to as QoL.

3. Measuring Quality of Life

The measurement of any attribute, physical or psychological, requires that the instrument being used is adequate for the specific indicators and the population being addressed. This is even more true in the assessment of a concept as complex as quality of life, particularly within the context of a disease condition. HRQoL may be assessed using generic or condition-specific measures. Generic measures may not be sensitive enough to detect clinically important changes as they are intended for use in different types of populations and diseases without focus on the particular constraints imposed on these populations by different diseases and treatments. By contrast, condition-specific measures, which tend to be more sensitive to small changes in clinical states, have item-contents that are focused on the particular patient concerns in a given condition.

Instruments may also be categorized into psychometric-based measures and preference-based measures depending on the methods used to obtain patient scores. Psychometric-based measures allow the calculation of a profile of scores for different domains of QoL that comprise the instrument while utility or preference-based measures allow the calculation of a single overall score which summarizes the rating of QoL across different domains weighted by the relative preferences of respondents, proxies or other judges. One or more types of measures may be selected for inclusion as outcome measures depending on the purpose of planned studies and the particular features of candidate instruments including their psychometric properties of reliability, responsiveness and validity.

The key criteria of importance in choosing and using HRQoL scales have been defined by the Scientific Advisory Committee of the Medical Outcomes Trust (1995) and by Patrick and Erickson (1993). Each proposed measure should be evaluated for its general descriptive characteristics, conceptual basis and domains and, most importantly, psychometric properties including responsiveness.

4. Measurement Issues

The key factors to be considered prior to using any instrument include the following:

1. Taxonomy (levels/spheres of HRQoL explored, generic or condition-specific, profile or index, single- or multi-dimensional, single- or multi-item).
2. Languages of development and adaptation.
3. Evidence in support of scale structure (data on factorial and principal components analysis).
4. Scoring/weighting of item-responses (what type of scaling of responses). Evidence in support of Likert, Guttman, or ratio scaling. Use of Thurstone's method of paired comparisons or other forms of preference-weighting.
5. Acceptability (respondent and interviewer burden).
6. Adaptability (ease of adaptation into shorter forms and incorporation into a battery of instruments along with other scales).
7. Reliability. The types of reliability usually cited are internal consistency, test-retest reproducibility, inter-rater reliability and split-half reliability.
    a. Cronbach's alphas of around 0.9 have been considered to provide good evidence of internal consistency reliability (Nunnally, 1978) although alpha coefficients of at least 0.7 are acceptable for group comparisons. However, very high alphas may also mean item redundancy, and values in the range of 0.7 have been suggested as an alternative.
    b. The object of reproducibility testing is to ensure that a measure yields consistent scores in both stable subjects across points in time (test-retest) and between observers (inter-rater).
    c. Test-retest reproducibility is an essential feature of instruments that are intended for use in both cross-sectional and longitudinal studies. This is in order to avoid random changes or differences being falsely interpreted as effects of treatment or patient factors. Here again care needs to be taken that very high stability of scores does not compromise sensitivity to change during trials.
    d. The retest interval needs to be taken into consideration in order to interpret information on reproducibility. High test-retest correlation indices obtained over a short period (e.g., less than 1 week) may simply be reflecting

memory rather than actual stability of patient's perceptions. We have also found that retest periods of test-retest data vary markedly with authors and instruments. Of course the retest interval must be shorter than the recall period if the item-questions do not relate to the current time. Otherwise a true change might have taken place thereby defeating the purpose of reproducibility testing.

8. Validity. This refers to the extent to which the instrument in question measures what it purports to measure. This includes content (or face) validity, construct validity and criterion validity. Content validity is the extent to which the measures appear to reflect the relevant conceptual issues from the points of view of respondents and experts. Two types of construct validity exist. They are convergent and discriminant validity.

    a. Convergent validity is said to exist if the measure being evaluated shows significant correlation with other measures of similar constructs in the expected direction and magnitude.
    b. Discriminant validity is the absence, as would be expected, of correlation with measures of constructs or concepts that are dissimilar, or the ability to distinguish between subjects with known socio-demographic or clinical disparities. The latter is also referred to as clinical or known group validity. The best evidence of construct validity combines both types of validity using multi-trait multi-method analysis (Campbell and Fiske, 1959).

The literature, primarily cites evidence of construct validity when related to scale development. Criterion validity requires comparison of the measure being tested to some external "gold standard" measure. Evidence of this form of validity is rarely provided in the literature since most authors cannot furnish these data as a gold-standard rarely exists for measures of subjective concepts such as QoL. Other authors' stated claims of criterion validity are often what may only be considered to be, at best, construct validity. This is a general problem in psychometric terminology which is yet to be adequately addressed.

Criterion validity is determined by correlation of the measure with some generally accepted gold standard which, in obvious contrast to physical and biochemical indices, seldom exists in the measurement of HRQoL. The best compromise here is to compare the scale being validated with some much longer measure, as has been done for the Medical Outcomes Study (MOS) short-forms, (SF-36) to obtain concurrent validity. The other form of criterion validity is predictive validity, which is the capacity of the measure to predict the value of some hypothesized future criterion such as hospitalisation, development of disability or death.

9. Responsiveness. The sensitivity or responsiveness to change is probably the most indispensable measurement property for instruments intended for use in clinical trials and/or other prospective studies. However, it remains the least studied of all psychometric properties.

Ideally, evidence of responsiveness must be founded on a significant change having taken place in an instrument's scores over time under the influence of a treatment (or factor) of known efficacy (or impact) preferably in the context of a randomized controlled study. The issue of significance or meaningfulness of observed change has been discussed in several reviews (Guyatt, Walter and Norman, 1987; Guyatt, Feeny and Patrick, 1991). The ability of instruments to detect improvement or change over time is expressed in the following ways:

a. *t*-tests: here the significance of change is based on the p-value; however, a significant p-value of, say <0.05, is a purely statistical inference implying that the probability that the observed change is due to chance is less than 5%. Whether that change is large enough to influence clinical or policy decisions is unknown.
b. Standardized response mean (SRM): this is the mathematical product of the mean change in scores divided by the standard deviation of score changes of subjects making up the sample population. The higher the SRM, the higher the responsiveness of the instrument.
c. Effect size (ES): this is expressed as the mean change in scores divided by the standard deviation of scores observed at baseline (Kazis, Anderson and Meenan, 1989).
d. Guyatt's responsiveness index: this is the ratio of mean change in scores of patients reporting improvement divided by the standard deviation of baseline scores of stable subjects.
e. Receiver Operating Characteristic (ROC) curve: what is being evaluated here is not only the sensitivity but also the specificity of observed change based on the change of an external criterion such as a clinical measure or a measure of, say, patient satisfaction. In actual practice, it requires plotting a graph with the true-positive rate as the *y*-axis and the false-positive rate as the *x*-axis. The aim is to decide whether the instrument's change in score represents a true improvement or deterioration, the external criterion being whatever has been decided to be the yardstick of "true" change.
f. Correlation Method: This is similar to the ROC in that an external anchor is the yardstick for evaluating responsiveness but here, the instrument score change is simply correlated with that of the criterion using a statistic such as a Pearson's product-moment or the intra-class correlation coefficients.

Each one of these indices should, ideally, allow the comparability of instrument sensitivities. It is not yet clear, however, which values should be generally accepted as cut-offs for establishing satisfactory responsiveness. Cohen (1977) suggested that an effect size of 0.2 to 0.49 is small, 0.5 to 0.79 is moderate and 0.8 or greater is large. Another issue, still unresolved, is that of the time over which change must be observed.

By and large, the responsiveness properties of instruments have not been formally addressed by most developers in the course of validation studies. Most users of HRQoL instruments have to resort to studies in which these instruments had been applied to discover relevant data.

5. Application of Quality of Life Assessment in Clinical Settings

Appropriate choice among existing instruments for application in research or practice settings depends on detailed attention to their measurement characteristics and other features based on published data. Ideally this should be performed using an explicit systematic approach that allows independent peer-review of findings with respect to each feature shown below.

1. Instrument name
2. Developers
3. Types of instruments (not mutually exclusive) generic, specific, utility, battery, profile, index
4. Language of development and language(s) of adaptation
5. Availability: where and under what conditions the instrument, the user's manuals and the various formats may be obtained
6. Stated purpose
7. Target population
    a. Socio-demographic characteristics of the population in which it was developed
    b. Clinical characteristics of the population in which it was developed
8. Taxonomy of measures
    a. Health status
    b. Functional status
    c. Quality of life
    d. Health-related quality of life
9. Conceptual model
    a. Dimensions
    b. Disease-specific domains
10. Scale Structure
    a. Item development
    b. Scaling assumptions
    c. Factor analysis
    d. Principal components analysis
11. Methodological/psychometric considerations
    a. Reliability: internal consistency/Cronbach's alpha coefficient, split-half reliability, test-retest reproducibility, Pearson's product-moment correlation, intra-class correlation coefficient, weighted Kappa/Kappa Coefficient, inter-rater reliability
    b. Validity: content validity (qualify, with data), construct validity (state correlation coefficients as appropriate), discriminant, convergent, criterion validity

   c. Responsiveness: longitudinal data, preferably in the setting of a randomized controlled trial, factor of change (treatment or disease progression), time interval, effect size/Guyatt's responsiveness index, paired *t* statistic, receiver operating characteristics (ROC) curve
   d. Scaling: Likert-type, visual analogue, dichotomous responses
   e. Weighting of scores: relative preference, statistical
12. Interpretability: considering the instrument's features (i.e., population sample, descriptive statistics, skewness, scaling assumptions, possible floor and ceiling effects, etc.) and how relevant are the scores to issues of patient care, clinical practice and healthcare management?
13. Modes of administration: self-administered, interviewer-administered, in-person or by telephone, paper-and-pencil or by computer/touch-screen
14. Burden: respondent, administrative
15. Adaptability (ease of adaptation to alternative forms and language versions)
   a. Alternative modes of administration
   b. Language/culturally adapted versions
   c. Literature evidence of cross-cultural validity
16. Applications
   a. Extent of use in published clinical studies
   b. Prior or potential usefulness for routine clinical practice

6. Using Existing Health-Related Quality of Life (HRQoL) Measures

Assessment of HRQoL may be envisaged in different scenarios including clinical trials, observational studies, economic evaluations and during routine clinical practice. HRQoL measures may be divided into discriminative and evaluative instruments for purposes of clinical application.. Discriminative instruments tend to have high reproducibility whereas the primary criterion of performance of evaluative instruments is their sensitivity to change or responsiveness. Evaluative instruments are most suited to measuring change over time especially in clinical trials, while discriminative instruments are more sensitive to point-in-time differences between subjects. The score distribution of discriminative instruments tend to correlate better with known clinical and socio-demographic features of individuals in the same group whereas the distribution of scores of evaluative instruments may be more correlated to changes taking place in a given group of subjects over time. Construct validity is, an indispensable requirement for instruments of either category; neither cross-sectional nor temporal variability of scores can be meaningful if it is not certain that instruments are actually capturing and measuring the concepts for which they are intended.

Other issues of practical importance in using HRQoL instruments include the ease of scoring, response scaling, time of administration, need for translation and cultural adaptation and relevance to the age-group being studied. For different uses, these should be considered on a case-by-case basis.

For practical purposes, considering their differing coverage of HRQoL concepts and psychometric properties, instruments may be used singly, in combination or in a modular structure. The addition of generic scales in randomized controlled trials can be used to support the absence of baseline differences in HRQoL between subjects and controls thereby confirming the comparability of groups for HRQoL, and hence the validity of any changes observed following the treatment period. Utility measures yield a single preference-weighted global HRQoL score, and are particularly useful for economic evaluations.

The principles discussed here should serve as general guidelines to those planning the assessment of HRQoL in research and practice settings. Before any assessment, contact should systematically be made with developers of candidate instruments who may supply further information about their scales and how appropriate they are for the proposed use.

REFERENCES

Bergner, M. (1993). The development, testing of the use of the Sickness Impact Profile. In: Walker, S.R. and Rosser, R.M. (eds.), *Quality of Life Assessment: Key Issues in the 1990's*. Lancaster: MTP.

Brazier, J.E., Jones, N. and Kind, P. (1993). Testing the validity of the EuroQoL and comparing it with the SF-36 health survey questionnaire. *Quality of Life Research* **2**, 169–180.

Campbell, D.R. and Fiske, D.W. (1959). Convergent and discriminant validation by the multitrait-multimethod matrix. *Psychological Bulletin* **56**, 81–105.

Cohen, J. (1977). *Statistical Power Analysis for the Behavioral Sciences*. New York: Academy Press.

Guyatt, G.H., Walter, S. and Norman, G. (1987). Measuring change over time: assessing the usefulness of evaluative instruments. *Journal of Chronical Disease* **40**, 171–178.

Guyatt, G., Feeny, D. and Patrick, D. (1991). Issues in quality of life measurement in clinical trials. *Controlled Clinical Trials* **12**, 81S–90S.

Hunt, S.M., McEwen, J. and McKenna, S.P. (1986). *Measuring Health Status*. London: Croom Helm.

Kazis, L.E., Anderson, J.J. and Meenan, R.F. (1989). Effect sizes for interpreting change in health status. *Medical Care* **27** (supplement), S178–S189.

Nunnally, J.C., ed. (1978). *Psychometric Theory, 2nd Edition*. New York: McGraw-Hill.

Patrick, D.L. and Erickson, P. (1993). *Health Status and Health Policy: Quality of Life in Health Care Evaluation and Resource Allocation*. Oxford: Oxford University Press.

Scientific Advisory Committee (1995). Instrument Review Criteria. *Medical Outcomes Trust Bulletin* **3**. Boston: Medical Outcomes Trust.

Torrance, G.W., Furlong, W., Feeny, D., Boyle, M. (1995). Multiattribute preference functions. Health Utilities Index. *Pharmacoeconomics* **7**, 503–520.

Ware, J.E. and Sherbourne, C.D. (1992). The MOS 36-item Short-Form Health Survey (SF-36). I. Conceptual framework and item selection. *Medical Care* **30**, 473–483.

Ware, J.E., Snow. K.K., Kosinski, M. and Gandek, B. (1993). *SF-36 Health Survey. Manual & Interpretation Guide*. Boston: The Health Institute.

METHODOLOGICAL ISSUES IN THE ANALYSIS OF QUALITY OF LIFE DATA IN CLINICAL TRIALS: ILLUSTRATIONS FROM THE NATIONAL SURGICAL ADJUVANT BREAST AND BOWEL PROJECT (NSABP) BREAST CANCER PREVENTION TRIAL

STEPHANIE LAND,[1] SAMUEL WIEAND,[1] RICHARD DAY,[1] TOM TEN HAVE,[2] JOSEPH P. COSTANTINO,[1] WEI LANG[3] AND PATRICIA A. GANZ[4]

[1]*University of Pittsburgh and the National Surgical Adjuvant Breast and Bowel Project,* [2]*University of Pennsylvania School of Medicine,* [3]*Wake Forest University School of Medicine,* [4]*UCLA Schools of Medicine and Public Health and the Jonsson Comprehensive Cancer Center*

We present two Quality of Life (QOL) endpoints collected in conjunction with the recently completed Breast Cancer Prevention Trial (BCPT) performed by the National Surgical Adjuvant Breast and Bowel Project. The analyses of these endpoints (depression and hot flashes) indicate the importance of randomization and give some insight about the impact of missing data in a large randomized trial.

1. Introduction

Quality of life (QOL) assessments have been increasingly included as secondary or primary endpoints in clinical trials (Tannock *et al.*, 1996; Moinpour *et al.*, 1998). The impetus for doing so comes from a desire to obtain patient-rated evaluations of treatments, especially in circumstances in which treatments have substantially differing toxicities or in which survival outcomes are not expected to be different (Ganz, 1994a, 1994b). Under such circumstances, an evaluation of the morbidity of treatment from the patient's or participant's perspective may be the most important endpoint. Although there is now a wide range of psychometrically validated scales for the measurement of QOL in clinical trials (Cella and Bonomi, 1995), there are considerable challenges to the implementation and collection of QOL data in these studies (Bernhard *et al.*, 1998), as well as equally formidable statistical and analytical concerns (Bernhard and Gelber, 1998). In this paper, we provide examples from the recently completed NSABP Breast Cancer Prevention Trial (BCPT) to highlight challenges that can arise in the analyses of such data, specifically focusing on the importance of randomization and the issue of missing data and its potential to affect the interpretation of QOL outcomes.

2. Background

The BCPT was a double-blinded, placebo-controlled clinical trial that was open for accrual from June 1, 1992, through September 30, 1997. During this interval 13,338 women at high risk for breast cancer were randomly assigned to receive either 20 mg/day of tamoxifen or placebo for a duration of five years. The primary objective of the trial was to determine if tamoxifen therapy reduces the risk of breast cancer among women.

M. Mesbah et al. (eds.), Statistical Methods for Quality of Life Studies, 71–85.

Secondary objectives related to the full benefit/risk profile of tamoxifen therapy in healthy women. Participants in the trial were screened for breast cancer at six-month intervals by clinical breast examination and at yearly intervals by bilateral mammography. At each screening, visit participants were also evaluated for several other endpoints including heart disease, fractures, thromboembolic disease, and endometrial cancer. Heart disease and fractures were included because it was theorized that tamoxifen might also reduce the risk of these problems. Thromboembolic disease and endometrial cancer were included because these were known side effects associated with tamoxifen. As an additional means to monitor the safety of tamoxifen in the trial, the incidence of all invasive cancers and the occurrence of all deaths were also included as endpoints.

The results of the BCPT have been reported (Fisher *et al.,* 1998), as has a study of the risk-benefit ratio for tamoxifen (Gail *et al.,* 1999). During follow-up, 175 participants randomized to receive placebo developed invasive breast cancer compared to only 89 randomized to receive tamoxifen, indicating an estimated 50% reduction in the risk of breast cancer from the use of tamoxifen. Other major findings include the detection of a preventive effect on osteoporotic fractures, no effect on heart disease, and a confirmation of the known side effects of endometrial cancer and thromboembolic disease. These overall findings will not be further discussed in this chapter, as we wish to focus on issues that relate to QOL studies.

Because the participants in this trial were healthy women, the monitoring of their QOL during the intervention was of particular importance. Thus, the NSABP included a concurrent QOL study designed to describe side effects of tamoxifen, to examine the relationship between side effects and QOL, to compare the side effects and QOL in placebo and treated subjects, and to examine the effects of symptoms on compliance with study medication. The BCPT QOL questionnaire was a 104-item battery that included four instruments: the Center for Epidemiologic Studies Depression Scale (CES-D) (Radloff, 1997); the Medical Outcomes Study 36-Item Short Form (SF-36) (Ware, Kosinski and Keller, 1994); a symptom checklist based on the Postmenopausal Estrogen Progesterone Intervention (Shumaker S., personal communication) specifically adapted for the BCPT trial; and the Medical Outcomes Study Sexual Problems Scale (Sherbourne, 1992). These instruments were selected because of their psychometric characteristics and validity, the availability of normative data in healthy women, and ease of self-administration. The latter was particularly important because the trial was conducted at several hundred clinical centers throughout North America and the battery of questions we asked was completed on multiple occasions in conjunction with study visits. The QOL assessment was scheduled to occur at baseline before administration of the study medication and at every clinical visit during the five years after randomization (at three months, at six months, and every six months thereafter). However, the trial was unblinded on March 31, 1998, following an interim analysis that showed a dramatic reduction in the incidence of breast cancer among the participants who received tamoxifen. The QOL follow-up was terminated at that time due to the potential loss of the control arm. In this manuscript, as in our prior analyses of QOL data from the trial (Day *et al.*, 1999, Ganz *et al.*, 1995, 1998), we used QOL data available from participants who were recruited to the trial during the first two years of the study (June 1, 1992 to May 31, 1994) as all of these women would have been expected to have 36 months of completed follow-up data at the time the study was terminated. The sample includes 11,064 women who represent 82.6% of the total accrual to the BCPT. We used only the first three years of follow-up.

3. The Effect of Tamoxifen on Depression

When the BCPT began, there was considerable concern that tamoxifen therapy might be associated with the development of depressed mood in women with breast cancer. Although Love *et al.* (1991) did not find such an effect when reporting symptoms associated with tamoxifen treatment in a randomized trial in postmenopausal women with breast cancer, several researchers subsequently reported results suggesting that administration of tamoxifen might lead to depression in some breast cancer patients (Cathcart *et al.*, 1993; Shariff *et al.*, 1995; Anelli *et al.*, 1994). The latter studies were relatively small (fewer than 400 patients) and none had a placebo comparison group. However, there was a potential scientific rationale for tamoxifen's association with depression. Estrogen had been shown to have a beneficial effect on mood in postmenopausal women (Halbreich, 1997; Gregoire, *et al.*, 1996), and it was considered plausible that tamoxifen might negate these positive effects of estrogen. Thus, careful measurement of depression, including a screening instrument to identify potential cases of depression, was important in the design of the BCPT QOL study.

The primary instrument used in the BCPT to study the change in depression level over time was the CES-D, a self-administered questionnaire (20 questions) that screens for depressive symptoms over the seven days prior to administration (Radloff, 1977). A participant's score is the sum of the responses for the 20 questions and can range from 0 (no depressive symptoms) to 60 (maximum depressive symptoms). The instrument is widely used because it is easy to administer and has excellent population-based normative data (Myers and Weissman, 1980; Roberts and Vernon, 1983; Boyd *et al.*, 1982). To assess the validity of the CES-D in the BCPT sample, we compared the baseline CES-D scores of BCPT participants with ten medical history items related to mental health that had been obtained at entry to the trial (Table 1). The first three items were obtained in the context of questions about diagnosed medical problems, although we did not verify that there had been a recorded diagnosis. There is nearly a linear relationship between the number of positives from the participant's mental health history and the CES-D score ($p < 0.0001$), providing considerable reassurance that the CES-D score from this study sample was highly associated with a clinical mental health history. Similarly, the association between the mean CES-D score and the three depression-related items, "ever had depression," "ever took antidepressants" (either item 4 or 6 positive), or "any two years depressed or sad", showed an increasing relationship between the CES-D score and the number of positives ($p < 0.001$). In addition, the baseline CES-D scores were well balanced across placebo and tamoxifen treatment assignment (Table 2). The ranges of CES-D scores shown in Table 2 are somewhat arbitrary; however, a cut-off of 16 (i.e., scores of 16 or more) is commonly used for classifying a person as depressed (Myers and Weissman, 1980; Roberts and Vernon, 1983; Boyd *et al.*, 1982), and Lyness *et al.* (1997) used the cutoff of 22 when screening for major depression.

In Figure 1, we present the mean CES-D scores by visit and treatment arm during the BCPT. The observed increase of depression among participants receiving tamoxifen is slightly less than the observed increase among participants receiving placebo, although the difference is not significant ($p = 0.24$). Thus, the increase in the depression score during the first six months of the trial does not appear to be related to the administration of tamoxifen. It is noteworthy that the dramatic increase in scores at months 3 and 6

Table 1. BCPT Participant History Mental Health Items Obtained at Entry to the BCPT

Item	% Yes
1. Ever had depression	15
2. Ever had nervous or emotional disorder	3
3. Ever had psychiatric problems	1
4. Current antidepressants	6
5. Current tranquilizers	16
6. Previous antidepressants	4
7. Previous tranquilizers	15
8. Two weeks sad, blue, depressed, disinterested	17
9. Any two years depressed or sad	9
10. Depressed or sad most of past year	5

Table 2. Baseline CES-D Scores

Score	Placebo (%)	Tamoxifen (%)
0-10	85.5	83.9
11-15	7.8	9.0
16-21	3.8	4.1
22-60	2.8	3.0

Figure 1. Change from baseline score for depression in participants in the BCPT. Depression is slightly increased in the placebo group, compared to the tamoxifen group (not statistically significant).

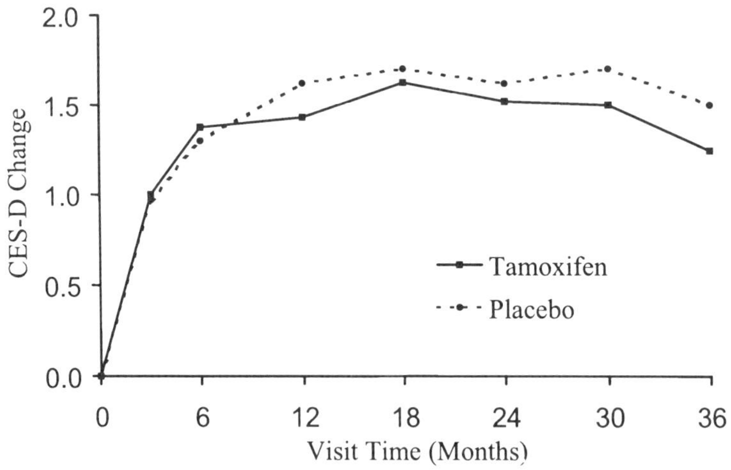

would almost certainly have been attributed to tamoxifen had there not been a placebo arm. This illustrates the danger of trying to establish a cause-and-effect relationship in a non-randomized setting.

We do not know why the CES-D depression scores increased for participants on both arms of the study (placebo and tamoxifen). It is possible that symptoms of worry and depression increased due to the controversy surrounding this trial, the fear and uncertainty of taking either placebo or active agent, an increased awareness of breast cancer risk, or a concern over potential therapy side effects. Alternatively, the raised scores might be partially attributed to "nocebo effect" (Hahn, 1997): if an individual fears or believes that a side effect may occur from a medication, he or she will report it. (As will be shown later, participants receiving placebo also reported an increase in hot flashes, but at a lesser rate than participants on tamoxifen.) Since neither group of women knew which pill they were taking, they may have reported increased symptoms because they feared the potential medication side effects described to them as part of the consent process. A third possibility is that the baseline scores were artificially low and the subsequent increase reflected a regression to the mean. We do not believe the baseline scores are much lower than would be expected for the educated, socioeconomically advantaged population in the trial. However, to the extent that the scores were artificially low, it could be either that women were less likely to enter the trial when they were experiencing depressive symptoms, or that they would under-report for fear of jeopardizing their inclusion in the trial. In any case, the phenomenon of an early increase in depressive symptoms appears to be independent of tamoxifen use.

However, we were concerned that there might be a treatment effect in the subset of subjects at higher risk of depression. Because 93% of the participants had baseline CES-D scores <16, and 85% had scores <11, such an effect might not be apparent in an analysis based on the entire population. To explore this possibility we divided the women into four groups of risk: zero, one to two, three to five, and six to ten "yes" responses to the mental health items listed in Table 1. There was no difference observed between tamoxifen and placebo participants in any of the four groups. Results were similar when the baseline CES-D score was used to create risk groups (CES-D scores from 0 to 11; 12 to 15; 16 to 21; or 22 or more). There was a suggestion that tamoxifen is beneficial in the high-risk group ($p = 0.04$), although this is likely to be a statistical artifact.

The problem of missing data is common in clinical trials that assess QOL (Bernhard *et al.*, 1998a). In the BCPT, this was exacerbated by the fact that the clinical centers were not required to collect QOL data when a participant went off the study medication. As will be seen, this led to a substantial problem of non-random missing data. Only 82 participants did not fill out the CES-D form at entry (an extremely low rate of missing baseline data), and these participants were excluded from subsequent analyses. (Questionnaires that were partially completed are considered missing in this report.) However, of the possible 76,874 post-entry forms that the 10,982 remaining participants were expected to submit during the three-year period, 13,752 (18%) were missing. At the end of the third year, slightly more than 30% were missing and participants who received tamoxifen were more likely to have missing data (33% versus 30% missing, $p < 0.001$). The first three rows in Table 3 present the number and percent of missing forms preceded by a protocol-specified event (such as second primary cancer, deep-vein thrombosis, ischemic heart disease, or death); missing forms preceded by early termination of therapy

Table 3. Number and Percent of Forms Missing by Status of Patient

	Placebo	Tamoxifen
Protocol Event	801 (12%)	791 (11%)
Stopped Therapy	3,347 (50%)	3,883 (55%)
Withdrew Consent	1,359 (20%)	1,297 (18%)
On Therapy	1,140 (17%)	1,134 (16%)
Total	6,647	7,105

Figure 2. The percent of missing questionnaires at each visit by baseline CES-D group (0-10, 11-15, 16-21, and 22-60) which is higher for subjects with higher baseline CES-D scores.

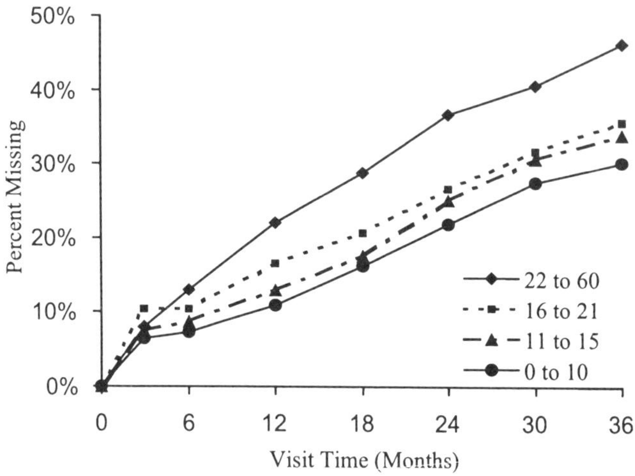

Table 4. Average CES-D Score* Prior to Missing vs. Observed Scores

	Before Missing Score	Before Observed Score
Tamoxifen Arm	7.78	6.50
Placebo Arm	7.70	6.44

*A score of 16 or higher is considered an indicator of depression.

for a reason not specified by the protocol; and missing forms preceded by consent withdrawal by the participant; the fourth row of this table shows the number of forms that were missing when the participant was still receiving therapy. Figure 2 displays the percent of missing forms in four groups based on baseline CES-D scores. Participants who began with an elevated CES-D score were more likely to have missing data ($p < 0.001$ at three years).

The average of the CES-D scores immediately preceding a missing score was higher than the average of the CES-D scores immediately preceding an observed score (Table 4), which raised the possibility that missing scores would have been higher than concurrently observed scores. The differences were almost identical in the tamoxifen and placebo arms, indicating that while the missing data might result in an underestimate of depression, the bias would be the same in both arms. When we considered other functions of preceding scores, we found that none had a stronger association with missing scores than did the immediately preceding score. In particular, the slopes between two scores preceding a missing score were not significantly different from slopes between two scores preceding an observed score. Therefore we considered some simple imputations based on the scores immediately preceding the missing scores.

In discussing the imputation methods, we will use the following notation. The baseline and seven post-entry CES-D scores for the j-th individual participant will be represented by $x_{0j},\ldots,x_{7j}$, where "missing" is a possible value for the CES-D score. Let $x^T_{i\cdot}$ ($x^P_{i\cdot}$) be the average CES-D among tamoxifen (placebo) participants with an observed CES-D score at the i-th visit. For $i = 1,\ldots,7$, we define $x^I_{ij} = x_{ij}$ if x_{ij} is observed. If x_{ij} is missing, we define $x^I_{ij} = x^I_{(i-1)j} + x^T_{i\cdot} - x^T_{(i-1)\cdot}$ for a tamoxifen participant and $x^I_{ij} = x^I_{(i-1)j} + x^P_{i\cdot} - x^P_{(i-1)\cdot}$ for a placebo participant, where the imputation proceeds sequentially. The mean CES-D curves are slightly higher than in Figure 1 (where no imputation is involved), but the differences between the two curves remain nearly identical to the differences seen in Figure 1.

Although Table 4 suggests that the imputed values defined above would be appropriate for replacing missing values, we cannot rule out the possibility that the missing values mask a greater increase in depression for tamoxifen participants than for placebo participants. For example, there might have been a subset of tamoxifen participants who became depressed as a result of the treatment and dropped out before this effect could be observed. However, we have no data available to verify this. To see just how great a differential (by treatment) would have been required to change the interpretation of the data, we performed three sensitivity analyses.

For the first sensitivity analysis, we imputed missing values as defined above, but for every missing value of a tamoxifen participant we added 0.5 units to the imputed value. The resultant mean values of CES-D at each assessment are almost the same between treatment arms. This is somewhat reassuring, since adding 0.5 units to each missing CES-D score for tamoxifen participants and none for placebo participants is extreme. As Table 3 indicated, the status of the participants with missing forms was similar on both arms. In instances in which institutions reported the reason participants went off study, only 3% reported depression as the reason for doing so.

The second sensitivity analysis was based on a partitioning of missing questionnaires into those that were missing for a variety of non-treatment related reasons and those that were missing for treatment-related reasons. Specifically, we assumed that if m questionnaires were missing (at a particular assessment time) in the placebo arm, and $m + x$ questionnaires were missing in the tamoxifen arm, then some fraction of the x questionnaires might be attributable to excess depression caused by tamoxifen. We calculated treatment group means (at each assessment time) as if some fraction r (for various candidate values of r) of the missing tamoxifen scores were replaced with the mean of all observations at that assessment that were at least 16, since these represent severe depressive symptoms. The remaining missing values in both arms were replaced with the mean of all observations at that assessment. At $r = 1/2$, the curves of imputed CES-D for the two treatment groups overlapped (data not shown). That is, there did not appear to be a tamoxifen-related increase in CES-D unless greater than half of the excess missing questionnaires were assumed to coincide with severe depressive symptoms.

Figure 3. (A) Increase in percent of participants whose CES-D score was at least 16, minus the percent at baseline. The percent increased in both arms. (B) Effect of missing data. Increase in percent of participants whose CES-D score was at least 16, after imputation with the previous observed score, adjusting for the difference in treatment arm means between the missed visit and the preceding visit. The imputed observations in the tamoxifen arm had an additional 3.2% added, and the resulting curves are nearly overlapping.

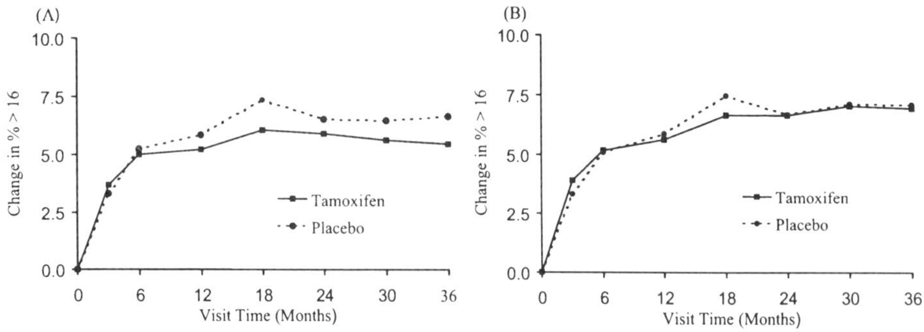

All of the analyses shown above were also carried out for a binary outcome of severe depressive symptoms, defined as any CES-D score ≥16. In Figure 3A, we plot the proportion of values classified as a "yes" as a function of time and again find no tamoxifen effect. Imputation of the missing values using preceding scores had minimal impact on our findings. For a sensitivity analysis, we performed the imputation with the additional assumption that 3.2% of the missing tamoxifen CES-D forms had a score ≥16, even though the prior score was <16. This would be roughly equivalent to assuming that all the tamoxifen participants who reported depression before dropping out of the study subsequently had a score ≥16, while none of the placebo participants reporting depression before dropping out had a score exceeding 15. The sensitivity analysis, presented in Figure 3B, indicates that under this fairly extreme assumption about the drop-outs, the two curves would essentially overlap.

As a final step in the sensitivity analysis, we considered a model-based method that adjusts for drop-out related to observed and unobserved CES-D outcomes through subject-level random effects. This approach, which may be used to adjust for other covariates, has been presented previously in other randomized trial contexts for continuous data (Schlucter, 1992; DeGruttola and Tu, 1994) and for binary data (Ten Have *et al.*, 1998), and in a cohort study context for ordinal data (Ten Have *et al.*, 2000). More specifically, we fitted an ordinal logistic model with random effects to the CES-D outcome data. The CES-D score was categorized as in Table 2. The models make the proportional odds assumption, that is, the odds ratio specified for a given cut-point of the ordinal CES-D scale is the same as the odds ratio specified for every other cut-point. This approach is not designed for intermittent missingness. Therefore, any participant's data subsequent to a missing form was deleted for the purpose of this analysis. The model comprised three components consisting of different covariate effects but sharing the same subject-level random effect structure. The first was an ordinal CES-D outcome component with treatment arm and time (7 degrees of freedom) as main effects, and their interaction (7 degrees of freedom). The second and third model components corresponded to separate discrete survival time logistic specifications for non-protocol and protocol specified drop-out. Each of these drop-out components included main effect covariates corresponding to treatment arm and time.

We present results based on two versions of each of these drop-out components. The first version includes as covariates the CES-D outcome before drop-out and its interaction with treatment arm and type of dropout (protocol vs. non-protocol). In the second version, each of these drop-out components excludes the CES-D outcome and its interactions. The ensuing results are based on these model specifications without baseline covariates. Including baseline age did not alter the results. The subject-level random effect structure shared by the CES-D and drop-out components induces a relationship between the CES-D observed and unobserved outcomes and the risk of drop-out. The magnitude of this relationship is characterized by the specification of separate variance components of the random effect for each of the three components in the model. Separate large variance components for the outcome component and for a drop-out component indicate a strong relationship between outcome and the respective form of drop-out. For comparison, we also present results based on the assumption that drop-out is missing at random (MAR). That is, drop-out is conditionally independent of the unobserved CES-D outcomes, conditioned on all observed data (Little, 1995). In summary, we have used these three models: (1) the random effects logistic model without a drop-out component, under the assumption that drop-out is missing at random (naïve model); (2) the random effects logistic model augmented with a discrete time survival logistic model for drop-out, which shares a random effect with the ordinal CES-D outcome (joint 1 model); and (3) model 2 with the last observed CES-D outcome added as a covariate (joint 2 model).

The likelihood ratio test of treatment arm differences in change across time (7 degrees of freedom) was not significant ($p = 0.14$). As Table 5 suggests, this result was robust with respect to the drop-out assumptions (e.g., MAR). More specifically, the estimates of the log treatment odds ratio at baseline and corresponding treatment-time interaction terms at each follow-up time differ very little across the three models. To evaluate the strength of the relationship between outcome and drop-out, we present the variance components of the random effect shared by the three components (outcome, two drop-out types: non-protocol- and protocol-defined) for two of the models, joint 1 and joint 2, in Table 6. Note that the naïve model only has the outcome component and therefore only one variance component. Table 6 shows that neither of the drop-out components in joint 1 and joint 2 models is related to the outcome through a random effect. This lack of relationship between outcome and drop-out is consistent with the fact that the log odds ratio estimates in Table 5 are very stable between the naïve and joint models. This suggests that the naïve random effects model accommodates the relationship between outcome and protocol-defined drop-out. That is, the MAR relationship under the naïve model characterizes the type of relationship between drop-out and outcome represented by the joint models. Of course, it may be that a different relationship exists that is not characterized by either the joint or naïve models.

In summary, our study data indicate that tamoxifen does not influence depressive symptoms among women who are at high risk for breast cancer, and there is no indication that missing data masked an effect. It appeared that the missing data did result in slight underestimates of the CES-D scores, which were increased following imputation.

Table 5. Effect of missing: For CES-D scores, estimates of baseline treatment log odds ratio and corresponding interactions between treatment and time for each follow-up time (standard errors in parentheses) for three models.*

Model	Base Tx LogOR	Tx by Time Interaction Log OR at Follow-up Times (months)						
		3	6	12	18	24	30	36
Naïve	0.17 (0.08)	−0.07 (0.09)	−0.11 (0.09)	−0.20 (0.09)	−0.18 (0.09)	−0.17 (0.09)	−0.26 (0.10)	−0.19 (0.10)
Joint 1	0.18 (0.08)	−0.08 (0.09)	−0.12 (0.09)	−0.21 (0.09)	−0.19 (0.09)	−0.18 (0.10)	−0.27 (0.10)	−0.20 (0.10)
Joint 2	0.17 (0.08)	−0.08 (0.09)	−0.12 (0.09)	−0.21 (0.09)	−0.19 (0.09)	−0.17 (0.10)	−0.27 (0.10)	−0.19 (0.10)

*Models: (1) The random effects logistic model without a drop-out component under the assumption drop-out is MAR (naïve model); (2) the random effects logistic model augmented with a discrete time survival logistic model for drop-out that shares a random effect with the ordinal symptom outcome (joint 1 model); (3) model (2) with the last observed symptom outcome added as a covariate (joint 2 model).

Table 6: For CES-D, estimates of variance components of random intercepts for three models.*

Model	Symptom Outcome Component	Non-Protocol-Specified Drop-Out	Protocol-Specified Drop-Out
Naïve	5.25	NA†	NA†
Joint 1	5.91	0.05	0.01
Joint 2	5.59	0.04	0.02

*Models: (1) The random effects logistic model without a drop-out component under the assumption drop-out is MAR (naïve model); (2) the random effects logistic model augmented with a discrete time survival logistic model for drop-out that shares a random effect with the ordinal symptom outcome (joint 1 model); (3) model (2) with the last observed symptom outcome added as a covariate (joint 2 model).
†NA: not applicable because naïve model does not include drop-out components.

4. Strategies for the Evaluation of Missing Data: Hot Flashes

Although tamoxifen did not appear to influence the CES-D score in this study, it clearly was associated with other symptoms. Numerous studies have shown that tamoxifen increased the number and severity of hot flashes in women being treated for cancer, and this effect was also seen in the high-risk women participating in the BCPT (Day *et al.*, 1999). Hot flash was the most commonly reported symptom on either arm of the BCPT.

In Figure 4 (solid lines), we present the score reported by these women for hot flashes at each cycle by treatment (possible values ranged from 0 = none to 4 = extreme). There is a clear increase in this symptom associated with tamoxifen throughout the study. (Note that participants taking placebo also report an increase in mean hot flash score,

Figure 4. The mean hot flash score after subtraction of each participant's baseline score, by treatment arm (solid lines) and the mean hot flash score after subtraction of each participant's baseline score, by treatment arm (dashed lines). Tamoxifen subjects experienced more severe hot flashes. For each subject, missing values were first imputed with previous observed values, adjusting for the difference in treatment arm means between the missed visit and the preceding visit. Imputation did not substantially change the comparison.

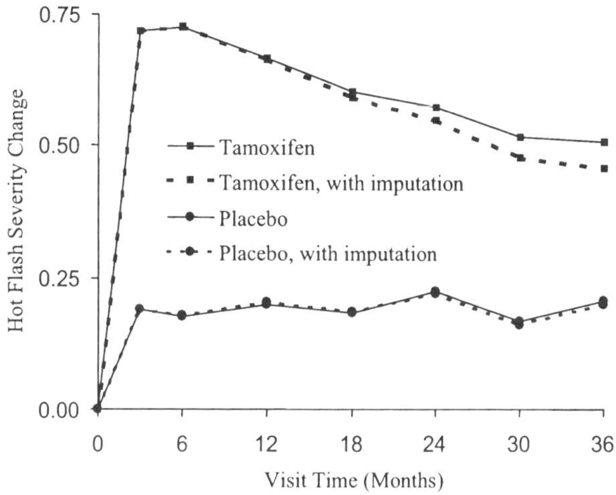

although this increase is not as great as for those taking tamoxifen. This may be another example of the nocebo effect.) Differences in hot flashes due to treatment are highly significant (p <0.001) at every visit. However, when hot flash scores immediately preceding a missing value were compared to the scores immediately preceding an observed value (Table 7), there was a differential effect according to treatment. We again did an imputation in which missing values were replaced by the prior score adjusted for the mean for the visit (as described previously for the CES-D analyses). There is still clear evidence of a tamoxifen effect (dashed lines in Figure 4), but the values for the tamoxifen curve are slightly lower than when the missing values are omitted, while the values for the placebo curve remain nearly unchanged, indicating that we might be slightly overestimating the treatment effect if we ignore missing values. For example, the difference in average scores is 0.30 at three years when missing data are ignored versus 0.26 following the imputation.

An alternative analysis of these data based on the informative drop-out model used for the CES-D revealed a significant difference between the treatment arms with respect to change at each follow-up time ($p < 0.001$). As with the CES-D non-significant treatment difference, this significant result was robust with respect to drop-out assumptions under the random effects ordinal logistic model. The logistic model requires the assumption that the relationship between symptoms and drop-out risk is in the same direction in both the placebo and tamoxifen groups and over time. As Table 8 indicates, this assumption did not hold for the hot flash data. Hence, we were unable to adjust for the observed drop-out pattern to obtain valid estimates of the treatment effect.

Table 7. Average hot flash score prior to missing versus observed scores

	Missing subsequent questionnaire	Observed subsequent questionnaire
Placebo	0.87	0.77
Tamoxifen	1.12	1.16

Table 8. Difference in Mean Preceding Missing HFS – Observed HFS. The logistic approach would be appropriate if the values all had the same sign

Visit (Month)	Placebo	Tamoxifen
3	0.0259	0.0384
6	0.1218	0.1418
12	0.1212	–0.0484
18	0.1037	–0.0952
24	–0.0272	–0.0850
30	–0.0594	–0.2230
36	0.0862	–0.1182

5. Conclusions

Several points became clear in the analysis of the CES-D data. Perhaps the most important is that one would be likely to conclude that tamoxifen increased depressive symptoms if all the participants had received tamoxifen, as this would appear to be the most likely cause of the immediate increase in depressive symptoms. However, the randomization allowed us to see that the effect increase was comparable when participants received placebo, ruling out tamoxifen as the cause. The fact that the prior scores associated with missing values were elevated in both arms indicated that the degree of depressive symptoms might have been underestimated slightly on both arms. However the elevation was the same in both arms, which made it unlikely that there was a differential drop-out effect by treatment. This partially explains why imputation analyses still led to the conclusion that tamoxifen did not result in increased depressive symptoms. Sensitivity analyses indicated that even if there were a fairly substantial treatment-related difference in the depressive symptoms among the drop-outs, accounting for this differential effect would not change the conclusion that the depressive symptoms were not treatment related.

The situation was slightly different for the hot flash outcome. There was a clear substantial effect of tamoxifen on the incidence and severity of hot flashes. Furthermore, there was evidence of a differential drop-out effect by treatment. Imputation indicated that this resulted in a small overestimate of treatment effect. The rather unusual relationship between drop-outs and treatment presented in Table 8 would require fairly flexible models if one were to estimate and make inference regarding the effect. In future methodology studies, we will address ways to handle this drop-out pattern.

ACKNOWLEGEMENTS

We would like to give special thanks to the participants in the BCPT and the data coordinators at the participating sites, without whom this QOL study would not have been possible. We also wish to note that this work was supported in part by NIH/NCI Grant U10 CA69974 and DAMD grant 17-97-1-7058. We thank Barbara C. Good, Ph.D., for excellent editorial comments. In addition, we thank Maria Harper, Ph.D., and Ginny Mehalik, M.A., for editorial assistance with the manuscript.

REFERENCES

Anelli, T.F., Anelli, A., Tran, K.N., Lebwohl, D.E. and Borgen, P.I. (1994). Tamoxifen administration is associated with a high rate of treatment-limiting symptoms in male breast cancer patients. *Cancer* **74**, 74–77.

Bernhard, J., Cella, D.F., Coates, A.S., Fallowfield, L., Ganz, P., Moinpour, C.M., Mosconi, P., Osoba, D., Simes, J. and Hürny, C. (1998a). Missing quality of life data in cancer clinical trials: serious problems and challenges. *Statistics in Medicine* **17**, 517–532.

Bernhard, J. and Gelber, R.D., eds. (1998b). Workshop on missing data in quality of life research in clinical trials: practical and methodological issues. *Statistics in Medicine* **17**, 511–796.

Boyd, J.H., Weissman, M.M., Thompson, W.D. and Myers, J.K. (1982). Screening for depression in a community sample. *Archives of General Psychiatry* **39**, 1195–1200.

Cathcart, C.K., Jones, S.E., Pumroy, C.S., Peters, G.N., Knox, S.M. and Cheek, J.H. (1993). Clinical recognition and management of depression in node negative breast cancer patients treated with tamoxifen. *Breast Cancer Research and Treatment* **27**, 277–281.

Cella, D.F. and Bonomi, A.E. (1995). Measuring quality of life: 1995 update. *Oncology* **9** (11-suppl), 47–60.

Day, R., Ganz, P.A., Costantino, J.P., Cronin, W.M., Wickerham, D.L. and Fisher, B. (1999), Health-related quality of life and tamoxifen in breast cancer prevention: a report from the National Surgical Adjuvant Breast and Bowel Project P-1 study. *Journal of Clinical Oncology* **17**, 2659–2669.

DeGruttola, V. and Tu, X.M. (1994). Modelling progression of CD4-lymphocyte count and its relationship to survival time. *Biometrics* **50**, 1003–1014.

Fisher, B., Costantino, J.P., Wickerham, D.L., Redmond, C.K., Kavanah, M., Cronin, W.M., Vogel V., Robidoux, A., Dimitrov, N., Atkins, J., Daly, M., Wieand, S., Tan-Chiu, E., Ford, L. and Wolmark, N. (1998). Tamoxifen for prevention of breast cancer: report of the National Surgical Adjuvant Breast and Bowel Project P-1 study. *Journal of the National Cancer Institute* **90**, 1371–1388.

Gail, M.H., Costantino, J.P., Bryant, J., Croyle, R., Freedman, L., Helzlsouer, K. and Vogel V. (1999). Weighing the risks and benefits of tamoxifen treatment for preventing breast cancer. *Journal of the National Cancer Institute* **91**, 1829–1846.

Ganz, P.A. (1994a). Long range effect of clinical trial interventions on quality of life. *Cancer* **74** (9-suppl), 2620–2624.

Ganz, P.A. (1994b). Quality of life measures in cancer chemotherapy: methodology and implications. *Pharmacoeconomics* **5**, 376–388.

Ganz, P.A., Day, R., Ware, J.E., Redmond, C. and Fisher, B. (1995). Base-line quality-of-life assessment in the National Surgical Adjuvant Breast and Bowel Project Breast Cancer Prevention Trial. *Journal of the National Cancer Institute* **87**, 1372–1382.

Ganz, P.A., Day, R. and Costantino, J. (1998). Compliance with quality of life data collection in the National Surgical Adjuvant Breast and Bowel Project (NSABP) Breast Cancer Prevention Trial. *Statistics in Medicine* **17**, 613–622.

Gregoire, A.J., Kumar, R., Everitt, B., Henderson, A.F. and Studd J.W. (1996). Transdermal oestrogen for treatment of severe postnatal depression. *Lancet* **347**, 930–933.

Hahn, R. A. (1997). The nocebo phenomenon: concept, evidence, and implications for public health. *Preventive Medicine* **26**, 607–611.

Halbreich, U. (1997). Role of estrogen in postmenopausal depression. *Neurology* **48** (5 Suppl 7), S16–19.

Little, R.J.A. (1995). Modeling the drop-out mechanism in repeated measures studies. *Journal of the American Statistical Association* **90**, 1112–1121.

Love, R.R., Cameron, L., Connell, B.L. and Leventhal H. (1991). Symptoms associated with tamoxifen treatment in postmenopausal women. *Archives of Internal Medicine* **151**, 1842–1847.

Lyness, J.M., Noel, T.K., Cox, C., King, D.A., Conwell, Y., Caine, E.D. (1997). Screening for depression in elderly primary care patients: a comparison of the Center for Epidemiologic Studies-Depression Scale and the Geriatric Depression Scale. *Archives of Internal Medicine* **157**, 449–454.

Moinpour, C.M., Savage, M.J., Troxel, A., Lovato, L.C., Eisenberger, M., Veith, R.W., Higgins, B., Skeel, R., Yee, M., Blumenstein, B.A., Crawford, E.D. and Meyskens, F.L. Jr. (1998). Quality of life in advanced prostate cancer: results of a randomized therapeutic trial. *Journal of the National Cancer Institute* **90**, 1537–1544.

Myers, J.K. and Weissman, M.M. (1980). Use of a self-report symptom scale to detect depression in a community sample. *American Journal of Psychiatry* **137**, 1081–1084.

Radloff, L.S. (1977). The CES-D Scale: a self-report depression scale for research in the general population. *Applied Psychological Measurement* **1**, 385–401.

Roberts, R.E. and Vernon, S.W. (1983). The Center for Epidemiologic Studies Depression Scale: its use in a community sample. *American Journal of Psychiatry* **140**, 41–46.

Schluchter, M.D. (1992). Methods for the analysis of informatively censored longitudinal data. *Statistics in Medicine* **11**, 1861–1870.

Shariff, S., Cumming, C.E., Lees, A., Handman, M. and Cumming, D.C. (1995). Mood disorder in women with early breast cancer taking tamoxifen, an estradiol receptor antagonist: an expected or unexpected Effect? *Annals of the New York Academy of Sciences* **761**, 365–368.

Sherbourne, C.D. (1992). Social functioning: sexual problems and measures. In: Stewart, A.L. and Ware, J.E. (eds.). *Measuring Functioning and Well-Being: The Medical Outcomes Study Approach*, Durham, North Carolina: Duke University Press.

Tannock, I.F., Osoba, D., Stockler, M.R., Ernst, D.S., Neville, A.J., Moore, M.J., Armitage, G.R., Wilson, J.J., Venner, P.M., Coppin, C.M. and Murphy, K.C. (1996). Chemotherapy with mitoxantrone plus prednisone or prednisone alone for symptomatic hormone-resistant prostate cancer: a Canadian randomized trial with palliative end points. *Journal of Clinical Oncology* **14**, 1756–1764.

Ten Have, T.R., Kunselman, A.R., Pulkstenis, E.P. and Landis, J.R. (1998). Mixed effects logistic regression models for longitudinal binary response data with informative drop-out. *Biometrics* **54**, 367–383.

Ten Have, T.R., Miller, M.E., Reboussin, B.A. and James, M.K. (2000). Mixed effects logistic regression models for longitudinal ordinal functional response data with multiple-cause drop-out from the Longitudinal Study of Aging. *Biometrics* **56**, 279–287.

Ware, J.E., Kosinski, M. and Keller, S.D. (1994). *SF-36 Physical and Mental Summary Scales: A User's Manual.* Boston: The Health Institute, New England Medical Center.

DISEASE-SPECIFIC VERSUS GENERIC MEASUREMENT OF HEALTH-RELATED QUALITY OF LIFE IN CROSS-SECTIONAL AND LONGITUDINAL STUDIES: AN INPATIENT INVESTIGATION OF THE SF-36 AND FOUR DISEASE-SPECIFIC INSTRUMENTS

SERGE BRIANÇON, BERNADETTE GERGONNE, FRANCIS GUILLEMIN, FABIENNE EMPEREUR AND SYLVIE KLEIN

University of Nancy

We studied the specificity and sensitivity to change of disease-specific questionnaires by assessing their relationship with generic questionnaires. The SF-36 and a disease-specific questionnaire were administered to 843 hospitalised patients on the day of admission and 15 days after discharge. The disease-specific questionnaire selected depended on the speciality of admission. The dimensions common to all questionnaires were studied. These were the physical, mental and social dimensions. Relationships were evaluated and compared for two groups of patients: those presenting with a disease for which the specific questionnaire was well matched, and those presenting with a disease for which it was not well matched. We hypothesised that correlations between generic and specific questionnaires would be lower when the disease-specific questionnaire was well matched. We found no significant differences in correlations at baseline; however, when considering changes in scores from baseline to follow-up, patients for whom the specific questionnaire was well matched had significantly lower correlations for the physical and mental dimensions. These results indicate that disease-specific questionnaires are not appropriate for use in cross-sectional studies, but are more sensitive to change than generic questionnaires and therefore more applicable to longitudinal investigations.

1. Introduction

Health status indicators are increasingly used to assess patient outcomes and supplement usual medical investigation. Notable among the numerous instruments developed over recent decades are several health-related quality of life (HRQoL) questionnaires. Measurement of HRQoL covers various dimensions describing different aspects of health as conceptualised and valued by the general public [1]. There is a distinction between generic and disease-specific instruments. The former are designed to be valid across respondents with a variety of clinical and sociodemographic characteristics [2] and are required to be sensitive to the effects on health of a particular condition or intervention, and of any other condition affecting health status [1,3]. They can provide a common measure by which to judge the health status of a heterogeneous population [1,2]. Disease-specific measures are designed to assess HRQoL in patients with a specific diagnosis. They achieve greater specificity by relating health status to the condition under study [1,4,5] and contain items that may be particularly meaningful to patients with that disease (potentially making them more sensitive to change) [2]. Both types of instruments are intended to be used at different levels [6]. At a population level, HRQoL may be incorporated into programme evaluation and policy. HRQoL measures are also commonly

M. Mesbah et al. (eds.), Statistical Methods for Quality of Life Studies, 87–99.

included in clinical trials. Finally, HRQoL may influence decision-making at the patient-practitioner level.

To date, most studies investigating or making use of HRQoL questionnaires have been conducted in distinct populations, such as patients exposed to a similar disease, with strict case definitions and inclusion or exclusion criteria. Similarly, generic and specific questionnaires have been compared in very homogeneous populations (even if the specific questionnaire was designed for use in a more heterogeneous sample) [2,7–11] to decrease inter-subject variability. The conclusions reached are sometimes contradictory: in some instances, generic instruments better capture information about the effects on overall health of unforeseen events or side-effects due to an intervention, whereas specific-disease instruments are more sensitive to change among patients [9–11]. Consequently, in spite of inherent difficulties, some authors recommend using both types [5,13]. Other studies [2,7] have found no important differences in measurement when discriminating between different types of patients. Generalisation of such results is difficult and, in practice, no one generic or disease-specific instrument has been clearly demonstrated to be superior to any other.

If HRQoL instruments are to be widely used in general practice, further information is required about the relationship between generic and specific questionnaires in heterogeneous populations. The purpose of the present study was to assess the specificity and sensitivity to change of disease-specific instruments in a heterogeneous population of patients who had been hospitalised. Specific instruments selected on the basis of the principal disease present were compared as a whole with the Short Form 36 (SF-36) generic instrument.

Hospitalisation is considered to be an important health intervention liable to affect the patient's quality of life. To confirm that disease-specific instruments are really specific and sensitive to change, we developed an original methodology comparing two groups of patients from different specialities: those with conditions for which the disease-specific questionnaire was well matched, and those with conditions for which it was not.

2. Methods

2.1 Study Design and Sample

The study group comprised adults aged 18 to 80 years admitted to the teaching hospital in Nancy, France, between April 1997 and April 1999. Both medical and surgical departments were involved, and subjects had disorders affecting the locomotor, respiratory, cardiovascular and urinary systems. Random clustered sampling was conducted on a weekly basis for organisational reasons: only patients admitted 3 days a week were eligible. Other eligibility criteria (checked on the day of admission) were as follows:

1. Patients were required to have come from home and to have an expected length of stay of more than 3 days (to increase the likelihood that hospitalisation would change HRQoL).
2. Patients were required to be able to complete a questionnaire unaided. Nurses and the investigator assessed this.
3. Patients included in previous HRQoL studies were not eligible. Of 1,763 eligible patients, 1,312 (74%) gave their consent and were enrolled.

2.2 Data collection

Investigators contacted eligible patients on the first day of hospitalisation to deliver the self-administered questionnaires and gather sociodemographic information on factors such as age, sex, education, activity, and way of life. Generic and disease-specific questionnaires (depending on the department of admission) were provided in the same booklet. One copy was given to patients on the day of admission, and a second was sent to their homes by mail 15 days after discharge. Of the 1,312 subjects enrolled, 978 (75%) returned both questionnaires. After discharge, medical records were reviewed for primary and secondary diagnoses, antecedents and surgical procedures. Coding was according to the International Classification of Diseases, 10th revision [14].

The generic instrument used, the SF-36, consists of 36 multiple-choice questions and is validated in French [6,15]. It measures health on eight multi-item dimensions: physical functioning, mental health, social functioning, physical role limitation, emotional role limitation, vitality, pain, and general health perception.

French versions of disease-specific instruments were used, the choice depending on the most common pathologies in the departments concerned:

Rheumatology and Orthopaedic Surgery: AIMS2-SF (Arthritis Impact Measurement Scale 2, Short Form), which is specific to arthritis. It is a 26-item questionnaire with five dimensions: physical, symptom, affect, social interaction, and role [16,17].

Pneumology and Thoracic Surgery: St George's Respiratory Questionnaire, which is specific for chronic obstructive respiratory diseases. It has 50 questions in four dimensions: impact, activity, symptoms, and global health [18,19].

Cardiology and Cardiac Surgery: Minnesota Living with a Heart Failure Questionnaire. This is a cardiac-failure-specific, self-administered questionnaire with 21 questions in five dimensions: physical, mental, social, incapacity, and global health [20,21].

Nephrology and Urology: KDQoL-SF (Kidney Disease Quality of Life). This instrument was developed for use in individuals with kidney disease and receiving dialysis. It measures 11 dimensions: effect of kidney disease, cognitive functions, quality of social interaction, burden of kidney disease, work status, symptoms, sexual function, sleep, social support, dialysis staff encouragement, and patient satisfaction [22]. No French version has yet been published.

Disease-specific instruments explore numerous different dimensions. Our study used three main dimensions commonly explored by all questionnaires: physical, mental and social domains. Table 1 shows how they correspond to the dimension names for each questionnaire.

The score for each dimension was computed according to the recommendations of the instrument's developers. We then linearly transformed these scores to a common range of 0 (worst quality of life) to 100 (best quality of life). The score for a particular dimension was computed only when a patient completed at least half of the relevant items. A total of 135 patients had at least one missing dimension score (on the SF-36 or the

Table 1. Correspondence between the named dimensions for each questionnaire and the physical, mental and social domains used in this study

Questionnaire	Dimension		
	Physical	Mental	Social
	Dimension as named for the questionnaire		
SF-36	Physical functioning	Mental health	Social functioning
AIMS2-SF	Physical symptoms	Affect	Social interaction
St. George's Respiratory	Impact	—	Activity
Minnesota Living with Heart Failure	Physical	Mental	Social
KDQol-SF	Effect of kidney disease	Cognitive function	Quality of social interaction

specific questionnaire) at admission or after discharge; 843 had valid scores for the three dimensions under study and were therefore retained for analysis. Two groups of patients were distinguished: those presenting with a disease for which the specific questionnaire was designed (25%) and those presenting with a disease in the same speciality but for which the specific questionnaires was not perfectly matched (75%). The distribution is presented in Table 2.

2.3 Analysis Plan and Method

Analysis was designed to assess relationships between generic and disease-specific measures across the two groups. Scores and changes in score (score at discharge minus score at admission) were calculated. Responsiveness was measured with the Standardised Response Mean (SRM) [13,23–25], which is the mean change in score divided by the standard deviation of individual changes in score. The sampling distribution (SRM mean and standard deviation) was estimated using a bootstrap procedure involving 200 bootstrap samples [26]. (Each bootstrap sample consisted of 843 observations randomly selected with replacement from the original sample of 843 patients.) A generic and specific SRM was obtained for each dimension (with 95% confidence intervals), and the SRM's for the two groups of patients were compared using a *t*-test.

A linear stepwise regression was performed to assess the effect of patient characteristics on admission scores and changes in score. Sociodemographic factors considered were sex, age, education, living alone (yes/no) and employment (yes/no). Medical factors considered were surgical treatment and speciality of admission. Further analyses were carried out with adjustment for factors significantly (i.e., $p < 0.05$) associated with at least one dimension and for factors that were non-significant but known from the literature to be potentially confounding.

Table 2. Description of the patient sample

Characteristic	Disease area: Locomotor (N = 254)	Respiratory (N = 248)	Cardiovascular (N = 211)	Urinary (N = 130)	All patients (N = 843)
	Percent of patients				
Age (years)					
< 30 years	8.3	4.8	1.4	6.2	5.2
30-39	20.4	4.1	5.7	7.6	10.0
40-49	24.4	16.5	13.3	25.4	19.4
50-59	18.2	25.4	19.4	13.1	19.8
60-69	19.6	30.7	31.8	26.9	27.1
> 70	9.1	18.5	28.4	20.8	18.5
Male gender	45.7	70.6	72.0	73.8	63.9
Level of education					
Primary school	43.0	46.5	48.1	38.1	44.6
Secondary school	46.6	42.8	39.8	46.8	43.8
University	10.4	10.7	12.1	15.1	11.6
Employed	43.7	30.6	21.8	39.2	33.7
Living alone	16.5	16.5	15.2	14.6	29.4
Surgery	26.8	19.4	29.4	46.2	33.7
Well-matched disease- specific questionnaire	35.0	35.9	9.5	14.6	25.7

Are disease-specific instruments more specific than generic instruments? We hypothesised that in cross-sectional studies a well-matched, disease-specific questionnaire would better detect the specific effects of the disease, and that one not well-matched to the disease would be more affected by other comorbid conditions and produce results closer to those achieved with the generic instrument. Thus, we expected that among patients given a specific questionnaire well matched with their condition, the correlation between admission scores of generic and specific questionnaires would be lower than among patients given specific questionnaires not well matched with condition.

Are disease-specific instruments more sensitive to change than generic instruments? The approach to this question was similar to that described in Section 2.4. In longitudinal studies, disease-specific questionnaires should better detect changes related to the disease for which they were designed, whereas generic questionnaires should detect the same changes only as a part of a change in general health. Poorly matched specific questionnaires should also be affected by other comorbid conditions and more strongly correlated with generic questionnaires. Thus, we expected that the correlation between generic and specific questionnaires would be lower among patients given a well-matched specific questionnaire than among those given a poorly-matched one.

To address these issues, we compared the two groups of patients (using *t*-tests) in terms of mean scores, mean changes in scores and standardised regression coefficients for the generic and specific scores. We then used analysis of covariance to adjust for patient characteristics. All analyses were carried out using BMDP software® [27].

3. Results

3.1 Mean Scores and Mean Changes in Score in the Global Sample

Mean admission scores and mean changes in scores (from admission to 15 days following discharge) are presented in Table 3 for the whole sample. Of the three dimensions, the physical dimension had the lowest mean score for both the SF-36 and the disease-specific measures. Standard deviations ranged from 20 to 29. Mean changes in physical and mental score were significantly higher with specific questionnaires than with the SF-36 ($p < 0.0001$).

Mean changes in scores over time for the whole sample were small, but variability was large; for example, for the physical dimension changes ranged from –80 to +90 for specific questionnaires and from –100 to +100 for the SF-36. Mean changes in score did not differ significantly between the SF-36 and the specific measures in each dimension.

Table 3. Summary statistics for scores at admission and for changes in scores from admission to 15 days following discharge ($N^{*} = 843$)

	Instrument type	
Dimension	SF-36	Disease-specific
Scores at admission		
	Mean (SD)	
Physical	54.1 (28.1)	61.6 (26.7)
Mental	58.2 (20.6)	70.1 (22.1)
Social	62.9 (25.4)	63.5 (23.4)
Change from admission to 15 days following discharge		
	Mean (SD)	
Physical	–0.05 (25.2)	–1.0 (20.3)
Mental	3.3 (17.2)	2.4 (18.2)
Social	1.6 (26.2)	0.1 (0.1)
Change from admission to 15 days following discharge (bootstrap SRM)		
	Mean (SD); 95% CI	
Physical	–0.03 (0.07); –0.17 to 0.11	–0.03 (0.07); –0.18 to 0.11
Mental	0.24 (0.07); 0.10 to 0.38	0.02 (0.09); –0.15 to 0.19
Social	–0.10 (0.08); –0.25 to 0.05	0.03 (0.07); –0.11 to 0.17

*As St George's questionnaire does not measure the mental dimension, only 595 patients were used in the analysis of this dimension.

SRM's were also low, with standard deviations (estimated with the bootstrap procedure) ranging from 0.7 to 0.9. SRM's were not significantly different from zero, and a paired *t*-test showed no significant difference between the SF-36 and the disease-specific SRM for each dimension.

3.1 Correlation between the SF-36 and Disease-Specific Measures in the Global Sample

Correlations between the SF-36 and the disease-specific admission scores and changes in scores are summarised in Tables 4 and 5. For the whole sample, the highest correlation was observed for the mental dimension, at 0.66 and 0.51 for scores at admission and for changes in score, respectively. In the physical dimension, correlation was good for the admission score but low for changes in score. Correlations were lowest in the social dimension. Adjustments had no major effect on correlation.

3.3 Relationships between the SF-36 and Specific Questionnaire Scores at Admission According to the Fit of the Specific Questionnaires (Table 4)

Compared to patients with conditions for which the disease-specific questionnaire was poorly matched, SF-36 scores at admission were significantly lower in the group of patients given well-matched questionnaires, indicating greater severity of disease. Similar differences were observed among specific scores. Adjustments tended to increase means in the well-matched group but decrease them in the poorly matched group. Correlations between SF-36 and disease-specific questionnaires were significantly higher in the well-matched group for the mental dimension ($p < 0.001$). Neither physical nor social dimension regression coefficients were significantly different between the two groups ($p = 0.98$ and 0.42, respectively).

3.4 Relationships between the SF-36 and Changes in Specific Questionnaire Scores According to the Adaptation of the Specific Questionnaires (Table 5)

Unadjusted changes in score did not differ significantly other than for the mental dimension from the SF-36 measure. With regard to disease-specific measures, changes in score were significantly different between the two groups of patients. Correlations between the SF-36 and disease-specific measures were significantly lower in the group of patients with a well-fitted specific questionnaire for the physical and mental dimensions ($p = 0.03$ and 0.0001, respectively). Correlations for the social dimension were weak and did not differ between the two groups.

4. Discussion

The main findings of this study can be summarised as follows. In the global sample, mean changes in HRQoL between admission and discharge were small. Generic and specific questionnaires were highly correlated. Correlations between generic and specific admission scores were similar among patients with a condition for which the specific questionnaire was well matched versus those with a condition for which it was not well matched. With regard to the mental dimension, the specific questionnaire was more highly correlated with the SF 36 when it was well matched.

Concerning changes in scores over time, relationships between specific

Table 4. Mean scores at admission and correlation (standardised regression coefficient) between generic and diseases-specific questionaires comparing the well-matched group versus the poorly-matched group

Instrument and dimension	Patient group: Poorly-matched	Well-matched	Total
Unadjusted estimates			
SF-36			
Physical	57.4	44.9	54.2
Mental	58.4	55.0	57.8
Social	64.2	59.3	62.9
Disease-specific			
Physical	66.1	48.7	61.6
Mental	71.9	63.2	70.1
Social	67.3	52.1	63.5
Standardised regression			
coefficient	0.52	0.47	0.53
Physical	0.70	0.73	0.71
Mental	0.38	0.28	0.37
Social			
Adjusted estimates*			
SF-36			
Physical	55.8	49.5	
Mental	57.9	57.1	
Social	63.8	60.4	
Disease-specific	64.8	52.4	
Physical	70.7	67.5	
Mental	65.9	56.1	
Social			
Standardised regression			
coefficient	0.53	0.37	0.50
Physical ($p = 0.98$)†	0.65	0.70	0.66
Mental ($p < 0.0001$)	0.30	0.27	0.30
Social ($p = 0.42$)			

*Adjusted for age, sex, surgery (yes/no), living alone (yes/no), employed (yes/no), speciality.

†The p-values are for the comparisons of the two groups, poorly-matched versus well-matched.

Table 5. Mean change in score between admission and 15 days after discharge and correlation (standardised regression coefficient) between SF 36 and disease-specific measures comparing the well-matched group versus the poorly-matched group

	Patient group		
Instrument and dimension	Poorly-matched	Well-matched	Total
Unadjusted estimates			
SF-36			
Physical	–0.9	2.5	0.0
Mental	2.7	7.4	3.8
Social	0.8	3.6	1.6
Disease-specific			
Physical	–2.0	1.9	–1.0
Mental	1.2	6.3	2.4
Social	–0.5	2.3	0.1
Standardised regression			
coefficient	0.39	0.25	0.36
Physical	0.52	0.43	0.51
Mental	0.27	0.24	0.26
Social			
Adjusted estimates*			
SF-36			
Physical	–1.0	2.7	
Mental	2.6	7.7	
Social	0.7	3.7	
Disease-specific	–2.1	2.4	
Physical	1.2	6.4	
Mental	–0.7	2.8	
Social			
Standardised regression			
coefficient	0.37	0.17	0.33
Physical ($p = 0.03$)†	0.52	0.10	0.51
Mental ($p < 0.0001$)	0.27	0.21	0.26
Social ($p = 0.83$)			

*Adjusted for age, sex, surgery (yes/no), living alone (yes/no), employed (yes/no), speciality.

†The p-values are for the comparisons of the two groups, poorly-matched versus well-matched.

questionnaires and the SF-36 were affected by the fit of disease-specific questionnaires in the physical and mental dimensions. When the disease-specific questionnaire was well matched, it correlated less well with the generic instrument, thus providing different or complementary information.

The sample was chosen to provide what we call a heterogeneous population of non-selected hospitalised patients. Patients unable to answer questionnaires unaided were excluded, potentially biasing the sample towards individuals with less serious disease. Nevertheless, the 843 subjects who remained in the analysis covered a broad spectrum of age, disease, and social origin and were thus suitable for the study of relationships between disease-specific instruments and the SF-36. Acceptability of the protocol was good; 74% of eligible patients gave their consent, and 75% of consenting individuals returned their second questionnaires. One hundred and thirty five patients (14%) failed to correctly complete all questions related to the three dimensions explored. Reasons for that may include complex questions and unclear presentation. If these kinds of questionnaires are to be used more widely and in large populations, it will be necessary to make them easier to understand.

Two novel approaches were used in the present study. First, we explored the application of disease-specific measures to disorders affecting several organ systems. Each score in each speciality was considered to be the disease-specific score as opposed to the generic one. The intention was to compare specific instruments as a whole with a generic instrument, the SF-36, in a large number of patients. Second, we studied the behaviour of disease-specific questionnaires that were not perfectly matched to the disease.

Correlations between the SF-36 and disease-specific admission measures in the whole sample were high for the mental and physical dimensions. This supports the consistent validity of these questionnaires, even following adjustment for patient characteristics. With regard to the social dimension, correlations were low, even when significant, suggesting that disease-specific questionnaires and the SF-36 do not measure the same concept. No significant difference in correlation in the physical dimension was found comparing the group of patients with a well-matched specific questionnaire to those with a poorly-matched one. In a so-called heterogeneous population containing individuals of various ages and social origins and with various comorbid conditions, specific questionnaires behave similarly whether well matched or not. With regard to the mental dimension, correlations are significantly higher when the questionnaire is well matched. Thus, in terms of specificity or discrimination, this study failed to demonstrate any advantage to disease-specific questionnaires when measuring quality of life in a heterogeneous population.

Large improvements or degradations in health status were observed in the three dimensions studied. For the whole sample, SRM comparisons failed to reveal any difference between SF-36 and disease-specific measures. Studies using SRM or other responsiveness indices are conducted among patients expected to change in the same direction (usually improvement) [8,24,28,29]. In heterogeneous populations, evolutions over time of HRQoL measures are too different for standard indices of responsiveness, such as SRM, to be used. In the present sample, major improvements as well as major deteriorations were observed. The second assessment was only 15 days after discharge, by which time patients who had undergone treatments such as surgery or chemotherapy might not have recovered completely or might have worsened. Thus, indices of responsiveness are not relevant to the study of sensitivity to change among generic and disease-specific measures in heterogeneous populations. Hence, SRM was not used to address sensitivity to change.

Correlations between generic and specific questionnaires were low for the physical dimension (0.33). When studied separately, well-matched and poorly-matched questionnaires were significantly different with regard to correlations with the SF-36. When the specific questionnaire matched well, correlations with the SF-36 were lower (0.17). That well-matched specific questionnaires do not measure the same changes as generic ones indicates that specific questionnaires are more sensitive to change, even in heterogeneous populations; similar observations were made in the mental dimension. These findings are interesting. Although the specificity of disease-specific questionnaires was not demonstrated in this heterogeneous population, sensitivity to change remained relevant for the physical and mental dimensions. Thus, it appears that specific questionnaires can be used to measure specific changes in score among non-selected hospitalised patients with conditions for which they are fitted; they provide complementary information, as demonstrated in a more restricted population.

In conclusion, generic and specific questionnaires show high correlation for physical and mental scores at admission, measuring the same concept and providing similar information. Disease-specific questionnaires do not seem appropriate for use in cross-sectional studies. Similar conclusions (that generic and disease-specific measures provide essentially the same information) have been drawn from studies involving diabetic patients [7] and individuals with arthritis [2]. Conversely, in longitudinal studies specific questionnaires provide different and complementary information to generic ones with regard to the physical and mental dimensions. Other authors [10–12] report similar findings. Disease-specific questionnaires appear more sensitive to change than the generic one studied.

ACKNOWLEDGEMENT

This work has been supported by a grant from French Ministry of Health, PHRC (Hospital Clinical Research Program) 1996. The authors would like to thank the research team of the service of clinical epidemiology and evaluation, the physicians and nurses of the study services and the administrative staff of CHU Nancy for their help with organisation. They would also like to thank all the patients for their participation.

REFERENCES

1. Kantz, M.E., Harris, W.J., Levitsky, K., Ware, J.E. and Davies, A.R. (1992). Methods for assessing condition-specific and generic functional status outcomes after total knee replacement. *Medical Care* **30**, 240–252.
2. Weinberger, M., Samsa, G.P., Tierney, W.M., Belya, M.J. and Hiner, S.L. (1992). Generic versus disease specific health status measure: comparing the Sickness Impact Profile and the Arthritis Measurement Scales. *Journal of Rheumatology* **19**, 543–546.
3. Bombardier, C., Melfi, C.A., Paul. J., Green, R., Hawker, G., Wright, J. and Coyte P. (1995). Comparison of a generic and a disease-specific measure of pain and physical function after knee replacement surgery. *Medical Care* **33** (supplement), AS131–AS144.

4. Parkerson, G.R., Broadhead, W.E. and Chiu-Kit, J.C. (1990). The DUKE Health Profile. A 17-item measure of health and dysfunction. *Medical Care* **28**, 1056–1071.
5. Patrick, D.L., Deyo, R.A. (1989). Generic and disease-specific measure in assessing health status and quality of life. *Medical Care* **27**, S217–S232.
6. Till, J.E., Osoba, D., Pater, J.L. and Young, J.R. (1994). Research on health-related quality of life: dissemination into practical application. *Quality of Life Research* **3**, 279–283.
7. Parkerson, G.R., Connis, R.T., Broadhead, W.E., Patrick, D.L., Taylor, T.R. and Tse, C.K. (1993). Disease-specific versus generic measurement of health-related quality of life in insulin-dependent diabetic patients. *Medical Care* **31**, 629–639.
8. Vickrey, B.G., Hays, R.D., Genovese, B.J., Myers, L.W. and Ellison, G.W. (1997). Comparison of generic to disease targeted health related quality of life measure for multiple sclerosis. *Journal of Clinical Epidemiology* **50**, 557–569.
9. Ware, J.E., Kemp, J.P., Buchner, D.A., Singer, A.E., Nolop, K.B., Goss, T.F. (1998). The responsiveness of disease-specific and generic health measure to change in the severity of asthma among adults. *Quality of Life Research* **7**, 235–244.
10. Gliklich, R.E. and Hilinski, J.M. (1995). Longitudinal sensitivity of generic and specific health measures in chronic sinusitis. *Quality of Life Research* **4**, 27–32.
11. Bessette, L., Sangha, O., Kuntz, K.M., Keller, R.B., Lew, R.A., Fossel, A.H. and Katz, J.N. (1998). Comparative responsiveness of generic versus disease-specific and weighted versus unweighted health status measures in carpal tunnel syndrome. *Medical Care* **36**, 491–502.
12. Garrat, A.M., Ruta, D.A., Abdalla, M.I. and Russell, I.T. (1998). Responsiveness of the SF 36 and a condition-specific measure of health for patients with varicose veins. *Quality of Life Research* **7**, 223–234.
13. Fortin, P.R., Stucki, G. and Katz, J.N. (1995). Measuring relevant change: an emerging challenge in rheumatologic clinical trials. *Arthritis and Rheumatism* **38**, 1027–1030.
14. World Health Organization (WHO, 1993). *International Classification of Diseases. 10th Revision*. Geneva: WHO.
15. Brazier, J.E., Harper, R., Jones, N.M., O'Cathain, A., Thomas, K.J., Usherwood, T. and Westlake, L. (1992). Validating the SF-36 health survey questionnaire: new outcome measure for primary care. *British Medical Journal* **305**, 160–164.
16. Guillemin, F., Coste, J., Pouchot, J., Ghezail, M., Bregeon, C., Sany, J. (1997). The AIMS2-SF: a short form of the Arthritis Impact Measurement Scales 2. French Quality of Life in Rheumatology Group. *Arthritis and Rheumatism* **40**, 1267–74.
17. Pouchot, J., Guillemin, F., Coste, J., Bregeon, C., Sany, J. and the French Quality of Life in Rheumatology Group. (1996). Validity, reliability and sensitivity to change of a French version of the Arthritis Measurement Scales 2 (AIMS) in patients with rheumatoid arthritis treated with methotrexate. *Journal of Rheumatology* **23**, 52–60.
18. Bouchet, C., Guillemin, F., Hoang Thi, T.H., Cornette. A. and Briançon, S. (1996). Validation of the St George's questionnaire for measuring the quality of life in patients with chronic obstructive pulmonary disease. *Revue des Maladies Respiratoires* **13**, 43–46 (French).
19. Jones, P.W., Quirk, F.H. and Baveystock, C.M. (1991). The St. George's Respiratory Questionnaire. *Respiratory Medicine* **85** (supplement B), 25–31.

20. Briançon, S., Alla, F., Méjat, E., Guillemin, F., Villemot, J.L., Mertes, P.M. and Zannad, F. (1997). Assessment of functional capacity and quality of life among cardiac failure patients. Transcultural adaptation and validation of the Goldman, Minnesota and Duke questionnaires. *Archives des Maladies du Coeur et des Vaisseaux* **90**, 1577–1585 (French).
21. Rector, T.S., Kubo, S.H. and Cohn, J.N. (1987). Patient's self-assessment of their congestive heart failure. Part 2: content, reliability and validity of a new measure, The Minnesota Living with Heart Failure Questionnaire. *Heart Failure* **3**, 198–209.
22. Hays, R.D., Kallich, J.D., Mapes, D.L., Coons, S.J. and Carter, W.B. (1994). Development of the Kidney Disease Quality of Life (KDQOL) instrument. *Quality of Life Research* **3**, 329–338.
23. Katz, J.N., Larson, M.G., Phillips, C.B., Fossel, A.H. and Liang, M.H. (1992). Comparative measurement sensitivity of short and longer health status instruments. *Medical Care* **30**, 917–925.
24. Anderson, J.J. and Chernoff, M.C. (1993). Sensitivity to change of rheumatoid arthritis clinical trial outcome measure. *Journal of Rheumatology* **20**, 535–537.
25. Liang, M.H., Fossel, A.H. and Larson, M.G. (1990). Comparison of five health status instruments for orthopedic evaluation. *Medical Care* **28**, 632–642.
26. Chavance, M. (1992). Le canif et les bretelles, Jackknife and bootstrap. *Revue d'Epidémiologie et de Santé Publique* **40**, 209–218.
27. Dixon, W.J. (1992). BMDP Statistical Software Manual, Version 7.0.
28. Hawley, D.J. and Wolfe, F. (1992). Sensitivity to change of health assessment questionnaire (HAQ) and other clinical and health status measures in rheumatoid arthritis. Result of short-term clinical trials and observational studies versus long-term observational studies. *Arthritis Care and Research* **5**, 130–136.
29. Kazis, L.E., Anderson, J.J. and Meenan, R.F. (1989). Effect sizes for interpreting hanges in health status. *Medical Care* **27**, S178-S189.

Chapter 2

Analysis and Interpretation of Multiple Endpoints

ANALYZING LONGITUDINAL HEALTH-RELATED QUALITY OF LIFE DATA: MISSING DATA AND IMPUTATION METHODS

DENNIS A. REVICKI

Center for Health Outcomes Research, MEDTAP International

Health-related quality of life (HRQL) outcomes are frequently incorporated into clinical trials of new medical treatments. Problems associated with missing data, multiplicity of outcomes, and longitudinal data structure complicate the statistical analysis of HRQL data. Various simple and complex imputation techniques and statistical methods have been evaluated to deal with missing at random or missing not at random HRQL data. I used simulations to examine how well four relatively simple imputation methods reproduce known population statistics. The findings suggest that all the imputation methods provide acceptable estimates of the missing HRQL data when less than 10% of the data is missing. The empirical Bayes method was best at reproducing population characteristics, even when missing data rates exceeded 25%. The remaining imputation approaches began to introduce bias into the imputed estimates when missing data rates exceeded 20% across treatment groups. Future research should compare empirical Bayes or multiple imputation with statistical analysis approaches to handling missing HRQL outcome data.

1. Introduction

Health-related quality of life (HRQL) outcomes are frequently incorporated into clinical trials comparing new medical treatments. HRQL data are multidimensional, and data collection occurs on multiple occasions within clinical trials. Clinical trials comparing treatments for chronic diseases, such as end-stage renal disease, cardiovascular disease, HIV disease, and cancer, often have missing data due to clinical events, mortality, and other reasons. Problems associated with missing data, multiplicity of correlated endpoints, and longitudinal data structure complicate the statistical analysis of HRQL data. Missing data is a critical issue in HRQL data analysis. The nature and extent of missing data, and differential missing data across groups, can introduce significant bias in the treatment comparisons.

The prevention of missing data, where feasible, is the best way of handling this problem [1]. However, missing data due to disease progression, treatment-related toxicity, hospitalization, death or other reasons are often unavoidable in clinical trials in chronic disease populations [2]. Several mechanisms underlying missing data have been identified: missing completely at random (MCAR), missing at random (MAR), and missing not at random (MNAR) [3]. For MCAR, the mechanism for missing HRQL scores is dependent only on baseline covariates and is independent of other HRQL assessments. Most missing HRQL data is MAR or MNAR. For MAR, the mechanism for missing HRQL scores is dependent on baseline covariates and the previous HRQL assessments. For MNAR, the missing data mechanism depends on the unobserved HRQL

M. Mesbah et al. (eds.), Statistical Methods for Quality of Life Studies, 103–112.

assessments. Informative missing data processes, MNAR, are most problematic for making treatment group comparisons. Bias introduced into the treatment comparisons is proportional to differences in mean HRQL scores between subjects with and without missing data and to the overall proportion of missing data [2]. It is not possible to test for MAR or MNAR without access to the missing data, and different statistical analysis models may result in biased estimates of treatment effects [4].

There is no accepted method for handling missing HRQL data in clinical trials. Two main families of methods have been recommended for handling missing HRQL data: (1) imputation methods and (2) statistical analysis models. Simple imputation techniques, such as the last observation carried forward (LOCF) or substitution of lowest HRQL scores, for missing values may bias treatment effects when there are significant missing data. Diehr and others [5] suggest several methods for incorporating missing due to death into the statistical analysis of HRQL data. However, these techniques modify continuous HRQL scores into categorical indicators, or they make assumptions about the relationship between different HRQL scores and the probability of healthy outcomes or death. Multiple imputation methods, based on survey research methodology, have been recommended for imputing missing values in HRQL studies [6–8]. However, there have been few applications of these multivariate imputation methods in clinical trials involving HRQL outcomes. Most statisticians agree that when there is a large percentage of missing data due to mortality, morbidity or toxicity, sensitivity analysis should be completed to address the impact of non-ignorable missing data on the HRQL findings [9–11].

The methods and findings of a simulation study are contained in this chapter. The simulation study is intended to evaluate different methods for imputing missing HRQL data due to mortality [12]. The study's objective was to compare four different imputation methods for missing values using simulation data that systematically varied mortality rates and change over time in HRQL scores. The simulated data set is based on a clinical trial in end-stage renal disease [13].

2. Methods

The plan for this study involved (1) generation of HRQL and mortality data for a clinical trial with 2 treatment groups; (2) censoring data based on a mortality indicator; (3) application of four imputation methods; and (4) a comparison of how well each imputation method recovered the true characteristics of the original simulated data [12]. The simulated data represented a clinical trial with subjects randomly assigned to one of two treatments where subjects were followed over 18 months with HRQL outcomes measured at baseline and every 6 months. For the simulations, it was assumed that one treatment group demonstrates superiority in mortality and HRQL outcomes. In this study, mortality rates were varied over a range of 0% to 30% and overall change in HRQL (from baseline) was varied from –20 to +20 points on a 0 to 100 point scale with higher scores representing better HRQL. These mortality rates were selected to reflect rates observed in HRQL studies of patients with chronic medical conditions. The rates of change in HRQL endpoints correspond to small, moderate and large changes and were selected to reflect the range of differences in HRQL observed in clinical trials. Baseline mean HRQL scores were specified as 70 (on the same 100 point scale), which is the mean physical function score for the SF-36 in the US general population aged 45 years or older [14]. All combinations of the simulation study parameters were examined. We completed 50 replications of each constructed baseline value, mortality, and HRQL change data file.

2.1 Imputation Methods

Three relatively simple imputation methods were evaluated, LOCF, arbitrary substitution (ARBSUM), and within-subjects modeling (WSMOD), and one more-complicated method, empirical Bayes (BAYES). For all the simulation methods, if an imputed value was less than 0, it was assigned a value of 0.

Last Observation Carried Forward: In the LOCF approach, the last non-missing HRQL score was used as the endpoint score for all subsequent missing scores. This technique assumes that HRQL scores do not change after the last observation.

Arbitrary Substitution: ARBSUB assumes that death is an indicator of worsening health and missing HRQL scores are assigned the previous complete score minus a standardized decrement. A 15 point decrement was used which corresponds to the difference between mean SF-36 physical function scale scores for persons reporting that their health was unchanged and those reporting their health worsened [14].

Within-Subject Modeling: For each subject with missing values but with a minimum of two non-missing assessments, estimates of the missing HRQL scores were based on the observed rate of change of the non-missing assessments. The predicted WSMOD estimates were then substituted for missing scores.

Empirical Bayes: The BAYES with informative censoring imputation method was developed based on previous work by Mori, Woodworth and Woolson [15]. This method groups subjects with $n - r$ sequential observations and r sequential missing observations due to death. For each subject, I estimated a slope that was a weighted average of the individual's slope for the available time points and the least squares estimate for the population slope. The population value was identical for all subjects with missing data and corresponded to the slope for that subject's treatment group. The weights associated with the population slope and the individual slope were $V_I / (V_I + A_I)$ and $1 - V_I / (V_I + A_I)$, respectively. V_I is the variance of an individual's slope and A_I is the variance of the population slope. A censoring parameter was incorporated into the population slope estimate. This allowed the population slope to be conditioned on censoring time, which in this example was equivalent to the number of observations per subject. If subjects who died earlier had a higher rate of HRQL decline over time, this steeper decline was reflected in the BAYES estimates for these individuals.

2.2 Development of Simulated Data Files

Simulated data were used to evaluate the selected imputation techniques. In these simulations, different patterns of missing HRQL data were specified according to a known mechanism for missing data. It was also possible to evaluate a range of missing data rates and changes in HRQL endpoints, and the impact of varying these parameters on the imputation methods.

The simulated data files were constructed as follows. First, a simple structural equation model was developed [16] for generating the longitudinal simulated data sets.

The model was developed to ensure a "known" relationship between mortality and HRQL that is consistent with observed empirical data [13]. A structural equation model with four latent (unobserved) variables was specified (see Figure 1). Each latent variable corresponded to unobserved health status at each measurement occasion. Each latent variable had two observed indicators, a mortality indicator and an observed HRQL variable (i.e., physical function). The latent variables were specified as continuous, normally distributed variables. For any two adjacent time points, corresponding latent variables had a correlation of 0.80. The mortality indicator had a loading of 0.995 and the HRQL indicator has a loading of 0.964 with the associated latent variable. The loading of the HRQL indicator was selected to correspond to the square root of the reliability of the SF-36 physical function scale [14]. The observed variables had associated error terms that were assumed to be independent of each other, and the variances of the latent variables were fixed at 1.0.

Second, the specified model was used to generate the base simulated data set. This was accomplished by invoking a random number generator to create the values for the latent variables with the associated restrictions. The observed variables were then generated by creating a linear combination of the latent variables with an appropriate randomly generated error term. In this way, the data were simulated with known population characteristics.

Simulated data sets were constructed for each treatment group where the change in HRQL over time and the mortality rates in each group were varied in pre-specified ways. This data set was the "complete" version of the simulated data set reflecting changes in HRQL, over 18 months, in ranges comparable to findings in clinical trials in chronic renal disease [13]. Finally, observations from the "complete" data sets were removed to reflect missing data due to death. Mortality for each individual subject was determined by a draw of a random number from the distribution of the mortality indicator. SAS was used to generate the simulated data sets [17].

Figure 1. Structural Equation Model for Simulated Data (Q1–Q4 = observed HRQL at times 1 through 4; M1–M4 = observed mortality indicator at times 1 through 4; H1–H4 = latent (unobserved) health status at times 1 through 4; e = error terms in the model for observed HRQL and mortality indicators)

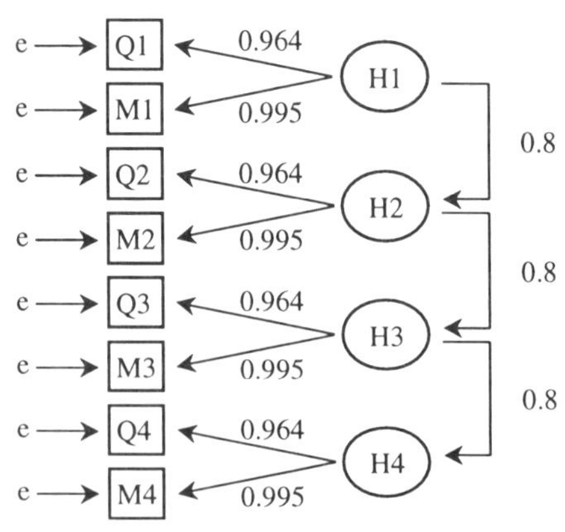

2.3 Data Analysis

Two approaches were used to compare the four imputation methods based on the simulated HRQL data. First, I calculated a pseudo root mean square residual (RMSR) for the differences between the true and imputed values for each simulation [18]. Second, I compared the ability of the imputation methods to recover the true population slopes for the treatment groups by examining the arithmetic difference between the true and estimated slopes by imputation method. I compared the RMSRs and differences between true and estimated slopes by imputation methods using ANOVA. The ANOVAs included factors for mortality rate (6 levels), HRQL change (11 levels), and imputation method (4 levels). Planned contrasts were made between the parameter estimates based on LOCF and the other imputation methods using *t*-tests. Given the large number of statistical comparisons, a Bonferroni-adjustment was used to determine statistical significance. A p-value < 0.0001 was considered statistically significant.

3. Results

3.1 RMSRs by Imputation Method

The overall ANOVA comparing RMSRs was statistically significant ($p < 0.0001$). Statistically significant main effects were found for mortality rate, change in HRQL, and imputation technique. All 2-way interactions were significant (mortality rate by imputation method; change in HRQL by imputation method; mortality rate by change in HRQL). The 3-way interaction between mortality rate, change in HRQL, and imputation method was not significant ($p = 0.999$). The greater the missing data due to mortality, the larger the RMSRs (data not shown; $p < 0.0001$).

Mean RMSRs for the main effects of mortality rates between the treatment groups are reported in Table 1. The RMSR data indicates that overall, BAYES provided the best estimates of the missing scores. In only one situation, where Group A mortality was 0% and Group B mortality was 10%, did ARBSUB have a lower RMSR, although not significantly different than BAYES. BAYES appears to generate the smallest RMSRs and WSMOD, the largest. The RMSRs from ARBSUB and LOCF tended to be smaller than WSMOD although larger than BAYES. Overall, RMSRs increase as the amount of missing data increases, regardless of the imputation method used.

When compared within rates of change in HRQL scores, BAYES generated the smallest RMSRs (7.05 to 7.34), and WSMOD generated the largest (9.81 to 10.16; Table 2). ARBSUB and LOCF produced RMSRs that were smaller than those from WSMOD and larger than those from BAYES. In many cases, RMSRs from ARBSUB and LOCF were not significantly different from each other.

3.2 Estimated Slopes by Imputation Method

An ANOVA was completed comparing the difference between true and estimated slopes, including main effects for mortality rate, HRQL change, imputation method and 2-way and 3-way interactions. The overall ANOVA model was statistically significant. Significant main effects were found for mortality rates, change in HRQL and imputation method. The only statistically significant interaction term was for mortality rate by imputation method. Over the range of mortality rates and missing data, the magnitude of the deviation from the true slope for BAYES and WSMOD are comparable (Table 3),

Table 1. Root Mean Square Residuals by Imputation Method and Mortality Rate Imputation Method*

Group A	Group B	Imputation Method				Comparison
		LOCF	ARBSUB	WSMOD	BAYES	
Mortality Rate		*Mean ± SD*				
0%	10%	4.58 ± 0.21	4.15 ± 0.27	5.45 ± 0.27	4.26 ± 0.18	ARBSUB = BAYES < LOCF < WSMOD
0%	20%	6.49 ± 0.22	6.35 ± 0.31	8.23 ± 0.26	5.98 ± 0.21	BAYES < ARBSUB = LOCF < WSMOD
0%	30%	7.94 ± 0.21	8.14 ± 0.33	10.40 ± 0.29	7.20 ± 0.24	BAYES < LOCF = ARBSUB < WSMOD
10%	20%	7.95 ± 0.20	8.02 ± 0.31	10.17 ± 0.30	7.57 ± 0.22	BAYES < LOCF = ARBSUB < WSMOD
10%	30%	9.18 ± 0.24	9.50 ± 0.41	11.99 ± 0.34	8.56 ± 0.30	BAYES < LOCF < ARBSUB < WSMOD
20%	30%	10.21 ± 0.27	10.96 ± 0.47	13.58 ± 0.29	9.52 ± 0.32	BAYES < LOCF < ARBSUB < WSMOD

*LOCF = last observation carried forward; ARBSUB = arbitrary substitution; WSMOD = within-subjects modeling; and BAYES = empirical Bayes; $p < 0.0001$, *t*-test for independent groups.

Table 2. Root Mean Square Residual by Imputation Method and Change in HRQL*

Group A	Group B	Imputation Method				Comparison
		LOCF	ARBSUB	WSMOD	BAYES	
Change in HRQL		*Mean ± SD*				
0	–10	7.87 ± 1.92	7.58 ± 2.13	9.88 ± 2.66	7.15 ± 1.77	BAYES < ARBSUB < LOCF < WSMOD
5	0	7.62 ± 1.86	8.04 ± 2.20	10.01 ± 2.69	7.21 ± 1.72	BAYES < LOCF < ARBSUB < WSMOD
5	–10	7.80 ± 1.87	7.55 ± 2.19	9.81 ± 2.62	7.06 ± 1.79	BAYES < ARBSUB = LOCF < WSMOD
10	0	7.55 ± 1.81	8.07 ± 2.24	10.03 ± 2.64	7.22 ± 1.73	BAYES < LOCF < ARBSUB < WSMOD
10	–10	7.77 ± 1.90	7.55 ± 2.23	9.82 ± 2.68	7.05 ± 1.77	BAYES < ARBSUB = LOCF < WSMOD
20	0	7.61 ± 1.89	8.35 ± 2.48	10.16 ± 2.77	7.34 ± 1.84	BAYES = LOCF < ARBSUB < WSMOD
20	–10	7.80 ± 1.93	7.79 ± 2.42	9.91 ± 2.78	7.19 ± 1.90	BAYES < ARBSUB = LOCF < WSMOD

*HRQL = health-related quality of life; LOCF = last observation carried forward; ARBSUB = arbitrary substitution; WSMOD = within-subjects modeling; and BAYES = empirical Bayes; $p < 0.0001$, *t*-test for independent groups.

Table 3. Comparison of Difference Between True Slope and Estimated Slope by Imputation Method and Mortality Rate

		Imputation Method*				
Group A	Group B	LOCF	ARBSUB	WSMOD	BAYES	Rank Order (Absolute Value)
Mortality Rate			*Mean*			
0%	10%	–0.0295[abc]	0.0191[acd]	–0.0100[cd]	0.0046[ab]	BAYES < WSMOD < ARBSUB < LOCF
0%	20%	–0.0517[abcd]	0.0497[abcd]	–0.0156[acd]	0.0110[abc]	BAYES < WSMOD < ARBSUB < LOCF
0%	30%	–0.0724[abcd]	0.0858[abcd]	–0.0205[abcd]	0.0114[abcd]	BAYES < WSMOD < LOCF < ARBSUB
10%	20%	–0.0707[abcd]	0.0829[abcd]	–0.0190[abcd]	0.0185[abcd]	BAYES < WSMOD < LOCF < ARBSUB
10%	30%	–0.0908[abcd]	0.1186[abcd]	–0.0242[abcd]	0.0190[abcd]	BAYES < WSMOD < LOCF < ARBSUB
20%	30%	–0.1016[abcd]	0.1612[abcd]	–0.0269[abcd]	0.0206[abcd]	BAYES < WSMOD < LOCF < ARBSUB

*LOCF = last observation carried forward; ARBSUB = arbitrary substitution; WSMOD = within-subjects modeling; and BAYES = empirical Bayes

[a] $p < 0.0001$, *t*-test between LOCF and other imputation methods

[b] $p < 0.0001$, *t*-test between BAYES and other imputation methods

[c] $p < 0.0001$, *t*-test between ARBSUB and other imputation methods

[d] $p < 0.0001$, *t*-test between WSMOD and other imputation methods

although BAYES underestimates the true slope while the WSMOD overestimates the true slope. The deviation for the LOCF and ARBSUB methods are comparable, with LOCF tending to overestimate the true slope and ARBSUB underestimating the true slope. In all cases, BAYES provided the closest estimate to the true slope, with WSMOD providing the next best estimate. In simulations with less missing data (i.e., rows 1 and 2 of Table 3). ARBSUB provided a better estimate of the true slope than LOCF, although the reverse was observed for simulations with more missing data.

4. Discussion

This is the first study that examines different methods for imputation of HRQL scores when data are missing due to death or other MNAR reasons [12]. Based on the RMSR findings, the ARBSUB or BAYES techniques appear to most closely estimate treatment group slopes and other parameters, regardless of amount of missing data and differences in changes in HRQL scores. LOCF and WSMOD consistently provided more biased parameter estimates and there were few differences between ARBSUB and LOCF. WSMOD still consistently had higher RMSRs. All of the methods introduce more variance when estimating missing HRQL scores with higher rates of missing data.

BAYES clearly was most successful at estimating the true slopes for changes in HRQL scores, regardless of extent of missing data and changes in HRQL. In most situations, BAYES slightly underestimated the true slope; in the case with the most missing data, it slightly overestimated the slopes. ARBSUB consistently overestimated the true slopes, across each of the mortality rates. With large amounts of missing data, ARBSUB resulted in HRQL outcomes that are significantly higher than would be observed if complete data were available. The WSMOD and LOCF techniques consistently underestimated the true slopes, and this problem was exacerbated as mortality rates increased.

Some recommendations can be made about imputing missing data in the analysis of between-group differences in HRQL outcomes based on the results of this study. First, when there is very little missing data (<10%) and comparable rates of mortality across treatment groups, all the imputation methods provide consistent estimates of treatment differences. Even when there is differential missing data due to mortality and relatively little missing data (<15% across groups), these imputation methods are fairly comparable, although there is a definite advantage for BAYES. When missing data rates exceed 20%, the BAYES method produced the least biased estimates. WSMOD is also recommended when missing data is less than 20%, since WSMOD slightly underestimates change in HRQL and therefore is somewhat more conservative compared with BAYES. WSMOD is not recommended for cases with missing data rates greater than 20%. When there are greater than 15% missing data, the LOCF and ARBSUB methods introduce significant bias in the HRQL estimates.

Missing HRQL data in clinical trials is often non-ignorable and improved methods for handling missing data are needed. Various imputation methods and statistical analysis methods have been evaluated for dealing with missing HRQL data that are MAR or NMAR. In this study, we used simulations to examine how well four relatively simple imputation methods reproduce known population statistics. The findings suggest that all the imputation methods provide acceptable estimates of the missing HRQL data when there is less than 10% of missing data. The empirical Bayes method was best at reproducing population characteristics, even when missing data rates exceeded 25%. The remaining imputation approaches began to introduce bias into the imputed estimated when missing data rates exceeded 20% across treatment groups. These results may be generalizable to other MNAR reasons for missing HRQL data, such as disease progression or hospitalization. It is unknown whether the empirical Bayes method produces unbiased estimates when missing data rates are 30% or more, or in situations where there are unbalanced or small sample sizes. Additional research is necessary to extend the findings of the current study. Mori, Woodworth and Woolson [15] demonstrated that under the linear random effects model, the statistical analysis procedure of Wu and Bailey [19] and the empirical Bayes imputation method produced results that were similar. Future research should compare the empirical Bayes or multiple imputation methods, and these imputation methods with statistical analysis approaches to handling missing HRQL outcome data.

HRQL data are increasingly used in clinical trials to more comprehensively assess the effectiveness of new medical treatments. Interest in incorporating HRQL data into product labeling and promotional efforts requires standards for research designs, measurement methods, and the statistical analysis of HRQL data [20]. It is important to evaluate and provide guidance on handling missing data in clinical trials involving HRQL endpoints. Given the range in various imputation methods and statistical analysis methods, each with differing assumptions and advantages and disadvantages in estimating treatment effects, statisticians and HRQL researchers must assist government regulatory agencies and clinicians in determining the best methods for addressing the missing data problem. It seems reasonable to adopt a minimal modeling perspective. Future research needs to focus on determining the most reasonable imputation or statistical model for MAR and non-ignorable missing HRQL data.

REFERENCES

1. Bernhard, J., Cella, D.F., Coates, A.S., Fallowfield, L., Ganz, P.A., Moinpour, C.M., Mosconi, P., Osoba, D., Simes, J. and Hurny, C. (1998). Missing quality of life data in cancer clinical trials: serious problems and challenges. *Statistics in Medicine* **17**, 517–532.
2. Curran, D., Molenberghs, G., Fayers, P.M. and Machin, D. (1998). Incomplete quality of life data in randomized trials: missing forms. *Statistics in Medicine* **17**, 697–710.
3. Little, R.J.A. (1995). Modeling the drop-out mechanism in repeated-measures studies. *Journal of the American Statistical Association* **90**, 1112–1121.
4. Fairclough, D.L., Peterson, H.F., Cella, D. and Bonomi, P. (1998). Comparison of several model-based methods for analyzing incomplete quality of life data in cancer clinical trials. *Statistics in Medicine* **17**, 781–796.
5. Diehr, P., Patrick, D.L., Hedrick, S., Rothman, M., Grembowski, D., Raghunathan, T.E. and Beresford, S. (1995). Including deaths when measuring health status over time. *Medical Care* **33** (suppl), AS164–172.
6. Rubin, D.B. (1987). *Multiple Imputation for Nonresponse in Surveys*. New York: John Wiley and Sons.
7. Lavori, P.W., Dawson, R. and Shera, D. (1995). A multiple imputation strategy for clinical trials with truncation of patient data. *Statistics in Medicine* **14**, 1913–1925.
8. Fairclough, D. Multiple imputation for non-random missing data in longitudinal studies of health-related quality of life. International Workshop on Statistical design,

measurements and Analysis of Health Related Quality of Life, University of South Brittany, Arradon, France, October 16-17, 2000.

9. Fayers, P.M. and Machin, D. (2000). *Quality of Life: Assessment, Analysis and Interpretation*. Chichester: John Wiley & Sons.
10. Molenberghs, G. Sensitivity analysis of longitudinal quality of life data. International Workshop on Statistical design, measurements and Analysis of Health Related Quality of Life, University of South Brittany, Arradon, France, October 16-17, 2000.
11. Fairclough, D.L. (1998). Methods of analysis of longitudinal studies of health-related quality of life. In: Staquet, M.J., Hays, R.D. and Fayers, P.M. (eds), *Quality of Life Assessment in Clinical Trials: Methods and Practice*. New York: Oxford University Press.
12. Revicki, D.A., Gold, K., Buckman, D., Chan, K., Kallich, J.D. and Woolley, M. (2001) Imputing physical function scores missing owing to mortality: results of a simulation comparing multiple techniques. *Medical Care* **39**, 61–71.
13. Besarab, A., Bilton, W.K., Browne, J.K., Egrie, J.C., Nissenson, A.R., Okamoto, D.M., Schwab, S.J. and Goodkin, D.A. (1998). The effects of normal as compared with low hematocrit values in patients with cardiac disease who are receiving hemodialysis and epoetin. *New England Journal of Medicine* **339**, 584–590.
14. Ware, J.E., Snow, K.K., Kosinski, M. and Gandek, B. (1993) *SF-36 Health Survey: Manual and Interpretation Guide*. Boston: The Health Institute, New England Medical Center.
15. Mori, M., Woodworth, G.G. and Woolson, R.F. (1992) Application of empirical Bayes inference to estimation of rate of change in the presence of informative right censoring. *Statistics in Medicine* **11**, 621–631.
16. Bollen, K.A. (1989) *Structural Equations with Latent Variables*. New York: John Wiley & Sons.
17. SAS Institute (1996). *SAS/STAT User's Guide, Release 6.03*. Cary, NC: SAS Institute.
18. Zar, J.H. (1996). *Biostatistical Analysis. 3rd Edition*. Upper Saddle River, NJ: Prentice Hall.
19. Wu, M.C. and Bailey, K.R. (1989) Estimation and comparison of changes in the presence of informative right censoring: conditional linear model. *Biometrics* **45**, 939–955.
20. Revicki, D.A., Osoba, D., Fairclough, D., Barofsky, I., Berzon, R., Leidy, N.K. and Rothman, M. (2000). Recommendations on health-related quality of life research to support labeling and promotional claims in the United States. *Quality of Life Research* **9**, 887–900.

COMPARISON OF TREATMENTS WITH MULTIPLE OUTCOMES

PASCALE TUBERT-BITTER,[1] DANIEL A. BLOCH[2] AND TZE L. LAI[2]

[1]*INSERM U. 472 and* [2]*Stanford University*

Treatment comparisons in clinical studies often involve several endpoints, particularly those related to quality of life of patients suffering from diseases like cancer and arthritis. We review traditional statistical methods for this problem and describe some new approaches. One approach is based on a new formulation of the null hypothesis that incorporates the essential univariate and multivariate features of the treatment effects. Another approach is based on assigning benefit scores to different regions of the toxicity-efficacy outcome space. A third approach involves patient thresholds for tolerating different treatments. Bootstrap methods are used to circumvent the analytic and computational complexities of the new approaches. We illustrate these approaches using data from patients with rheumatoid arthritis. In this setting, quality of life involves trade-offs between efficacy and toxicity of treatments.

1. Introduction

Clinical studies on quality of life typically involve multivariate outcomes. When a new treatment is compared with a standard one, the multivariate nature of the response variable poses subtle statistical problems. A commonly used approach to circumvent these problems is to perform a univariate comparison for each response variable and then to combine the univariate comparisons into an overall test by using Bonferroni's inequality. This approach is too crude and conservative, and because it ignores correlations between the response variables, it often results in lower statistical power, particularly when response variables are highly correlated.

The problem of constructing one-sided tests for comparing multivariate treatment effects has received much attention in the biostatistics literature during the past two decades. Section 2 reviews that literature. The methods developed have been based on the multivariate normal distribution and a "reduced" form of the null hypothesis. In Section 3 we consider the "full" (instead of "reduced") null hypothesis and general non-normal joint distributions of the treatment effects (whose sample means and covariance matrices are no longer sufficient statistics). This leads to new formulations of the testing problem that are more appropriate for clinical studies of chronic diseases and cancer, in which treatment effects involve efficacy, toxicity and related measures of quality of life. These more appropriate formulations pose challenging statistical problems, whose complexity we resolve by making use of bootstrap tests. Section 4 presents illustrative examples comparing drugs prescribed to rheumatoid arthritis patients, for whom quality of life involves trade-offs between efficacy and toxicity of available treatments.

M. Mesbah et al. (eds.), Statistical Methods for Quality of Life Studies, 113–128.

2. A Review of One-Sided Tests of Multivariate Treatment Effects

We consider the case of two treatments to be compared on the basis of J outcomes. Typically, these outcomes are several measures of efficacy and toxicity. They may also include other aspects of the therapeutic response. The classical method to compare J means simultaneously between two groups is Hotelling's T^2 test. However, this test is not appropriate when there is a specific directional hypothesis on the difference between the means. In this section we review tests that have been proposed to compare a new treatment to a standard treatment when the former is expected to be better than the latter. To each of these statistical tests corresponds a set of multivariate one-sided hypotheses on the means. Most of these methods are based on the multivariate normal distribution.

To fix ideas, let μ_{ij} be the mean of the j-th outcome for treatment i ($i = 1,2;\ j = 1,\ldots,J$) and $\Delta_j = \mu_{1j} - \mu_{2j}$ for which $\Delta_j > 0$ indicates an improvement on the j-th outcome of the new treatment ($i = 1$) over the standard one ($i = 2$). Let $\mathbf{X}_i^{(k)} = (X_{i1k},\ldots,X_{iJk})'$ denote the multiple outcome response for patient k receiving treatment i, $k = 1,\ldots,n_i$. The difference between the sample means is denoted by $\hat{\Delta}_j = \bar{X}_{1j} - \bar{X}_{2j}$, where $\bar{X}_{ij} = \frac{1}{n_i}\sum_{k=1}^{n_i} X_{ijk}$, $i = 1,2$, $j = 1,\ldots,J$.

The treatment effect estimator $\hat{\mathbf{\Delta}} = (\hat{\Delta}_1,\ldots,\hat{\Delta}_J)'$ is assumed to be normally distributed with covariance matrix $\mathbf{C}$. For the purpose of describing the tests, $\mathbf{C}$ is assumed to be known. This condition can be easily relaxed. If $\mathbf{X}_i^{(k)}$, $i = 1,2$ have a common covariance matrix Σ, then $\mathbf{C}$ is estimated by

$$\frac{n_1+n_2}{n_1 n_2}\hat{\Sigma}, \quad \text{where} \quad \hat{\mathbf{\Sigma}} = \frac{1}{n_1+n_2-2}\sum_{i=1}^{2}\sum_{k=1}^{n_i}(\mathbf{X}_i^{(k)} - \bar{\mathbf{X}}_i)(\mathbf{X}_i^{(k)} - \bar{\mathbf{X}}_i)',$$

and $\bar{\mathbf{X}}_i = (\bar{X}_{i1},\ldots,\bar{X}_{iJ})'$. When the covariance matrices of the two populations are not equal, an unbiased estimate of $\mathbf{C}$ is given by

$$\mathbf{V} = \frac{\mathbf{V}_1}{n_1} + \frac{\mathbf{V}_2}{n_2}, \quad \text{where} \quad \mathbf{V}_i = \frac{1}{n_i - 1}\sum_{k=1}^{n_i}(\mathbf{X}_i^{(k)} - \bar{\mathbf{X}}_i)(\mathbf{X}_i^{(k)} - \bar{\mathbf{X}}_i)'.$$

2.1 The O'Brien Test

O'Brien's statistic (1984) is based on the null hypothesis that the treatment differences for the J outcomes are all equal; specifically H_0: $\Delta_j = 0$ for all j versus the alternative hypothesis H_1: $\Delta_j = \lambda$ ($\lambda > 0$) for all j. It is a linear combination of treatment effects and is obtained as a GLS (generalized least squares) test statistic: $\text{GLS} = \mathbf{e}'\mathbf{C}^{-1}\hat{\mathbf{\Delta}}/\sqrt{\mathbf{e}'\mathbf{C}^{-1}\mathbf{e}}$, where $\mathbf{e} = (1,\ldots,1)'$. The null hypothesis is rejected when GLS exceeds the $1-\alpha$ quantile of the standard normal distribution. Tang, Geller and Pocock (1993) extended the O'Brien ordered alternative hypothesis to H_1: $\Delta_j = \lambda\delta_j$, $j = 1,\ldots,J$ for some specified vector $\boldsymbol{\delta} = (\delta_1,\ldots,\delta_J)'$ with the test statistic $\boldsymbol{\delta}'\mathbf{C}^{-1}\hat{\mathbf{\Delta}}/\sqrt{\boldsymbol{\delta}'\mathbf{C}^{-1}\boldsymbol{\delta}}$. A case often considered is the equality of the J standardized differences Δ_j/σ_j, where σ_j^2 is the j-th diagonal element of Σ.

In his paper, O'Brien also considered a nonparametric procedure where the $n_1 + n_2$ values of X_{ijk} are ranked separately for each fixed j and then summed. The treatments are then compared by using a two-sample t-test on the rank sums.

2.2 The Approximate Likelihood Ratio Test

Tang, Gnecco and Geller (1989a) considered the same null hypothesis as did O'Brien (1984) with a broader alternative hypothesis H_1: $\Delta_j \geq 0$ for all j and $\Delta_j > 0$ for some j. The likelihood ratio test for this alternative had been derived by Kudô (1963) and Perlman (1969); however, its computation is difficult. The ALR (approximate likelihood ratio) test is obtained by transforming $\hat{\mathbf{\Delta}}$ to a vector of independent standardized normal variables, and is given by

$$\mathrm{ALR} = \sum_{j=1}^{J} \max(u_j, 0)^2 \quad \text{where} \quad (u_1, \ldots, u_J)' = \mathbf{A}\hat{\mathbf{\Delta}} \quad \text{with} \quad \mathbf{A}'\mathbf{A} = \mathbf{C}^{-1}.$$

The distribution of ALR under the null hypothesis with known covariance matrix is a chi-bar-squared distribution (Robertson, Wright and Dykstra, 1988) and critical values are tabulated in Tang, Gnecco and Geller (1989a). For example, for $J = 2$ and $\alpha = 0.05$, the null hypothesis is rejected if ALR > 4.23.

2.3 The Jennison-Turnbull Tests

Jennison and Turnbull (1993) considered the case $J = 2$ and used the test statistic

$$\mathrm{JT}_1 = \min_{1 \leq j \leq J} \frac{\hat{\Delta}_j + \varepsilon_j}{\sqrt{c_{jj}}} \tag{1}$$

to test the null hypothesis H_0: $\Delta_1 \leq -\varepsilon_1$ and $\Delta_2 \leq -\varepsilon_2$, where $\varepsilon_j > 0$ signifies that one is indifferent to either treatment with respect to the j-th outcome ($j = 1, 2$) if $|\Delta_j| \leq \varepsilon_j$. They also considered the case $\varepsilon_1 = \varepsilon_2 = 0$ in (1), which we shall denote below by JT_2 and which was also proposed earlier by Laska, Tang and Meisner (1992). Moreover, they used the test statistic

$$\mathrm{JT}_3 = \min_{1 \leq j \leq J} \frac{\hat{\Delta}_j + \varepsilon_j/2}{\sqrt{c_{jj}}} \tag{2}$$

to test the more complicated null hypothesis H_0: $\max(\Delta_1, \Delta_2) \leq 0$, or $\Delta_1 > 0$ and $\Delta_2 \leq -\varepsilon_2$ or $\Delta_2 > 0$ and $\Delta_1 \leq -\varepsilon_1$. We shall discuss the rationale behind this null hypothesis in a more general context and propose an alternative test statistic in Section 3.1.

2.4 The Thall-Cheng Test

Thall and Cheng (1999) were motivated by the antagonistic relationship between efficacy and safety as inherent to anti-cancer treatments. They assume that a two-dimensional parameter $\mathbf{\Delta} = (\Delta_1, \Delta_2)'$ accounts for the treatment efficacy and safety where, as before, positive values of Δ_1 and Δ_2 are desirable. The Δ_j can be the difference between the means, as before, or more generally, the difference between some parameters, or transformations thereof, of the two populations; e.g., $\Delta_j = \sin^{-1}(\sqrt{\theta_{1j}}) - \sin^{-1}(\sqrt{\theta_{2j}})$ for $j = 1, 2$, where $\theta_{ij} = P(X_{ijk} = 1)$ for a binary variable. The method requires specifying *a priori* a series of target points $\boldsymbol{\xi}_1, \ldots, \boldsymbol{\xi}_k$ in the $\boldsymbol{\Delta}$-space that "constitute clinically meaningful improvements over the null hypotheses $0 = (0, 0)$." These targets $\boldsymbol{\xi}_k = (\xi_{k1}, \xi_{k2})'$ must be defined so that $(0, 0)$ is outside the convex hull of

$$\bigcup_{k=1}^{k} \{\boldsymbol{\Delta}\colon \Delta_1 \geq \xi_{k1} \text{ and } \Delta_2 \geq \xi_{k2}\}.$$

The null hypothesis is of the form H_0: $\Delta_1 \leq 0$ and $\Delta_2 \leq 0$. Thus, a target parameter $\boldsymbol{\xi}_k$ with $\xi_{k2} < 0 < \xi_{k1}$ represents a trade-off target between a targeted improvement in the efficacy and an acceptable drop in safety. It is assumed that $\sqrt{n}(\hat{\boldsymbol{\Delta}} - \boldsymbol{\Delta})$ is asymptotically bivariate normal with mean $(0, 0)'$ and covariance matrix $\mathbf{B}$, where a consistent estimator $\hat{\mathbf{B}}$ of $\mathbf{B}$ is available. The corresponding rejection region of the test is obtained by a monotone search whereby the alternative region is shifted toward $\mathbf{0}$ along the 45° line $\Delta_1 = \Delta_2$ in order to satisfy the type I error probability requirement.

2.5 The Follmann Test

In the case $J = 2$, Follmann (1995) proposed to use a "risk score" $\alpha_1\hat{\Delta}_1 + \alpha_2\hat{\Delta}_2$, where the weights α_1 and α_2 are chosen so that $\alpha_1\hat{\Delta}_1 + \alpha_1\hat{\Delta}_2$ correlates well with the occurrence of an event. For example if surrogate endpoints are used in place of mortality, which is the endpoint of real interest, to save time or economize the sample size, then the risk score weights can be determined by logistic regression of the surrogate endpoints on mortality using an ancillary data set. Under the null hypothesis $\Delta_1 = \Delta_2 = 0$, the risk score has an asymptotically normal distribution with mean 0 and variance $(\alpha_1, \alpha_2)\mathbf{C}(\alpha_1, \alpha_2)'$, from which Follman derives his rejection region.

2.6 Group Sequential Extensions

The multiple endpoint problem is an active area of research in group sequential methods for clinical trials. Interim analyses in clinical trials often involve serveral outcome variables, see Pocock, Geller and Tsiatis (1987) for an example in which an active drug for treating chronic respiratory disease was compared to placebo with respect to three lung function measurements. Adaptation of O'Brien's test to a group sequential setting was described by Tang, Gnecco and Geller (1989b) and Tang, Geller and Pocock (1993) who also developed group sequential tests based on the ALR described in Section 2.2. A computational difficulty with ALR statistics is that they are not asymptotically normally distributed and therefore simulation methods are needed to generate appropriate stopping boundaries. As pointed out in Section 2.1, O'Brien (1984) also considered nonparametric rank-sum statistics besides parametric statistics that lead to the GLS. Su and Lachin (1992) proposed a group sequential test based on a summary rank statistic and Lin (1991) used rank statistics for interim analysis of multivariate survival data.

Jennison and Turnbull (1993) developed group sequential extensions of JT_1, JT_2 and JT_3, and Cook and Farewell (1996) have argued that there are situations where the overall (experiment-wise) Type I error rate may not be relevant and have advocated the use of tests on different endpoints with reference to marginal instead of overall error rates. Cook (1996) proposed a "coupled error spending" function approach in which separate marginal error spending functions are specified for different outcome variables.

3. Alternative Formulations of the Testing Problem and Bootstrap Tests

3.1 Comparing Drugs Based on their Mean Response Vectors

To begin with, we still assume the multivariate outcome $\mathbf{X}_i^{(k)}$ to be independent normal so that $\bar{\mathbf{X}}_i$ and $\mathbf{V}_i$ are sufficient statistics for $i = 1, 2$. Although treatment 1 is clearly the better treatment if $\mu_{1j} > \mu_{2j}$ for $j = 1, \ldots, J$, this requirement is difficult to sustain, particularly when J is not small. Since the μ_{ij} are actually unknown and have to be estimated from the data, the multiplicity of comparisons often makes it difficult to demonstrate that μ_{1j} is significantly larger than μ_{2j} for every j, with an overall significance level α (which is typically 0.01 or 0.05). We therefore regard Treatment 1 as the preferable treatment if it can be demonstrated that

$$\mu_{1j} > \mu_{2j} \text{ for some } j \text{ and } \mu_{1j} > \mu_{2j} - \varepsilon_j \text{ for all } j, \tag{3}$$

or equivalently, if the null hypothesis H_0: $(\mu_{11}, \ldots, \mu_{1J}, \mu_{21}, \ldots, \mu_{2J}) \in \Theta_0$ is rejected, where

$$\Theta_0 = \left\{ \max_{1 \le j \le J} \Delta_j \le 0 \right\} \cup \left\{ \max_{1 \le j \le J} \Delta_j > 0 \text{ and } \Delta_j \le -\epsilon_j \text{ for some } j \right\}. \tag{4}$$

In this formulation, (3) defines the alternative hypothesis H_1 and asserts treatment 1's "superiority" for at least one of the endpoints and "non-inferiority" for the remaining endpoints, with $\Delta_j > 0$ for superiority and $\Delta_j > -\varepsilon_j$ for non-inferiority relative to the j th endpoint.

Although the null hypothesis $\Delta_1 = \cdots = \Delta_J = 0$ considered by O'Brien (1984) and by Tang, Gnecco and Geller (1989) represents an extreme point, under stochastic ordering, of the null hypothesis $\max_{1 \le j \le J} \Delta_j \le 0$ (saying that treatment 1 is no better than treatment 2 for each response), (4) has another component (for which $\max_{1 \le j \le J} \Delta_j > 0$ but some Δ_j falls below $-\varepsilon_j$) that is not stochastically ordered with $\mathbf{\Delta} = 0$. For example, in the case of $J = 2$ and $\mathbf{C} = \mathbf{I}$, the ALR statistic in Section 2.2 can be written as $\sum_{j=1}^{2} \max(\hat{\Delta}_j, 0)^2$. Therefore, as long as one of the $\hat{\Delta}_j$ exceeds 2.06 ($\approx \sqrt{4.23}$), the null hypothesis defined by (4) is rejected at $\alpha = 0.05$ no matter how negative the other $\hat{\Delta}_j$ might be (e.g., –3). This implies that the tests of O'Brien (1984) and Tang, Gnecco and Geller (1989) can have type I error probabilities much larger than α at certain points of (4) even though their error probabilities at $\mathbf{\Delta} = \mathbf{0}$ are constrained to not exceed α, as confirmed by a simulation study reported in Bloch, Lai, and Tubert-Bitter (2001).

Let 1_A denote the indicator variable of an event A (i.e., $1_A = 1$ if A occurs and $1_A = 0$ otherwise). Bloch, Lai and Tubert-Bitter (2001) proposed the following test statistic to test the null hypothesis (4):

$$T = \left(\hat{\mathbf{\Delta}}'\mathbf{V}^{-1}\hat{\mathbf{\Delta}}\right) 1_{\{\hat{\Delta}_j > c_j \text{ for all } j\}}, \tag{5}$$

where c_j and the critical value of T are described below. Let $u_p^{(j)}$ denote the p-th quantile of the sampling distribution of $\left(\hat{\Delta}_j - \Delta_j\right)/\sqrt{v_{jj}}$ and let $u_p^{(0)}$ denote the p-th quantile of

$$\left(\hat{\mathbf{\Delta}} - \mathbf{\Delta}\right)' \mathbf{V}^{-1} \left(\hat{\mathbf{\Delta}} - \mathbf{\Delta}\right) 1_{\left\{\left(\hat{\Delta}_j - \Delta_j + \varepsilon_j\right)/\sqrt{v_{jj}} > u_p^{(j)} \text{ for all } j\right\}}.$$

Suppose $u_{1-\alpha}^{(0)}, u_{1-\alpha}^{(1)}, \ldots, u_{1-\alpha}^{(J)}$ were known. Consider the test that rejects H_0 if

$$\left(\hat{\Delta}_j + \varepsilon_j\right)/\sqrt{v_{jj}} > u_{1-\alpha}^{(j)} \text{ for all } j \text{ and } \hat{\mathbf{\Delta}}'\mathbf{V}^{-1}\mathbf{\Delta} > u_{1-\alpha}^{(0)}.$$

Then from the definition of Θ_0 and $u_{1-\alpha}^{(j)}$, $u_{1-\alpha}^{(0)}$, it follows that this test has type I error probability $\leq \alpha$ over Θ_0. Since the underlying distribution of $(\hat{\mathbf{\Delta}}, \mathbf{V})$ is not known in practice, $u_{1-\alpha}^{(0)}, \ldots, u_{1-\alpha}^{(J)}$ are unknown and we cannot implement this "ideal" test. Nevertheless, we can estimate these quantiles from the bootstrap distribution as follows. For $i = 1, 2$ let F_i denote the empirical distribution of $\mathbf{X}_i^{(1)}, \ldots, \mathbf{X}_i^{(n_i)}$, putting weight $1/n_i$ on each of the $\mathbf{X}_i^{(k)}$. Generate n_i independent random vectors from F_i for $i = 1, 2$, yielding the bootstrap sample $\{(X_{i1k}^\star, \ldots, X_{iJk}^\star)' : k = 1, \ldots, n_i;\ i = 1, 2\}$. With the bootstrap sample in place of the original sample, compute $\bar{X}_{ij}^\star, \hat{\Delta}_j^\star$ and $\mathbf{V}^\star$. For $j \geq 1$, let $\hat{u}_{1-\alpha}^{(j)}$ denote the $1 - \alpha$ quantile of the sampling distribution of $\left(\hat{\Delta}_j^\star - \hat{\Delta}_j\right)/\sqrt{v_{jj}^\star}$. Moreover, let $\hat{u}_{1-\alpha}^{(0)}$ denote the $1 - \alpha$ quantile of

$$\left(\hat{\mathbf{\Delta}}^\star - \hat{\mathbf{\Delta}}\right)' (\mathbf{V}^\star)^{-1} \left(\hat{\mathbf{\Delta}}^\star - \hat{\mathbf{\Delta}}\right) 1_{\left\{\left(\hat{\Delta}_j^\star - \hat{\Delta}_j + \varepsilon_j\right)/\sqrt{v_{jj}^\star} > \hat{u}_{1-\alpha}^{(j)} \text{ for all } j\right\}}. \tag{6}$$

The quantiles $\hat{u}_{1-\alpha}^{(1)}, \ldots, \hat{u}_{1-\alpha}^{(J)}, \hat{u}_{1-\alpha}^{(0)}$ can be computed, in succession, by using Monte Carlo simulation that generates B bootstrap samples. The bootstrap test rejects H_0: $\theta \in \Theta_0$ if

$$\left(\hat{\Delta}_j + \varepsilon_j\right)/\sqrt{v_{jj}} > \hat{u}_{1-\alpha}^{(j)} \text{ for all } j \text{ and } \hat{\mathbf{\Delta}}\mathbf{V}^{-1}\mathbf{\Delta} > \hat{u}_{1-\alpha}^{(0)}. \tag{7}$$

This is tantamount to using the critical value $\hat{u}_{1-\alpha}^{(0)}$ for the test statistic (5) with $c_j = \sqrt{v_{jj}}\hat{u}_{1-\alpha}^{(j)} - \varepsilon_j$.

The bootstrap test is nonparametric in nature. Unlike the tests considered in Section 2, the bootstrap test does not assume the $\mathbf{X}_i^{(k)}$ to be normal (or to belong to some other prespecified parametric family). Asymptotic theory in Bloch, Lai and Tubert-Bitter (2001) shows that the bootstrap tests have comparable or better power in comparison with parametric tests reviewed in Section 2. Although both the null and the alternative hypotheses are highly composite, the bootstrap test is able to adapt to the actual alternative, whatever it may be, while maintaining a type I error probability, no more than $\alpha + O(\tilde{n}^{-1/2})$, where $\tilde{n} = \min(n_1, n_2)$. A simulation study reported in Bloch, Lai, and Tubert-Bitter (2001) demonstrates this in a variety of scenarios with $J = 2$. In particular, the case of normal $\hat{\Delta}_1$ and $\hat{\Delta}_2$ reveals that the bootstrap test has power comparable to that of ALR and GLS (derived under normal theory) except for alternatives close to the null hypothesis (4) but not near the boundary point $(0,0)$. Other scenarios considered include (i) normal $\hat{\Delta}_1$, with $\hat{\Delta}_2$ being the difference between Poisson treatment effects, (ii) $\hat{\Delta}_j$ being a mixture of two normals, and (iii) $\hat{\Delta}_j$ being a mixture of a normal and a centered exponential, $j = 1, 2$.

In the null hypothesis (4), the treatment difference Δ_j is regarded as non-inferior if $\Delta_j > -\varepsilon_j$. Sometimes it is difficult to specify ε_j purely on biological grounds without consideration of the variability of the measurements. Letting $\sigma_j^2 = \mathrm{var}(X_{1jk} - X_{2jk})$, an alternative specification of the non-inferiority zone is $\Delta_j > -\delta_j \sigma_j$, leading to the following form of the null hypothesis (4):

$$\Theta_0 = \left\{ \max_{1 \le j \le J} \Delta_j \le 0 \right\} \cup \left\{ \max_{1 \le j \le J} \Delta_j > 0 \text{ and } \Delta_j \le -\delta_j \sigma_j \text{ for some } j \right\}. \quad (8)$$

To perform the bootstrap test in this case, let $\hat{u}^{(j)}_{1-\alpha}(-\delta_j)$ be the $1-\alpha$ quantile of the sampling distribution of $\left(\hat{\Delta}_j^\star - \hat{\Delta}_j - \delta_j \hat{\sigma}_j\right) / \sqrt{v_{jj}^\star}$, where $\hat{\Delta}_j^\star$ and $v_{jj}^\star$ are the same as defined previously and

$$\hat{\sigma}_j^2 = \frac{1}{n_1 - 1} \sum_{k=1}^{n_1} \left(X_{1jk} - \bar{X}_{1j}\right)^2 + \frac{1}{n_2 - 1} \sum_{k=2}^{n_2} \left(X_{2jk} - \bar{X}_{2j}\right)^2$$

is an unbiased estimate of σ_j^2. Let $\hat{u}^{(0)}_{1-\alpha}$ denote the $1-\alpha$ quantile of

$$\left(\hat{\mathbf{\Delta}}^\star - \hat{\mathbf{\Delta}}\right)' (\mathbf{V}^\star)^{-1} \left(\hat{\mathbf{\Delta}}^\star - \hat{\mathbf{\Delta}}\right) 1_{\left\{(\hat{\Delta}_j^\star - \hat{\Delta}_j)/\sqrt{v_{jj}^\star} > \hat{u}^{(j)}_{1-\alpha}(-\delta_j) \text{ for all } 1 \le j \le J\right\}},$$

in analogy to (6). Analogous to (7), the bootstrap test rejects H_0 if

$$\frac{\hat{\Delta}_j}{\sqrt{v_{jj}}} > \hat{u}^{(j)}_{1-\alpha}(-\delta_j) \text{ for all } 1 \le j \le J \text{ and } \hat{\mathbf{\Delta}} \mathbf{V}^{-1} \hat{\mathbf{\Delta}} > \hat{u}^{(0)}_{1-\alpha}.$$

Bloch, Lai and Tubert-Bitter (2001) have shown that this bootstrap test again has first-order correct type I error probability, with Θ_0 given by (8).

3.2 Comparing Drugs Based on Functionals Other than Means

When the underlying distribution of $\mathbf{X}_i^{(k)}$ is non-normal, $\bar{\mathbf{X}}_i$ and $\bar{\mathbf{V}}_i$ are no longer sufficient statistics, and $\hat{\mathbf{\Delta}}$ and $\mathbf{V}$ may no longer be appropriate summary statistics for comparing the multiple outcomes of the two treatments. Tubert-Bitter, Bloch, and Raynauld (1995) have introduced two other statistical methods for comparing multivariate treatment effects. One method is based on assigning benefits for patient values to lie in different regions of the J-dimensional outcome space, with particular consideration for $J = 2$ (including one efficacy variable and one toxicity variable). A second method is based on a trivariate assessment including one efficacy variable, one toxicity variable and the indicator of whether or not a patient continues taking the drug throughout the study period.

With the first method, the comparison between treatments is based on dividing the toxicity-efficacy plane into $T \times E$ cells. Let b_{jk} $(j = 1, \ldots, T;\ k = 1, \ldots, E)$ denote the benefit score for a patient's bivariate value to lie in the (j, k)-th cell, assumed to be equal for all $n_i(j, k)$ subjects treated with drug i $(i = 1, 2)$ with values in this cell. Marginally, the benefit scores are required to be monotonic; we assume without loss of generality that smaller values of either toxicity or efficacy outcomes are more beneficial than larger ones (i.e., the efficacy outcome measures the residual severity of the disease, so that low values indicate the drug is effective). However, there is only a partial ordering with respect to patients' bivariate values since in a particular cell efficacy may be better but toxicity worse, or vice versa, than in another cell. Any choice of benefit scores is allowable subject to the monotonicity requirements. Let B_i represent the expected benefit of treatment i and let $\Delta = B_1 - B_2$. With this formulation, assuming the sample scores to be normally distributed, Tubert-Bitter, Bloch, and Raynauld (1995) propose using a two-sample t-test basing the multivariate comparison of drugs on $\hat{\Delta} = \hat{B}_1 - \hat{B}_2$ where $\hat{B}_i$ is the sample mean of scores with drug i $(i = 1, 2)$. Often nonparametric test such as the Wilcoxon two-sample test may be more appropriate than the t-test.

To set out the ideas of the second formulation, let $\mathbf{X}_i^{(k)} = (X_{i1k}, X_{i2k}, 1_{ik})$ denote the three responses of the k-th subject receiving drug i, $k = 1, \ldots, n_i$, where the first and second responses are the toxicity and efficacy outcomes and 1_{ik} is the indicator variable taking the values 0 if the k-th patient continues taking the drug (and therefore tolerates the drug) throughout the study period, or the value 1 otherwise. With this method a nonparametric discriminant function is constructed whereby the toxicity-efficacy plane is divided into two regions: one where patients' indicators are likely to take the value 0 (type 0) and one where patients' indicators are likely to take the value 1 (type 1). As tolerance of a drug clearly increases with effectiveness of the treatment and decreases with toxicity, we require the discriminant function be monotone in the sense that the maximum tolerable toxicity is a monotone decreasing function of the efficacy outcome. Bloch and Silverman (1997) present a dynamic programming solution for finding the nonparametric monotone function that minimizes the total misclassification cost incurred when classifying the two types of patients. For drug i, the monotone discriminant function f_i takes into account the partial ordering that we wish to impose: patients having bivariate values below the curve f_i should have greater efficacy and/or lower toxicity than patients having values above f_i. It is an "indifference curve" to continuing or stopping taking drug i and the region below f_i is regarded as the "tolerance region" for patients who are treated with the drug. Tubert-Bitter, Bloch, and Raynauld (1995) and Bloch and Silverman (1997) propose to use the area of the tolerance region as a way to evaluate the efficacy-toxicity outcomes of a treatment, after $\mathbf{X}_{i1}$ and $\mathbf{X}_{i2}$ are transformed by their empirical distribution functions to lie in $[0, 1]$. Thus the area of the tolerance region is between 0 and 1, facilitating the comparison of treatments. In particular, letting A_i represent the expected area of the tolerance region for drug i and letting $\hat{A}_i$ denote the observed proportion of area below f_i $(i = 1, 2)$, Tubert-Bitter, Bloch, and Raynauld (1995) propose to use the bootstrap method to estimate the standard error, s_i, and to provide confidence intervals for A_i $(i = 1, 2)$. Independently for each drug, a large number, B, of bootstrap replications of $\hat{A}_i$ are obtained, which we denote by $\hat{A}^{\star}_{ib}$ $(b = 1, \ldots, B)$. A nonparametric statistical comparison of size of tolerance regions between drugs could be based on the percentile distribution of the differences in estimated areas, $\hat{A}^{\star}_{1b} - \hat{A}^{\star}_{2b}$.

We are currently working on other functionals for comparing the multivariate distributions of $\mathbf{X}_i$ $(i = 1, 2)$ that incorporate the essential features of efficacy and toxicity outcomes and the information provided by patient drop-out. We believe that a relatively small number of suitably chosen functionals can capture the key treatment effects of the two treatments under comparison, and that bootstrap methods can be used to resolve the analytic and computational difficulties of the nonlinearity of these functionals and the complexity of the null and alternative hypotheses associated with them.

4. Examples from Arthritis Treatments

The multi-centered database ARAMIS (Arthritis, Rheumatism and Aging Medical Information System) contains information from patients in the United States and Canada with rheumatic and musculoskeletal diseases, especially on outcomes measuring the impact of disease and effects of treatments. The patients' data are collected upon entry and longitudinally, with quality of life and toxicity measurements collected every six months. Different efficacy measurements such as pain reduction or functional improvement as well as the occurrence of adverse events are recorded.

We shall focus on three drugs that are used to treat rheumatoid arthritis (RA). RA is a chronic, systemic, inflammatory disorder of unknown etiology characterized by the manner in which it involves joints. RA usually results in progressive destruction of articular cartilage, ligaments, tendons and bone in body joints. Hand, wrist, knee and foot joints are the most commonly affected. Symptoms usually begin gradually over a period of months. Specific joints begin to exhibit pain, tenderness, swelling and redness. Pain increases gradually as RA progresses and is usually accompanied with increased limited ability to walk, climb stairs, open jars or doors, or to perform other basic tasks. Reducing joint pain and/or reducing or perhaps reversing the progression of functional incapacitation while minimizing undesirable side effects are among the main objectives of treatment.

4.1 Illustration of Some Methods of Section 2 and Section 3.1

Methotrexate (MTX) and Sulfasalazine (SSZ) are referred to as "disease modifying agents" because of their abilities to reduce joint inflammation and retard joint destruction. To compare these drugs, we choose the change in functional ability, measured by a disability index (DI) as the measure of efficacy of treatment and a toxicity score as a measure of toxicity of treatment. The DI is scaled from 0 to 3, where 0 represents no disability and 3 represents no ability to perform any basic tasks such as dressing and grooming, arising, eating, walking, jumping, reaching, and doing errands and chores (Ramey, Raynauld and Fries, 1992). Normal functioning adults over 50 years of age average less than 0.2 DI units compared to an average of about 1.2 DI units for RA patients. With ineffective treatments, RA patients' DI scores increase about 0.1 units per year (Wolfe, Hawley and Cathey, 1991). The toxicity score (TS) we used is an annualized measure of the number of serious adverse events experienced by a patient. Serious adverse events may include blood and liver abnormalities, mucosal ulcers, skin rashes, nausea and vomiting. A zero TS indicates no serious adverse event.

In the ARAMIS database, during the 1990s, SSZ and MTX were newly prescribed to 137 (SSZ) and 601 (MTX) RA patients who then continued taking the drug for at least one year. Table 1 contains summary statistics of the efficacy (measured by the change δDI in the disability index units per year) and toxicity values used for the study. The summary statistics are the sample sizes n_1 and n_2, toxicity scores (TS), and δDI (as a measure of efficacy) for the two treatments. These statistics appear to indicate that SSZ is less effective but less toxic than MTX; that is, the average increase of .07 DI units per year with SSZ exceeds the increase of .02 DI units per year with MTX, but the average TS of .09 with SSZ is less than the corresponding average of .19 with MTX. The percentages of patients experiencing a serious toxic event are markedly different (10.2% for SSZ versus 25.6% for MTX).

Table 1. Summary statistics of efficacy (δDI) and toxicity (TS) for Sulfasalazine (SSZ) and Methotrexate (MTX)

	n	TS	(s.e)	δDI	(s.e)
SSZ					
All	137	0.09	(0.03)	0.07	(0.03)
No Serious Toxicity	123	0.00		0.08	(0.03)
Serious Toxicity	14	0.92	(0.16)	–0.06	(0.04)
MTX					
All	601	0.19	(0.02)	0.02	(0.01)
No Serious Toxicity	477	0.00		0.02	(0.01)
Serious Toxicity	154	0.74	(0.05)	0.03	(0.02)

Bloch, Lai and Tubert-Bitter (2001) apply various one-sided multivariate tests described in Sections 2 and 3.1 to these data. Let $\hat{\Delta}_1$ be the difference in average TS between SSZ and MTX, and $\hat{\Delta}_2$ be the corresponding difference in δDI between the two treatments. Thus in the notation of Section 2, we let $-\bar{\mathbf{X}}_1$ (or $-\bar{\mathbf{X}}_2$) denote the mean vector to (TS, δDI) values of MTX (or SSZ); the minus sign is used here because a lower TS (or δDI) value is preferred to a higher one. Taking a non-inferiority zone of the type $\hat{\Delta}_1 > -\hat{\sigma}_1/2$ (for TS) and $\hat{\Delta}_2 > -\hat{\sigma}_2/2$ (for δDI), Table 2 summarizes the p-values of the Jennison-Turnbull tests JT_1, JT_2 and JT_3 and those of O'Brien and ALR tests and the bootstrap test. As pointed out in Bloch, Lai and Tubert-Bitter (2001), we believe the validity of the bootstrap test but not of the other tests because of the following reasons: (i) the data are very non-normal, and the nonparametric bootstrap test does not rely on normal theory; and (ii) JT_1 and JT_3, like ALR and GLS, have type I error probabilities that do not respect the null hypothesis (4). Although JT_2 respects the null hypothesis, it is overly conservative and cannot accommodate the marked increase in efficacy of MTX with its larger toxicity score.

Table 2. One-sided multivariate tests applied to the study in Table 1

Test	Test statistic	One-sided P-value
O'Brien (GLS)	–0.39	*
Tang *et al.* (ALR)	3.77	$0.05 < p < 0.10$
JT_1	$\min(5.54, 8.86)$	< 0.000001
JT_3	$\min(1.39, 5.32)$	0.082
JT_2	$\min(-2.76, 1.77)$	*
Bootstrap	9.95	0.014

*The value of the test statistic belongs to the region defined by the null hypothesis.

4.2 Illustration of Methods of Section 3.2

We next consider an example in Tubert-Bitter, Bloch and Raynauld (1995) that compares Methotrexate (MTX) with Intramuscular Gold (Gold), which is also a disease modifying agent and was commonly used in the treatment of RA in the 1980s and early 1990s. Skin rashes, a drop of white cell counts and proteinuria are well-known adverse reactions to Gold. To compare these drugs, we chose change in pain experienced by the patient as the measure of efficacy of treatment and a validated toxicity index (TI) as a measure of toxicity (Fries, Williams, Ramey and Bloch, 1993). TI values are available for all ARAMIS RA subjects' treatment courses before 1993 but not for subsequent years; therefore TS and not TI was used in the preceding example of Bloch, Lai and Tubert-Bitter (2001). Pain is measured on a scale from 0 to 3 where 0 represents no pain and 3 represents extreme pain. TI is a summary index of all side effects for a patient on a particular drug. The index includes components of symptoms, laboratory abnormalities and hospitalizations attributable to the medication.

In the ARAMIS database during the 1980s and early 1990s, Gold and MTX were newly prescribed to 205 Gold and 300 MTX patients who were followed for at least one year. Of these patients, 122 on Gold and 160 on MTX stopped their treatments within a year. Summary statistics of the efficacy (change in the pain scale) and TI values, and of the outcome defined as stopping the treatment within the one year study period or not, indicate that MTX is more effective but more toxic than Gold and that the worst outcome occurred in the group stopping treatment within a year (Tubert-Bitter, Bloch and Raynauld, 1995).

4.2.1 Comparison of Toxic-Therapeutic Benefits

Tubert-Bitter, Bloch and Raynauld (1995) partitioned the toxicity-efficacy plane into 16 cells, where the cell boundaries equalled the quartiles of change in pain scale and TI (for all 505 patients). Two choices of the scores b_{jk} were used to illustrate the comparison of the toxic-therapeutic benefit of the two drugs. A simple choice satisfying the monotonicity requirements is $b_{jk} = T + E - (j + k - 1)$. In our application, $T = E = 4$. Hence $b_{11} = 7$, $b_{12} = b_{21} = 6$, $b_{13} = b_{22} = b_{31} = 5$, and so on, with $b_{44} = 1$ representing the smallest benefit, for patients with bivariate values in the most toxic and least efficacious quartile. The numbers of patients with bivariate values equal to b_{jk} are contained in Table 3. The estimated benefits of MTX ($\hat{B}_1$) and Gold ($\hat{B}_2$) are 4.050 and 4.015, respectively. Hence $\hat{\Delta} = 0.035$. The pooled estimate of the standard error of $\hat{\Delta}$ is 0.144. The value of the t-statistic is 0.243, and its one-sided significance is 0.40. Thus, we do not reject the hypothesis that $B_1 = B_2$. A second choice selects the b's so that the benefit in cell (j, k) is much greater than for cell (j', k'), where $j' + k' = j + k + 1$, by choosing $b_{jk} = 2^{T+E-(j+k)}$. Then $\hat{B}_1$ and $\hat{B}_2$ equal 15.54 and 12.80, respectively, and the value of the t-statistic equals 1.86; its one-sided attained significance (p-value) is 0.03. We recommend choosing the b's in collaboration with the investigating clinician so they reflect medical expertise as to what is appropriate to the specific application being studied.

Table 3. Frequency distributions of toxic-therapeutic benefits for 300 MTX and 205 Gold patients

Treatment	Benefit score							Total
	7	6	5	4	3	2	1	
MTX	26	40	55	68	49	37	25	300
Gold	9	19	48	57	38	30	4	205

4.2.2 Comparison of Tolerance Regions

For each drug, the area of the tolerance zone, transformed (on the ranked scale) to be between 0 and 1, is another summary statistic of interest. The best monotone discriminators for the ranked data for MTX and Gold are shown in Figures 1A and 1B, respectively. The area for each drug is transformed to be between 0 and 1 by dividing by the square of the sample size. The proportion of area in the tolerance region equals $\hat{A}_1 = .623$ for MTX and $\hat{A}_2 = .274$ for Gold. Such analysis was not performed by Tubert-Bitter, Bloch and Raynauld (1995) in their analysis of these data since the monotone discriminant function of Bloch and Silverman (1997) had not been developed at that time. We can use the bootstrap method to estimate standard errors

Figure 1. Best monotone discriminators based on the ranked efficacy and toxicity of methotrexate (A, top), and gold (B, bottom) data. The reduction of pain measures efficacy and the Toxicity Index measures toxicity. The dots and squares represent patients who continued and those who stopped taking the drug during the study period, respectively.

(A) MTX

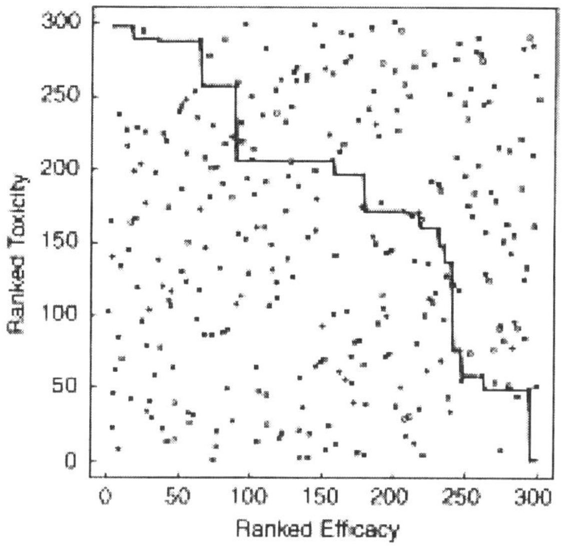

(B) Gold

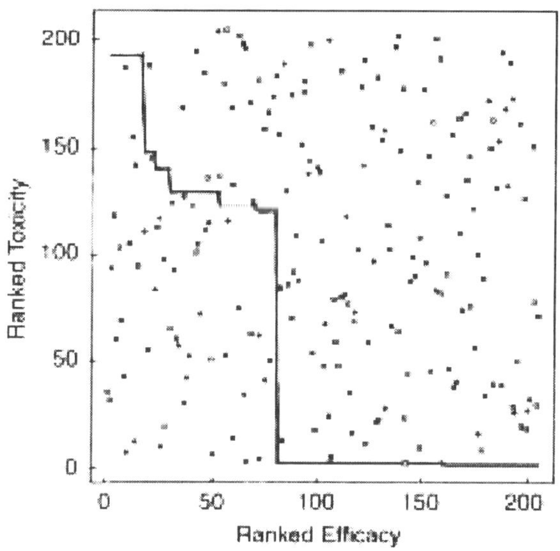

and provide 95% confidence intervals for A_1 and A_2. Using 2,000 bootstrap replications of the statistics $\hat{A}_1$ and $\hat{A}_2$, the standard deviation of the bootstrap replications equals $s_1 = 0.096$ for MTX and $s_2 = .152$ for Gold. The bias-corrected and accelerated 95% percentile intervals (Efron and Tibshirani, 1993) are (0.510,0.770) for MTX and (0.128,0.581) for Gold. Assuming the distributions of $\hat{A}_1 - \hat{A}_2$ to be approximately normal and using the bootstrap estimates of standard deviation, the studentized difference has the value $(0.623 - 0.274)/\sqrt{(0.096)^2 + (0.152)^2} = 1.94$; its one-sided p-value level equals 0.026, showing that MTX is preferable to Gold.

5. Summary

Although bootstrap tests may be computationally intensive, they have many advantages in comparing treatments with multiple endpoints. Testing one-sided or other order-restricted alternatives in the presence of unknown population covariance matrices has been a challenging problem in multivariate analysis. Perlman and Wu (1999) have provided a review and critique of recent developments in the problem of comparing multivariate means that (i) show likelihood ratio tests to be inadmissible and (ii) propose new tests which require even more complicated numerical integration tasks than likelihood ratio tests for multivariate normal observations. The bootstrap test offers a practical way to circumvent such difficulties. Moreover, the bootstrap's flexibility makes it particularly useful when the formulation involves other functionals (than means) of the multivariate distribution of the J responses in the comparison of treatments. An example is the area of the "tolerance region" considered in Sections 3.2 and 4.2.2. Bootstrap methods should allow new approaches to multiple-endpoint testing that incorporate the essential univariate and multivariate features of the treatment effects.

ACKNOWLEDGEMENTS

The authors thank Bonnie Chung and Sarah Robeson for secretarial assistance. This work was supported in part by grants 5PO1 AR43584-05 (ARAMIS 2000) from the National Institutes of Health, Y1-DA-8021-02 from the National Institution on Drug Abuse to the VA Cooperative Studies Program, and DMS-00-72523 from the National Science Foundation.

REFERENCES

Bloch, D.A., Lai, T.L. and Tubert-Bitter, P. (2001). One-sided tests in clinical trials with multiple endpoints. *Biometrics* **57**, 1039–1047.

Bloch, D.A. and Silverman, B.W. (1997). Monotone discriminant functions and their applications in rheumatology. *Journal of the American Statistical Association* **92**, 144–153.

Cook, R.J. (1996). Coupled error spending functions for parallel bivariate sequential tests. *Biometrics* **52**, 442–450.

Cook, R.J. and Farewell, V.T. (1996). Multiplicity considerations in the design and analysis of clinical trials. *Journal of the Royal Statistical Society Series A* **159**, 93–110.

Efron, B. and Tibshirani, R.J. (1993). *An Introduction to the Bootstrap.* New York: Chapman and Hall.

Follmann, D. (1995). Multivariate tests for multiple endpoints in clinical trials. *Statistics in Medicine* **14**, 1163–1175.

Fries, J.F., Williams, C.A., Ramey, D.R. and Bloch, D.A. (1993). The relative toxicity of disease-modifying antirheumatic drugs. *Arthritis and Rheumatism* **36**, 297–306.

Jennison, C. and Turnbull, B.W. (1993). Group sequential tests for bivariate response: interim analyses of clinical trials with both efficacy and safety endpoints. *Biometrics* **49**, 741–752.

Kudô, A. (1963). A multivariate analogue of the one-sided test. *Biometrika 50*, 403–418.

Laska, E.M., Tang, D.I. and Meisner, M.J. (1992). Testing hypotheses about an identified treatment when there are multiple endpoints. *Journal of the American Statistical Association* **87**, 825–831.

Lin, D.Y. (1991). Nonparametric sequential testing in clinical trials with incomplete multivariate observations. *Biometrika* **79**, 523–529.

O'Brien, P.C. (1984). Procedures for comparing samples with multiple endpoints. *Biometrics* **40**, 1079–1087.

Perlman, M.D. (1969). One-sided testing problems in multivariate analysis. *Annals of Mathematical Statistics* **40**, 549–567.

Perlman, M.D. and Wu, L. (1999). The emperor's new tests (with discussion). *Statistical Science* **14**, 355–381.

Pocock, S.J., Geller, N.S. and Tsiatis, A.A. (1987). The analysis of multiple endpoints in clinical trials. *Biometrics* **43**, 487–498.

Ramey, D.R., Raynauld, J.P. and Fries, J.F. (1992). The health assessment questionnaire 1992: status and review. *Arthritis Care Research* **5**, 119–129.

Su, J.Q. and Lachin, J.M., (1992). Group sequential distribution-free methods for the analysis of multivariate observations. *Biometrics* **48**, 1033–1042.

Tang, D.I., Gnecco, C. and Geller, N.L. (1989a). An approximate likelihood ratio test for a normal mean vector with nonnegative components with applications to clinical trials. *Biometrics* **49**, 23–30.

Tang, D.I., Gnecco, C. and Geller, N.L. (1989b). Design of group sequential clinical trials with multiple endpoints. *Journal of the American Statistical Association* **84**, 776–779.

Tang, D.I., Geller, N.L. and Pocock, S.J. (1993). On the design and analysis of clinical trials with multiple endpoints. *Biometrics* **49**, 23–30.

Thall, P.F. and Cheng, S.C. (1999). Treatment comparison based on two-dimensional safety and efficacy alternatives in oncology trials. *Biometrics* **55**, 746–753.

Tubert-Bitter, P., Bloch, D.A. and Raynauld, J.P. (1995). Comparing the bivariate effects of toxicity and efficacy of treatments. *Statistics in Medicine* **14**, 1129–1141.

Wolfe, F., Hawley, D.J. and Cathey, M.A. (1991). Clinical and health status measurements over time: prognosis and outcome assessment in rheumatoid arthritis. *Journal of Rheumatology* **18**, 1290–1297.

THE USE OF SOFT ENDPOINTS IN CLINICAL TRIALS: THE SEARCH FOR CLINICAL SIGNIFICANCE

JANET WITTES

Statistics Collaborative

Measures of health-related quality of life and other "soft" endpoints have appeal to clinical trialists because of their direct relevance to the patient. Unfortunately, while one can define "statistical significance" precisely, what constitutes "clinical significance" remains elusive. A very small difference in a scale, while statistically significant, may have little relevance to the individual patient. Cardiologists have developed a number of soft endpoints, for example, the Killip Scale and the New York Heart Association Score, that define easily recognizable and distinguishable scenarios. Clinical trials in cardiology have used these scores as entry criteria or, occasionally, as primary endpoints and the field has been able to interpret results clinically. Many other fields rely on scales that lack verbal tags to clinical scenarios. The clinical community often cannot interpret data from such scales, even though the scales themselves are quite reliable, precise, and sensitive to change. Without meaningful approaches to defining clinical significance, such scales are unlikely to become acceptable in clinical trials except, perhaps, as exploratory endpoints. This paper discusses several approaches to defining clinical significance, such as attaching changes in scale to changes in risk as defined epidemiologically, matching levels of scale to objective levels of function, using expert panels and groups of patients to calibrate the scales, and adopting the increasingly popular metric "reliable change."

1. Introduction

Imagine yourself about to design a randomized clinical trial. You have available an instrument that measures health-related quality of life (HRQoL) or some other soft endpoint of interest. You know how to scale your instrument and how to score it. The literature claims your instrument is "validated" and therefore possesses the requisite properties of a good instrument. In particular, refereed papers have touted its reliability, reproducibility, and responsiveness to change. It comes with construct validity, face validity, content validity, and a host of similar desirable properties. You believe you must now deal with only one problem: how to interpret summary statistics from your instrument in the context of a randomized clinical trial. In the back of your mind, however, lurks the question of what exactly the word "validation" means with respect to your instrument.

This paper addresses several issues faced by designers of randomized clinical trials in this position. My perspective comes from the way in which statisticians relate to others involved in trial design. Many of the ideas and comments in the paper will not be new to statisticians, but I include them because statisticians frequently work with people whose vocabulary and world-view differ considerably. Statisticians do think differently from psychometricians and from clinicians. Further, when talking to others about soft endpoints, we must recognize that we sometimes use identical words to refer to quite different concepts.

M. Mesbah et al. (eds.), Statistical Methods for Quality of Life Studies, 129–140.

I use "HRQoL" or "soft endpoint" interchangeably to mean a subjective, or at least partially subjective, measure of the status of a patient in one or more broadly-defined psychosocial domains. Several of the ideas apply more generally to the broader class of patient-reported outcomes.

The paper starts with problems faced by the trialist fortunate enough to be using an already "validated" scale. It then addresses the typical set of questions faced by the trialist presented with a widely-used, published, purportedly validated scale that has obvious or subtle statistical or scaling problems embedded within it.

2. Uses for Measures of Health-Related Quality of Life in Randomized Clinical Trials

Randomized clinical trials use measures of HRQoL for several quite different purposes. The purpose of the measure should affect the way to analyze the data and interpret the results clinically. I deal explicitly with four of those purposes. The HRQoL may be (a) the primary or a secondary endpoint of the study or (b) part of a composite primary or secondary endpoint. It may constitute (c) a descriptor of the survivors in a study with high mortality rate, or more generally, the measured subset when some clinical endpoint censors data from a group of participants, or (d) an indicator of a clinical event that has either occurred or is imminent. Sadly, a fifth common use for HRQoL is to simply collect data without concrete plans for analysis. I have rarely seen valuable information gleaned when this last reason is the sole justification for the use of soft endpoints. The purpose of measuring HRQoL should determine how to define the endpoint, how to assess clinical relevance, and how to deal with missing data.

3. A Soft Endpoint as the Primary Endpoint

In diseases for which the endpoint of interest is HRQoL, ideally all patients should have a measure at the specified assessment times. For example, the Huntington's Disease Collaborative Group has recommended using the Unified Huntington's Rating Scale [1], a multidomain assessment of the patient's functional status, as the primary endpoint in clinical trials. Similarly, pain is the outcome of primary interest in studies of alleviation of joint pain [2]. In this situation, the endpoint is simply some predefined score calculated from the responses on the instrument.

When a very large proportion of the participants contribute data regarding the outcome of interest, then use of a soft endpoint poses no statistical problem in addition to the problems inherent in the use of a hard endpoint. The additional difficulties are nonstatistical, for they stem from the need to translate the numbers observed to measurements that have interpretable clinical meaning.

When a soft endpoint serves as the primary endpoint of the trial, each person randomized should have a score for that endpoint. Suppose, for example, the trial is studying a medication for back pain, and the primary endpoint is self-assessed level of back pain on a visual analogue scale six weeks after randomization. Although, ideally, each person should have an outcome measured at six weeks, in practice some people will have missing data. Many people recommend that in the case of a missing endpoint, one should carry forward the last measurement, even if the last measurement occurred at baseline. I believe that approach fails to address the question posed by the study. The study aims to compare the treatment groups with respect to status of the participants at six weeks. In the absence of data on the primary endpoint, we should use methods that do not overstate the efficacy of the test drug and in many cases the last-value-carried-forward method does just that. Gould [3] describes a partial ordering of outcomes coupled with a rank test. He proposes assigning all deaths the worst score, and all failures to return for the final measurement a rank below all those who have a measured value. Within the deaths and drop-outs, he ranks the individuals according to time of drop-out. In a less stringent application, one could apply this method only to deaths and to those who drop out because of toxicity or lack of efficacy. For those people who fail to return because they have moved, one might consider dropping them from analysis or applying a method of multiple imputation [4].

4. Soft Endpoints as Part of a Composite Endpoint

Sometimes, the primary interest is HRQoL or another soft endpoint, but one or more clinical events may censor the data relating to the soft endpoint of interest. The most obvious case occurs when the patients being studied have a high mortality rate. If the mortality rate is of moderate size, then an approach such as imputation, worst-case analysis, worst-reasonable case analysis, or sensitivity analysis provides a sensible proxy for the measurements of interest. When the mortality rate is high, say over 20 percent of the randomized population, such statistical manipulations are insufficient. One cannot simply compare those who are still present because survivors are not randomly chosen. On the other hand, the types of imputation methods listed above can mask a true effect of the treatment. Late-stage cancer provides a commonly cited example. Designers of a trial to study an intervention to palliate pain or suffering in, for example, cancer-associated anemia, must define an endpoint that accounts for mortality. The endpoint may measure those alive and well at some specified time or it may integrate HRQoL with mortality. See Bernhard and Gelber [5] for discussions on handling missing values in studies with HRQoL as an outcome.

Mortality, though the most obvious, is not the only censorer of soft endpoints. Another life-changing clinical event like a stroke, a surgical intervention, or even a change in medical therapy may render irrelevant the soft endpoint of primary interest. One strategy for maintaining the balance between treatment groups conferred by randomization is to incorporate the clinical event as part of a definition of the endpoint. Consider, for example, two different antihypertensive drugs where the outcome of interest is some measure of patient-assessed HRQoL. Failure to maintain adequate control of blood pressure may lead to a change in medications. A possible endpoint in this scenario is time to either some prespecified change in HRQoL or a change in medication.

Several authors have discussed methods for incorporating HRQoL evaluations with censored data. They argue that treatment in terminal diseases should improve the time during which one is alive with good quality of life. In particular, Gelber, Gelman and Goldhirsch proposed an approach (Q-TWiST) that is now frequently used in cancer clinical trials [6]. See also Cole, Gelber and Anderson [7] for a summary of approaches and Murray and Cole [8] for methods of sample size calculations.

5. Soft Endpoints are Descriptors of Survivors

Combining a soft endpoint with mortality or with another clinically meaningful censoring mechanism risks failing to address the clinical question often on the patient's mind: "If I take this drug and the drug adds time to my life, will I feel worse than if I had not taken this drug?" In other words, the patient wants to know whether the extra misery the therapy causes is worth the price of additional days or weeks of life it confers. We must address this type of question conditionally. Again, cancer is the archetype. Is an expected increase in life by a few days (or weeks, or months) worth the toll in pain and toxicity of the chemotherapy? Similarly, in meningococcal septic shock, is the benefit of increased probability of survival worth an increased exposure to the chance of gangrene, amputation, and deafness? Lachenbruch [9] and Shih and Quan [10] describe bivariate models for examining the soft endpoint conditional on not experiencing the censoring endpoint. These models, while very useful, must be employed with caution when not experiencing an endpoint is correlated with the outcome score.

6. Soft Endpoints to Indicate Underlying Change

In some cases, a change in a soft endpoint indicates progression of disease or serves as a harbinger of imminent progression. Both clinicians and patients recognize that quite subtle changes the patient perceives (e.g., "I don't seem to remember names so well," or, "I don't seem to get so tired when I walk upstairs.") may presage or indicate a real change in function too subtle for many instruments to identify. Small deteriorations in cognitive function measured by sensitive psychological tests may indicate progression of neurological disease. With tests used for such purposes, many psychometricians recommend the "reliable change" statistic to indicate progression. Reliable change compares a given observed change with a multiple, usually based on a normal distribution, of the test-retest reliability. For example, suppose the test-retest correlation is ρ and the population standard deviation σ. Then one might declare that a person has "changed" if his absolute change in score from baseline to follow-up exceeds $1.64\sigma(1 - \rho)^{1/2}$. The sign of the change indicates whether the person has progressed or improved. If the underlying distribution of the score is normal, then this measure would identify as a progressor anyone whose change in score falls above the 95th percentile of deterioration or improvement. The appeal of this method is that it calls deterioration (or improvement) any change that is reasonably certain to be real even if the change is not itself clinically important. As described below, the method has some problems.

7. Types of Scales and Scores

This paper reserves the word "scale" for the instrument itself and "score" for the way to assign a number to the responses on the scale. Some psychometricians refer to the latter as the "measurement model".

Scales for HRQoL come in many different forms and the associated scoring systems vary considerably. Unidimensional ordinal or continuous scales have a natural scoring system. Consider, for example a visual analogue scale (VAS) for pain. The respondent places a mark on a line to denote where on a scale from 0, none, to 10, worst imaginable, he judges his pain to fall. One natural score is simply the distance along the line. In my experience, nearly all statistical analyses of VAS and similar scales assume linearity although linearity often does not make intuitive sense. In fact, we know from Stephen's [11] work on perceptual distances that many perceived continua are better scored on logarithmic or power function scales.

Sometimes success is defined in terms of a threshold either of follow-up or of change. Consider a VAS scale for shoulder pain. One may define success as having a score of 0 (or, perhaps, something like less than two) at follow-up or showing a decrease of, say, at least three from baseline.

Many HRQoL scales are multidimensional. The typical multidimensional scale in the medical literature consists of a list of questions that pertain to the disease under study. Some of the questions fall into clinically coherent categories, or domains. A published description of the scale may make a statement about reproducibility of the questions and about Cronbach's α, but that is often the only formal exploration of the scale's validity and, more importantly, its utility in a clinical trial. Published instructions often indicate that the scores from individual questions should be added together to arrive at a total score. Psychometricians and statisticians have developed complicated methods for scoring multidimensional scales, but these approaches are often not used in medical studies. Cox, *et al.* have argued that simple scoring is often preferable to more complex schemes [12]; however, simple addition of the answers to individual questions makes sense only if those who developed the instrument used a number of questions that balance sensible preconceptions of the importance of various manifestations of the disease under study. The aforementioned Huntington's Rating Scale provides a case in point. I am deconstructing it not because it is a particularly bad example of a so-called "validated" scale, but rather because I believe it is, unfortunately, quite typical of the scales in the medical literature. The scale is composed of four sections. The first section is a 21-question assessment of characteristics of motor function. Each question is scaled from 0 to 4, and the responses to all questions are added together. If the body happens to have only one of a specific type of part, like a mouth, then the instrument includes only one relevant question. If the body has more than one part, like four limbs or two hands, then a question for each part appears. Thus, limb function "counts" four times as heavily as mouth function. Nowhere do the publications describing the scale or its validation justify this type of weighting. An alternative weighting scheme might specify calculating mean scores for each like part of the body and then adding these means to construct a total score. The second section of the instrument contains several tests of verbal fluency. Although the tests have very different structures, the individual questions are still added together to obtain a total score. The third section is a scale from 10 to 100 representing overall well-being. The final section is a two-part questionnaire that deals with activities of daily living. The first, very short part has ten questions; it is scored from 0 (worst) to 10 (best). The second, longer part asks detailed questions about some, but not all, of the topics raised in the first part. Again, scores for the two parts are added together to compute a total score on this section. Lastly, the scores on all four sections are added together to compute the final score (even though for two of the sections "good" is a high score and for the other two sections "good" is a low score). Even a cursory look at the instrument shows it to have many problems. Surely adding scores that work in opposite directions cannot be correct. Even reversing the scales so that "good" is always high does not answer the questions of redundancy or peculiar weighting.

When a total score or a weighted total score is used as the outcome variable, the comparison between treated and control tests the difference between the mean, or median, between the groups. For multidimensional scales, another method of scoring defines success as either improvement in all measures, improvement in all domains, improvement in at least k of the d domains measured, improvement in at least k of the d measured domains but no worsening in any single domain, or improvement in at least k of the d measured domains but no worsening in the total score. A still more stringent criterion requires a specific amount of improvement to constitute success. Such definitions are often *ad hoc*. A publication may describe the instrument and the way the authors validated it, but fail to describe the scoring system. For example, in our manuscript concerning a new scale for oral mucositis [13], the journal was interested in the specific questions on the scale and their interrelationships; they deleted our discussion of the scoring system and its development. As one who examined the statistical properties of the scale, I did not believe that simply adding the components always leads to sensitive measure of change because the instrument measures some types of manifestation of disease more than others. The readers of the publication, however, are unlikely to realize that we recommend different scoring systems for different types of clinical questions.

Still another method for using these scores is to measure time to a specific deterioration in the score. The comparison between treatment and control is then based on survival methods. This method either censors the death or defines death as deterioration, that is, death is a surrogate for HRQoL [14].

A researcher about to use a "validated" scale needs to be aware that stamping a scale with the word "validated" means that the developers have tested the language of the scale and its scoring system in at least one specific situation. Modifying the questions, changing their order, translating the questions to another language, altering the scoring system, applying the scale to a new disease, employing the scale to assess the effect of a treatment that differs in mechanism from the interventions used to validate the scale, or incorporating the scale into a battery of other scales may require new validation to assess rigorously the properties of the modified scale in the new context. Slight changes are unlikely to affect the properties of a scale materially, but the user of the revised scale should question carefully whether the modifications change the properties enough to require a pretest of the revision.

A common problem in the practical application of published "validated" scales is that the description of the scoring method may not contain any guidance about how to handle missing data on the questionnaire. As mentioned above, scales often have questions that represent several domains. The number of questions within the domains may vary. The possible answers may differ from question to question. In a multiquestion instrument, different ways of handling missing data can produce quite different results. Often the methods used are *ad hoc*. In the absence of directions from the developers of the scale, the best the user can do is decide prospectively the rules for handling missing questions.

8. Clinical Relevance of the Measure of Success

The previous section addressed the ways in which researchers performing randomized clinical trials typically define success when they are comparing treatment groups with respect to HRQoL. Although feeling better has value in itself, a scale becomes more interpretable in the presence of some objective anchor that associates a given change on the scale with a specific change in level of function. For example, one might provide a rule of thumb that says something like, "A ten-point improvement in this scale has different meanings for different people. For a person previously unable to walk unaided, a ten-point improvement corresponds roughly to the ability to walk 20 feet without mechanical support. For a person previously on mechanical ventilation five hours a day, a ten-point improvement corresponds to no longer needing mechanical ventilation." We used this type of translation in a description of a scale we developed for amyotrophic lateral sclerosis (ALS, or "Lou Gehrig's disease") and it has provided helpful guidance to the clinicians who use the scale [15].

9. Relevance of the Instrument to the Population under Consideration

To provide interpretable data in a clinical trial the instrument being used must have both cultural and clinical relevance to the population under study. Many disease-specific instruments are developed in relatively small groups of patients with homogeneous cultural backgrounds. Some measures, most notably those that assess cognition, are developed in healthy populations. Moving from culture to culture, or from language to language, or from the healthy to the ill, may lead to unanticipated differences in interpretation.

Many developers of scales carefully translate them from language to language, and even dialect to dialect. The process often includes a back-translation. (Does a question written in English but translated into Spanish retain its meaning in English when it is translated back from Spanish to English? If it does not, then presumably the original English to Spanish translation was flawed). Translation, however, is not sufficient when the differences in performance of the tests stem from the very structure of the language itself. The following cautionary pair of graphs (Figure 1) shows the results of a test of verbal fluency developed in English but translated into other languages. The test gives subjects two minutes to list all words they can recall in certain specified categories. The first graph in the panel shows the distribution of scores at baseline superimposed with the best-fitting normal curve. The clear bimodality suggested to the investigators that two types of patients had entered the trial, some neurologically normal (the right mode) and some neurologically impaired (the left mode). The investigators were puzzled by fact that no nonverbal test in the same study group had shown marked bimodality. Given the nature of the disease, if the populations were composed of normal and impaired subjects, one would expect to see impairment reflected in the nonverbal tests. In fact, the bimodality is consistent with, and more parsimoniously explained by, the properties of the languages in the study. English has a much larger vocabulary than the other languages used. As seen in the second panel, the respondents to the non-English version of the test listed many fewer words than those who answered in English. These graphs show a typical experience when the size of the vocabulary of the language itself is related to the performance on the test. (I have deliberately modified the graphs and eliminated the scales to preserve confidentiality of the data.)

Another quite serious problem arises when one applies standard measures of function or cognition to an ill population. As an example, consider three tests all administered to the same group of patients who are suffering from a progressive disease that affects both cognitive and general neurologic function (see Figure 2.). The three tests are a performance test developed for a cognitively unimpaired population (e.g., a test of arithmetic ability; Figure 2A), a timed test developed for a neurologically unimpaired population (e.g., the number of seconds it takes to fill a pegboard; Figure 2B), and a test developed specifically for a cognitively impaired population (Figure 2C). All three panels come from the same population of ill patients. Scores from all three tests are normally distributed in the populations for which the tests were developed

Figure 2A shows a test of performance. The histogram represents the observed (somewhat modified) data with the best-fitting normal distribution superimposed. The

Figure 1. Scores on a test of verbal fluency*

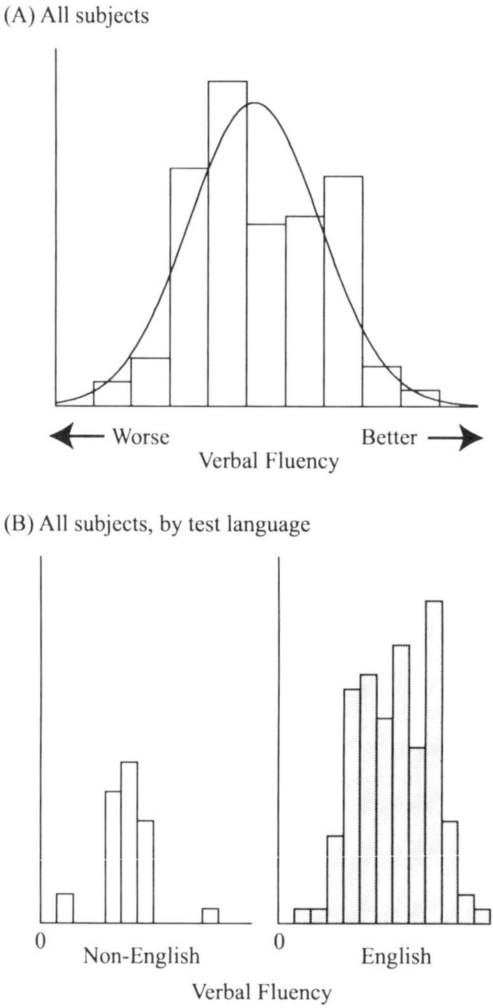

*Panel (A) shows the distribution of a test of verbal fluency administered in a multinational clinical trial. The tests have been "validated" in all languages used in the trial. The distribution is purported to be Gaussian. The bars show the observed distribution and the curve shows the best fitting normal density. The clinicians initially "explained" the bimodality as reflective of two groups of participants, one with normal and and one with impaired neurologic function. Panel (B) shows the data classified according to the language of the test. Those who took the test in English (US, UK, and Canada outside Quebec) scored consistently higher than those who took the test in another language. A parsimonious explanation of the results is that the difference reflects the fact that English has a much larger vocabulary than the other languages in which the test was administered.

Figure 2. Some distributions of soft endpoints*

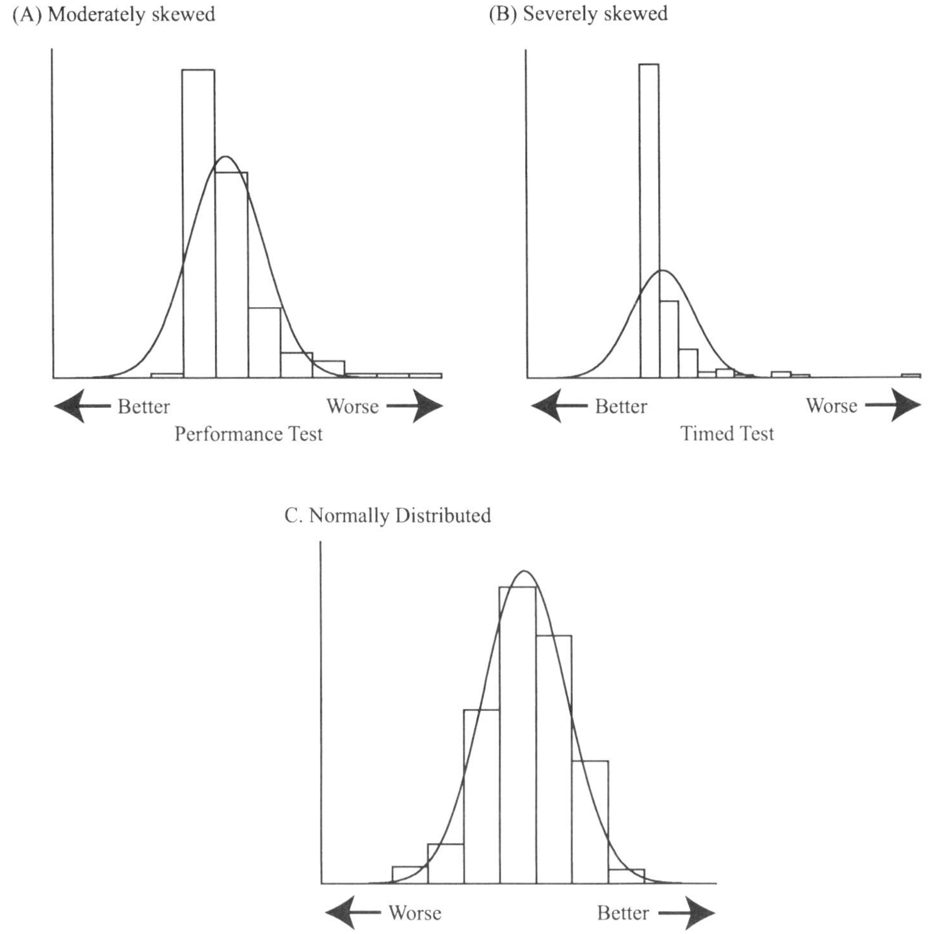

*Panels (A) and (B) show the scores on a test of cognitive performance and a timed test, respectively, in a cognitively impaired population. The healthy population in whom the tests were developed had normally distributed scores on both tests. Panel (C) shows the distribution of scores in the same study group on a third test; this test was developed in a population of cognitively impaired patients. The ratio of variance in the trial cohort to variance in the validation sample was 19 for Panel (A), 225 for Panel (B), and 0.8 for Panel (C).

distribution among patients is quite skewed with a small lump of probability in the tail representing worse functioning. This level of impairment is quite rare in a normal population. Of special interest is the ratio of the variance in the trial cohort to the variance in the healthy, or validation sample. In this case, the ratio is 19, representing a sizable increase in variability.

Figure 2B shows results, again slightly modified to preserve confidentiality, typical of timed tests. Here the distribution shows extreme skewness. In fact, a population of healthy people would be expected to finish the task within the time represented by the modal bar of the histogram. In the patient population, however, many people work more slowly and some take dramatically longer to complete the task than any healthy person. Here the ratio of variances is approximately 225.

By contrast, Figure 2C shows results from a cognitive test developed on the type of patients studied. A Gaussian curve fits the empirical distribution well; the variance in the sample is close to that in the sample used to validate the scale (variance ratio of 0.8).
These examples serve as warnings for those who are thinking of adopting reliable change to indicate progression. Recall that reliable change assumes normal distributions and assumes that the variance calculated in the validation process applies to the population of patients. Most statistical inference depends on behavior of distributions at their centers so that standard statistical tests are quite robust to deviations from normality. Reliable change, however, refers to the tails of the distributions, the very place where the failure of normality typically occurs. In the cases represented by the first two graphs, the reliable change is very small relative to the standard deviation in the patient population of interest. Thus, a very large proportion of patients will experience a change large enough to be deemed "reliable". One may avoid this problem by calculating reliable change for the population of interest. In other words, one should consider "reliable change" as a function not only of the test itself but as a function of both the test and the population to which it is being applied. Even so, the sample size used to calculate the reliable change must be large enough to be precise in the tails of the distribution of interest. Temkin, *et al.* [16] discuss other difficulties with reliable change.

10. Defining Clinical Significance

Understanding the clinical significance of a specific change on a scale, or of the difference between means in the treated and control groups of a clinical trial, is important for at least two very different reasons, one scientific and one regulatory. From a scientific point of view, the ability to understand what a number means helps with study interpretation. Suppose in a trial of back pain the control and treatment groups report mean pain scores of 7.2 and 6.8 on a VAS scale, respectively, and the difference is statistically significant. In thinking about prescribing the treatment, a clinician should know how much difference in pain is worth the expense and the risk of taking the drug. Such risk-benefit assessment requires understanding of the functional and emotional meaning of difference in the score.

From a regulatory point of view, a trials whose endpoint is a HRQoL measure may lead to an "overpowered" study, that is, a study with a sample size so large that a clinical trial can detect a very small clinically insignificant effect of therapy. In that case, when a clinical trial shows statistically significant benefit, a regulatory agency may feel pressured into approving a treatment that makes little clinical difference to the patient. Specifying *a priori* what constitutes a clinically significant benefit and designing the trial to show that the treatment confers at least the prespecified degree of benefit leads to a trial that can show convincing evidence that the treatment is clinically useful.

If the trial aims to assess the clinical benefit of a therapy through the use of an instrument that measures HRQoL, the user of the instrument has several approaches to defining clinical significance. One approach, widely employed in cardiology, is to associate changes in the scale to changes in risk of clinical events. In several commonly used scales in cardiology, for example, the Killip scale and the New York Heart Association scale, many epidemiologic studies have investigated the relationship between a one-point change on the scale and the probability of experiencing a major clinical event within the next year or the next five years. If reduction of risk by x percent corresponds to what cardiologists consider a clinically meaningful change in risk and if a y-point change in score on the scale is associated with an x percent reduction in risk, then one may regard a y-point change in score as a clinically relevant change.

An approach mentioned above matches levels of change in the scale to objective levels of change in function or to changes on other commonly used methods of assessment. For example, the standard method for evaluating bladder function in post-menopausal women is to ask subjects to report micturitions and urgency on a daily diary. The designers of a clinical trial in post-menopausal women with bladder dysfunction may worry lest daily diaries prove too onerous in a long-term clinical trial. A new instrument designed to replace the diary would have to demonstrate that changes on the new scale matched in some interpretable way a clinically meaningful change in frequency or urgency of micturition.

In the absence of any instrument to measure the construct of interest, some investigators use expert panels and groups of patients to calibrate the new scale and to define clinically relevant change.

11. Conclusion

Adopting soft endpoints in a clinical trial demands that the investigators understand the properties of the instrument they use. Questionnaires can be costly and intrusive. Data collected for no reason adds to the burden on the study. Thus, those of us who collect data on HRQoL owe clinicians, patients, and policy-makers an interpretable description of the meaning of the scales.

Users of published instruments, even those that purport to be "validated", should consider carefully the properties of the scale itself, the method of scoring, and the way in which to handle missing data. Of particular concern is the applicability in a new situation of an instrument designed for a different context.

Used carefully, measures of HRQoL provide important insight into the benefit, or harm, of a therapy. Patient may view improved HRQoL as the most important aspects of therapy; thus, it is incumbent upon the clinical research community to make these measurements with due diligence.

REFERENCES

1. Huntington Study Group (1996). Unified Huntington's Disease Rating Scale: reliability and consistency. *Movement Disorders* **11**, 136–142.
2. Heald, S., Riddle, D. and Lamb. R. (1997). The Shoulder Pain and Disability Index: the construct validity and responsiveness of a region-specific disability measure. *Physical Therapy* **77**, 1079–1089.

3. Gould, A. (1980). A new approach to the analysis of clinical drug trials with withdrawals. *Biometrics* **36**, 721–727.
4. Little, R.J.A. and Rubin, D.B. (1987). *Statistical Analysis with Missing Data*. New York: John Wiley and Sons, Inc.
5. Bernhard, J. and Gelber, R., eds. (1998). Workshop on missing data in quality of life research in clinical trials: practical and methodological issues. *Statistics in Medicine* **17**, 511–796.
6. Gelber, R., Gelman, R. and Goldhirsch, A. (1989). A quality-of-life-oriented endpoint for comparing therapies. *Biometrics* **45**, 781–795.
7. Cole, B., Gelber, R. and Anderson, K. (1994). Parametric approaches to quality-adjusted survival analysis. *Biometrics* **50**, 621–631.
8. Murray, S. and Cole, B. (2000). Variance and sample size calculations in quality-of-life-adjusted survival analysis (Q-TWiST). *Biometrics* **56**, 173–182.
9. Lachenbruch P (2001). Comparisons of two-part models with competitors. *Statistics in Medicine* **20**, 1215–1234.
10. Shih, W. and Quan, H. (1997). Testing for treatment differences with dropouts present in clinical trials–a composite approach. *Statistics in Medicine* **11**, 1225–1239.
11. Stephens, S. (1957). On the psychophysical law. *Psychological Reviews* **64**, 153–181.
12. Cox, D.R., Fitzpatrick, R., Fletcher, AE, Gore, SM, Spiegelhalter, D.J. and Jones, D.J. (1992). Quality of life assessment: can we keep it simple? *Journal of the Royal Statistical Society, Series A* **155**, 353–393.
13. Sonis, S.T., Eilers, J.P., Epstein, J.B., LeVoque, F.G., Liggett, W.H., Jr., Mulagha, M.T., Peterson, D.E., Rose, A.H., Schubert, M.M., Spijkervet, F.K. and Wittes, J. (1999). Validation of a new scoring system for the assessment of clinical trial research of oral mucositis induced by radiation or chemotherapy. *Cancer* **85**, 2103–2113.
14. Wittes, J., Lakatos, E. and Probstfield, J. (1989). Surrogate endpoints in clinical trials: cardiovascular diseases. *Statistics in Medicine* **8**, 415–425.
15. The ALS CNTF Treatment Study (ACTS) Phase I-II Study Group (1996). The Amyotrophic Lateral Sclerosis Functional Rating Scale. Assessment of activities of daily living in patients with amyotrophic lateral sclerosis. *Archives of Neurology* **53**, 141–147.
16. Temkin, N.R., Heaton, R.K., Grant, I. and Dikonen, S.S. (1999). Detecting significant change in neuropsychological test performance: a comparison of four models. *Journal of the International Neuropsychological Society* **5**, 357–369.

Chapter 3

Item Response Theory and Rasch Models

PARAMETRIC AND NONPARAMETRIC ITEM RESPONSE THEORY MODELS IN HEALTH RELATED QUALITY OF LIFE MEASUREMENT

IVO W. MOLENAAR

University of Groningen

Compared to the measurement of other latent traits like attitudes or abilities, measurement of quality of life poses somewhat more and somewhat different methodological challenges. This paper discusses issues like unidimensionality, number of answer categories per item, information source and the choice between general and group specific questionnaires. It is argued that item response theory can make a useful contribution to quality of life measurement. The parametric Rasch model and the nonparametric Mokken model are viewed as particularly promising.

1. Introduction

The interplay of statistical and substantive aspects of a research problem is a fascinating aspect of statistical consultation. I have worked in this area for forty years, and during that period I have observed major progress in statistical models for mental measurement. This remains, however, inherently more difficult than measuring physical properties. Nobody seems to object to measuring height, body temperature, or blood pressure. The use of scale scores for quality of life, or intelligence, or neuroticism, on the other hand, frequently leads to claims that such sensitive aspects of a human being cannot be measured, or should not be measured, or at least are not fairly measured by the current questionnaires or scales. People often dislike being judged, mental properties are vaguely defined, the instruments to measure them appear arbitrary and contrived, and they exhibit large temporal variations and large measurement errors compared to rulers, thermometers and instruments for blood pressure.

Nevertheless, mental measurement has a long history. Already in 1860 Fechner studied psychophysical scales for perceptions, like loudness of noise or brightness of light. In 1902 Binet measured intelligence of children with standardized instruments, and in 1904 Spearman used a form of factor analysis to distinguish general intelligence from specific subdomains such as verbal, spatial or arithmetic. In 1929 Thurstone published a paper with the triumphant title "Attitudes can be measured!" Next, the multivariate normal calculus with its means, variances and correlations was successfully applied in what became known as Classical Test Theory, culminating in the book by Lord and Novick (1968).

The rise of item response theory (IRT) began slowly. Already in 1945 Rasch developed ideas for an intelligence test to be used by the Danish army (and still used by the Danish army). Three other important years are 1960, when Rasch published his most famous book, 1968, when Lord and Novick invited Birnbaum to add some chapters about IRT to their volume on mental measurement, and 1974, when Fischer's book in German appeared with a convincing demonstration of the superiority of IRT compared to classical

M. Mesbah et al. (eds.), Statistical Methods for Quality of Life Studies, 143–154.

test theory and convincing proofs for the main properties of the Rasch model and its extensions. The reader is referred to Wainer (1990) or Andersen and Wølk Olsen (2001) for more history and to Fischer and Molenaar (1995) or Van der Linden and Hambleton (1997) for thorough overviews of modern IRT.

Anticipating a further explanation given below, it may be stated that the core of mental measurement is the following. Each subject is confronted with a skillfully chosen selection of items (which are tasks or statements) and his/her scores per item are combined into an overall number assessing his/her position on the latent (i.e., not directly observable) trait one wants to measure. This paper deals with measurement in the sense of assigning numbers to persons according to fixed rules in order to represent a specific property (in our case health related quality of life, QoL), or a subaspect of QoL. Note that QoL measurement may also involve utility assessment or rank ordering of scenarios, but that is a different problem not discussed here.

2. Some Dilemmas in Measuring QoL

Unidimensionality of a given test or scale is almost always viewed as desirable: one wants to measure one mental property at a time, without interference from other latent traits. It cannot be taken for granted, however, that a given item set satisfies this requirement. In Molenaar (1992) one finds the example of six items measuring children's arithmetic ability, namely $2 + 2$, $18 + 23$, 8×23, $87/13$, $a + b - 3a$ and $\log(64)/\log(2)$. It is clear that these items can be ordered on the latent continuum from easy to difficult, and that a child who correctly solves x of the items ($x = 0,1,\ldots,6$) will almost always solve the x easiest ones. The socalled Guttman scalogram technique then positions this child between the x-th and the $(x + 1)$-st item and predicts that a positive answer occurs if and only if the child dominates the item, that is, the child's ability exceeds the item's difficulty. This deterministic model is the precursor of the more advanced IRT models.

Even here, however, one can argue that being able to subtract, to divide or to manipulate logarithms are *different latent traits*, and that some children might be good in division but weak in subtraction. This is even more so when one considers personality traits like rigidity or neuroticism, or political attitudes like concern for the environment or views on redistribution of wealth. It has long been recognized that HRQoL too has several aspects or facets that may jeopardize our attempts to explain responses by locating all items and persons on just one latent trait. In such cases, an investigator should strike a balance between simplicity and completeness. One can perhaps reach agreement on an item set in which the important subaspects of a concept are all well represented, and then one summary score can still be reported for each respondent. This is, for example, how a teacher makes an exam, and uses it to report student progress in a broad domain like biology or geography. If the subaspects are too different and too important, however, one may choose to report scores on each subdomain separately (like botany, zoology, ecology and theoretical biology). The drawback is that this requires a longer test, because now each subdomain should be adequately measured, and subtests consisting of only one or two items are rarely reliable and valid enough to do so.

Looking at some widely used instruments like the EORTC QLQ-C30, SF36, CaW-QLI, SIP or EuroQol 5D, it emerges that one often reports *both overall scores and subdomain scores*. As stated by Diaz *et al.* (1999), "The CaW-QLI is based upon the theory that QoL is a complex multidimensional construct. This implies that each domain can measure a distinct aspect of QoL which, at the same time, is related to the same underlying construct." (This construct being the general QoL.)

For someone familar with psychometric models in achievement testing or personality assessment, it is surprising and frightening to see that many QoL scale constructors try to measure some subdomains by *two questions or even just one*! Medical doctors, who are used to duplicate measurements in laboratory work, should be ready to appreciate that self reports on the daily life of patients, who moreover live in different circumstances, are far more unstable than chemical measures. Without the converging evidence from, say, half a dozen items referring to the same subdomain, it is hard to believe that a difference between two subdomain scores is systematic and meaningful, not just random noise. If one uses one or two specific items for a subdomain, it may be questionable whether their content adequately covers the subdomain one intends to measure. If one only poses one or two general questions like "how would you rate your overall health during the past week", the answer may contain a lot of measurement error, both over time and between respondents. It is probably more reliable to use as an overall measure the average of subdomain scores, perhaps weighted by importance (with weights supplied by the test constructor, or in one case, according to each patient separately).

Another choice to be made is the *number of answer categories* per item. IRT is most suited to handle a limited number of ordered categories, which should have clear content labels. Some QoL questionnaires use dichotomous item scoring, like yes/no or agree/disagree. This may cause respondent frustration when neither answer is felt to be an adequate description. It has often been found that it also causes respondent variation, in the sense that some respondents alsmost always choose yes whereas others only do so when they are quite convinced. Moreover, it is well established that dichotomizing items which sample an underlying continuum results in additional mesurement error. Finally, for k items scored 0,1 the only possible sumscores are $0,1,\ldots,k$. If the same k items each have $m > 2$ categories, the scale values run from 0 to $k(m-1)$ and allow a finer distinction between respondents. IRT models for dichotomous items, however, were initially more widely available, are more easy to interpret and they more often fit empirical data. Now that models and software for polytomous items have become widespread, however, this author would recommend to offer three to five answer categories. The use of even more categories often leads to respondent problems (choice becomes problematic and erratic), analysis problems (sparsely used categories may cause statistical instability) and interpretation problems (too much accuracy is suggested, just like in reporting a correlation in five decimals).

In QoL measurement, often a *written questionnaire* is given to the patient. There is no a priori reason to exclude oral interviews (face to face or by telephone). In some clinics one has seated the patient in front of a computer that presented the questions and recorded the answers. Such variants can avoid post hoc data entry from a printed questionnaire, a dull job that produces coding errors. Via immediate feedback impossible or implausible answers can be checked. Also, routing instructions (if you live by yourself skip questions 11 to 15, if you live with a partner skip question 16) lead to less errors in an automated setting. From the extensive literature on data collection methods, and on computer assisted data collection, we just quote De Leeuw and Collins (1997), De Leeuw, Hox and Snijers (1995) and Richman *et al.* (1999).

In some cases the patient is not accessible and *another person* must reply on his/her behalf, which raises the question whether that makes a difference. Diaz *et al.* (1999) have studied 183 individuals with schizophrenia or schizoaffective disorder. They report that the W-QLI is the only currently available scale that solicits information about the client from three sources: the client, a professional care provider and a family member (whenever possible). The paper does not discuss agreements or differences, unfortunately. Theunissen *et al.* (1998) presented the 56 items of the TACQoL (seven 8-item subscales) to 1,105 children aged 8 to 11 years and found Pearson correlations between child and parent reports ranging from 0.39 to 0.62, while the children reported a significantly lower HRQoL than their parents. This illustrates that it is important, even though sometimes difficult, to obtain information from the patient him/herself when at all possible.

A final dilemma is whether one should try to develop a *general instrument* or use different ones for different patient groups. For comparability it is ideal to use the same questions, across nations, across illnesses, across personal living conditions. It is regularly found, however, that such all purpose questions are rather vague, or are almost meaningless for important groups of respondents. Whether one has a job, whether one is hospitalized, if so, what services this hospital provides, if not, whether one has access to professional or informal help at home, whether one has a partner, parents, children or other individuals who give social support, whether one lives in a subculture where everyone seems to have the right to be healthy or a subculture in which suffering is viewed as part of normal life, whether one suffers all the time, periodically, or hardly, which activities one undertook before the illness and which ones remain possible, are all aspects may matter a lot. Perhaps the best solution is to strive for a kernel of common items supplemented with some group-specific ones. Thus one could report about the kernel in large scale comparative surveys, and about the more valid and more meaningful group-specific scales for comparisons within the group, or within the individual over time. It will be argued below that IRT models are particularly useful in finding a common metric for measuring persons who have partly responded to different questions.

3. What IRT Has to Offer

Whenever a questionnaire is designed, its measurement quality should be thoroughly researched, particularly if widespread use is intended,. In Molenaar (1995) it was argued that measurement quality has several important aspects, not unlike the quality of a book or the quality of a car. Here I just mention that validity, reliability, and ease of use for both researcher and respondent are among those aspects. Note that the demands may be conflicting: a short scale is easier for the respondent but less reliable than a long one. Different research groups may have different research goals and thus their best choice of a scale may also differ. Just like with books or cars, the different choices made by consumers could still benefit from critical reviews in which it is established how the products being considered perform on the most important quality aspects.

Finding out to what extent a scale or subscale meets quality desiderata usually requires a dedicated research effort, in which substantive expertise plays the first violin but it is accompanied by statistical and psychometric instruments. General statistical tools like correlations, means and variances, and tests of hypotheses about these unknown parameters, are frequently used. It is even more useful, however, to postulate a formal measurement model, estimate its model parameters, and establish whether the observed data are in agreement with the model.

Examples of such models are classical test theory and factor analysis. There is a growing appreciation, however, that item response theory forms a class of measurement models that is more adequate for the questions that arise about assessment of latent traits such as educational achievement, QoL, attitudes or personality traits. Frequently one wants to decide whether all items form a unidimensional scale, against the alternative that they form clusters or subscales (either predefined by the test constructor or found from the data; IRT has both confirmatory and exploratory procedures). Moreover, IRT can handle both dichotomous and polytomous answer formats per item, without artificially relating them to underlying continuous variables. Missing data, either by the design or by a decision of an individual respondent, can be incorporated in the models; in socalled adaptive testing respondents are presented those items that are best suited for them, and yet the final scores of different respondents can be translated to person parameters located on one and the same continuum. Quality indices can be found both per item and per subscale, both for the group of all respondents and for meaningful subgroups. It is an important issue whether all items of the scale function in the same way for such meaningful subgroups; this detection of differential item functioning tries to avoid the use of items that are biased with respect to gender or ethnicity, for example.

The main statistical advantage of IRT is that the earlier psychometric methods mainly model the total score on the test, whereas the basic building block of IRT is the positive response probability for each specific item-person combination. For simplicity, this section mainly deals with dichotomously scored items; for multicategory items, one must replace item-person by item-category-person here. Persons, items and categories have their unknown parameters which can be estimated from the data. As was announced at the end of the previous section, this feature of IRT allows to position respondents on a common scale even when they have been given partly different items, for example because they had a different disease or a different living situation.

Thus one can *explain* why certain person-item combinations have turned out positive or negative. Even more important, one can *predict* what a given person would do on other items not presented to him/her. This aspect is useful for imputation of missing observations and for the test equating problem in which one predicts someone's score on a parallel test measuring the same latent trait. One can also predict what a different person would do when confronted with the given items. Such predictions assist in assessing whether a given test would exhibit adequate score variation for a new group of testees, and if not, which items from a previously calibrated *item bank* could replace the less adequate ones. One can also collect evidence whether certain persons give rather unexpected answers to some items, and this *person fit* research helps to find persons who cheated on an examination, who gave a wrong interpretation to some questions, or who live under circumstances not envisaged by the test constructors.

For large scale operations in educational testing and personnel selection such methods are regularly and successfully used. Their application to QoL scales is at least worth considering. In Sections 4 and 5 I attempt to present the background for two IRT models that have already been used in QoL measurement. Due to space limitations combined with the advanced statistical level of this material, it is unavoidable that this attempt will not make everyone happy. Some readers with a strong statistical background will regret that I skip some elegant proofs and some important aspects. Some readers with less mathematical expertise will have to bear with a partly less accessible character of these two sections.

4. The Rasch Model

The model proposed by Georg Rasch (1960), a Danish mathematician, is not only one of the oldest but also one of the most promising and widely used IRT models. Rasch insisted that measurement should be *specifically objective*. In short this means that inferences about persons should not depend on the choice of the items, and inferences about items should not depend on the selection of the persons. We must refer to the literature for details, but it will be clear that such properties are very relevant in QoL measurement where both instruments and respondent groups can be very different, and very heterogeneous. For dichotomously scored items, one makes the following four assumptions:

(a) There exists a unidimensional latent trait θ.
(b) Scores per item are independently distributed given θ.
(c) The item response function $P(X_i = 1 \mid \theta)$ is nondecreasing in θ.
(d) The total score ΣX_i is a sufficient statistic for θ.

Then it can be proven that $P(X_i = 1)$ is a logistic function of $\theta - \delta$, where δ denotes the item parameter, after a trivial transformation of the latent trait. The transformation may be trivial but the proof is not; the reader is referred to Fischer (1995).

In the usual situation where n different subjects have responded to k different items, one typically adds statistical independence between subjects to this list of assumptions. This additional assumption implies that the researcher should avoid that one subject is influenced by the answers of another subject, a situation that is undesirable both in examinations and in measurement of attitudes and personality traits. It can be proven (Mokken, 1971; Ellis and Van den Wollenberg, 1993) that postulates (a), (b) and (c) already imply nonnegative correlations between item pairs; such correlations are even strictly positive if the item response functions are strictly increasing and there is some variation in the latent trait values. Note that the local independence under (b) means that only the latent trait level causes this global positive between item association. This rather strong postulate plays the same role as independence of residuals in regression analysis. It not only excludes learning effects during test taking, but also group influence on item response functions other than via a different distribution of latent trait values. Clearly it is also violated when more than one latent trait determines the responses, because two items tapping different subdimensions would be less correlated and two items tapping the same subdimension would be more correlated than expected in the unidimensional case. This idea has led to the clustering of items via the DETECT index, see Zhang and Stout (1999a, 1999b).

The Rasch model has attractive properties. When n subjects have responded to k items, one arranges the data in the usual rectangular array of n rows, one for each person, and k columns, one for each item. The probability of this observed data matrix under the model, is a function of the unknown person and item parameters, called the likelihood. As indicated below, this is used to estimate the parameters and to infer the plausibility of the model assumptions. Now it can be shown that under the Rasch model, unlike under any other IRT model, this likelihood has a special form that statisticians call an exponential family, with row sums as sufficient statistics for person parameters and column sums as sufficient statistics for item difficulties. This not only justifies the use of the total number correct score in inference about persons, but this also achieves the specific objectivity mentioned before (item-free person inference and person-free item inference), at least in principle. In practice, of course, the estimation of the person parameters in a test of limited length, and in particular the precision of the estimates, is strongly influenced by the choice of the items. Indeed this is exploited by considering the Fisher information matrix obtained from the second derivatives of the loglikelihood, and choosing items located close to the estimated latent trait value in order to improve precision. This is a core issue in optimal test design and adaptive testing, for which we refer to literature such as Wainer (1990), Van der Linden and Hambleton (1997) or Fischer and Molenaar (1995). It illustrates the intuitive finding that items that are far too difficult or far too easy for a respondent have a very predictable outcome and are thus rather non-informative.

The use of the Rasch models also has unattractive aspects. Parameter estimation is not as easy as it normally is in an exponential family. In the joint estimation of all n person parameters and all k item locations, the latter are inconsistently estimated for $n \to \infty$, because of the growing number of nuisance parameters (Neyman and Scott, 1948). Ad hoc correction factors have been proposed, but they are far from optimal. A common solution to the problem is to estimate the item parameters by conditional maximum likelihood (CML) in which the person parameters are eliminated from the likelihood by conditioning on their sufficient statistics, followed by simple maximum likelihood for the person parameters plugging in the item parameter estimates. This leads to considerable bias for the person parameter estimates that can be mostly eliminated by a correction procedure due to Warm (1989). Tsutakawa and Johnson (1990) have studied the effect of the plug-in operation; it is minor in the usual case of few items and many respondents. Another popular procedure integrates across the person parameters, via marginal maximum likelihood (MML) in which either a normal distribution of the latent trait is assumed (Andersen, 1980) or a set of weights and nodes is estimated (Lindsay, Clogg and Grego, 1991). For all estimation methods, constraints are needed for identifiability of all parameters, and in rare cases the estimation breaks down.

Tests for fit of the Rasch model are also somewhat problematic. The basic assumptions listed above are phrased in terms of the non-observable latent trait. Examining their observable consequences is possible in principle. One mostly uses one or two overall tests, which have low power for at least some alternatives, combined with many local tests, each powerful against a specific alternative, but so numerous that some significant results will emerge even if the Rasch model holds. Moreover, for most test statistics only the asymptotic distribution is known, and it may be misleading in the case of sparse data. In the last decade a growing number of resampling and Markov chain Monte Carlo methods have been successfully used to overcome the latter problem.

Rasch models for multicategory data assume that the conditional probability of scoring x on an item, given that one scores either $x - 1$ or x, is a logistic function of the difference between the person parameter and a location for the item category. This so-called partial credit model has been well researched, by extension of the estimation methods and fit tests mentioned above for the dichotomous model. It poses occasional problems like zero frequencies for certain categories. The main problem, however, is that the model is very restrictive. For observed dichotomous data, this author has often been able to find a fitting Rasch model. For real world polytomous data, it is rare to find a good model fit. Verhelst and Glas (1995) have extended the model to include integer valued postulated slope values that may differ across items, not across categories, and their OPLM software allows this extension as well. Rather frequently, however, one finds that such an extension does not cure the model misfit. It appears that also for real valued estimated slopes and a positive lower asymptote (the so-called 2PLM and 3PLM), the polytomous case is much harder than the dichotomous one.

5. Mokken's Nonparametric Model

Mokken (1971) has studied how far one can get with IRT given only the first three assumptions of unidimensionality, local independence and monotonicity of item response functions. He calls this the model of monotone homogeneity (MH); other names are sometimes used by later authors like Grayson (1988), Stout (1990), Ramsay (1991), Ellis and Van den Wollenberg (1993), Sijtsma (1998) or Junker (2001). Without the sufficiency postulate, one does not obtain logistic curves or an exponential family. Indeed it is both the strength and the weakness of the MH model that item response curves are not restricted to be members of the logistic, normal ogive, or any other parametric family. This makes it more widely applicable. The price to be paid is that the location of items and persons is only determined at the ordinal level, and the same holds for response probabilities per item-person combination. Grayson (1988) proves for this MH model for dichotomous items that the total score, although no longer a sufficient statistic, stochastically orders persons with respect to latent trait values, and vice versa. This means that the natural inference from higher total score to higher θ values may be wrong due to measurement error, but is correct in principle.

Mokken's second model, called double monotonicity (DM), adds to MH the requirement that any two item response functions may not intersect. This allows us to infer the order of the items, from easy to difficult, regardless of the composition of the person sample. Similarly, because two subsets of items have total scores that both stochastically order respondents, both subsets should produce at least in principle the same ordering of persons. Here, however, the measurement errors will be larger because one tends to have far more persons than items. Be this as it may, the DM model can be viewed as satisfying an ordinal version of the specific objectivity promoted by Rasch.

Both MH and DM models have been extended to polytomous items, using the graded response modeling in which it is assumed that $P(X_i \geq x \mid \theta)$ is nondecreasing in θ for each item i and each category score x (and also nonintersecting, for DM). As is discussed by Hemker *et al.* (1996, 1997) and Sijtsma and Van der Ark (2001), the polytomous case may show occasional exceptions to the stochastic ordering of the latent trait by the total score. It is perhaps more important that they show that the partial credit Rasch model is the only polytomous model without such exceptions. The nonparametric graded response model discussed in this section can be shown to contain most other parametric and nonparametric IRT models for polytomous items as special cases. Thus it is the easiest model to fit, and will often fit where the polytomous Rasch model fails.

The software package MSP 5.0 for Windows incorporates both MH and DM Mokken models for both dichotomous and polytomous items (up to 9 answer categories). Its manual (Molenaar and Sijtsma, 2000) summarizes the theory, shows how to use the software, and includes a discussion of various diagnostics designed to test monotonicity, non-intersection and the absence of group differences. The latter feature is successfully used in an analysis of the EORTC QLQ-C30 in which seven groups of Norwegian cancer patients are compared (Ringdal *et al.*, 1999).

It was argued in Section 2 that during scale construction or scale validation it is important to find out whether all items can be viewed as measuring the same unidimensional latent trait, versus the alternative that there are subsets of items measuring different subdimensions. Within the framework of the Rasch model, such issues can be studied via the R2 test or in a confirmatory sense by the Martin Löf test, see, for example, Glas and Verhelst (1995). In nonparametric IRT, on the other hand, two easy clustering procedures are available. MSP offers the search and search extended options for bottom up clustering as described by Mokken (1971) or Molenaar and Sijtsma (2000). DETECT, described by Zhang and Stout (1999a, 1999b), is a stand-alone DOS program that uses a genetic algorithm to find the optimal partition of a given item pool into one or more unidimensional clusters. Both allow the user some flexibility in how strictly unidimensional each cluster should be. MSP uses estimates of interitem covariance divided by maximal possible covariance given the marginals, the socalled Loevinger (1948) H coefficient. DETECT uses skillful combinations of estimated conditional covariances given total testscore or restscore excluding the two items currently considered. Both algorithms tend to produce rather similar solutions for many realistic datasets. It will be interesting to use them for the study of the dimensionality structure of some well known QoL intruments, both in a confirmatory and in an exploratory setting.

6. Concluding Remarks

The measurement of health related quality of life has become a regular component of many clinical trials and epidemiological studies. It also attracts attention of organisations involved in health related policy making and policy evaluation. Therefore it is of increasing importance to measure QoL as well as one can. It has been argued in this paper that existing psychometric methods, and in particular item response theory, can offer valuable assistance in the construction and improvement of QoL instruments. In Section 4, information was given about the Rasch model. This is an example of a parametric model, in which the probability of a positive answer for all items can be found by the same algebraic formula (in this case the logistic curve), which differs only in some simple constants, the item parameters. Section 5 has presented the less demanding nonparametric Mokken model, in which the probability of a positive answer can vary freely as long as it satisfies some order constraints. Both models can also be used for items with more than two ordered categories, which are often used in QoL research. It can be recommended to use the more elegant and more informative Rasch model when it fits the data. Otherwise, the Mokken model hopefully does, and then at least at the ordinal level many nice properties of item response theory still hold. Two caveats, however, should be added to our plea in favor of IRT.

In the first place, not all tools, models and methods that were found to be useful in measuring latent traits like intelligence, academic achievement, personality traits or attitudes, can be blindly transferred to the domain of QoL measurement. It requires a dialogue between an interested group of psychometricians and statisticians on one side, and an interested group of substantive experts in the medical and psychosocial domain on the other side, to find out what one would like to achieve and what knowledge from psychometrics can do to achieve this. When I wrote "valuable assistance" in the preceding paragraph that was no coincidence. We need to study what is similar and what is different when we pass from standard psychometrics to QoL research. On the other hand, IRT models have already proven their usefulness in a large range of disciplines in which rather different latent traits are measured, and there is no reason to believe that

QoL would be the exception where IRT has nothing to say. On the contrary, the literature of the past decade shows that the dialogue has already begun.

Secondly, this paper has focused on what IRT can do in order to learn from the answers of a sample of persons to a given set of items. This entails the risk of creating the false impression that the process of *creating* such a set of items is less important, or even trivial. For some strange reason the general public, and even some researchers, are willing to believe that much technical knowledge is required to construct an instrument to analyze an MRI scan or even an instrument to measure blood pressure, whereas it appears so be easy to write a couple of statements adequately describing QoL aspects. That is a dangerous illusion, which has already led to many disappointing research outcomes. The use of an inadequate questionnaire is not unlike visual perception using somebody else's dirty eyeglasses instead of one's own clean ones: you see far less than under more favorable circumstances. Unreliable and invalid measurements can hardly be expected to produce reliable and valid research conclusions. This paper was not the appropriate place to detail the many steps that should be taken before a set of items can be used on a large sample of respondents. That aspect of social science methodology should be studied as well as the formal psychometric aspects that were discussed above. Let me just mention that I have read with much pleasure two papers in which these more substantive aspects of QoL measurements have been discussed in some depth: Fayers *et al.* (1997) and Hawthorne, Richardson and Osborne (1999).

REFERENCES

Andersen, E.B. (1980). Comparing latent distributions. *Psychometrika* **45**, 121–134.

Andersen, E.B. and Wølk Olsen, L.(2001). The life of Georg Rasch as a mathematician and as a statistician. In: A. Boomsma, M.A.J. van Duijn, and T.A.B. Snijders (eds.), *Essays on Item Response Theory*. New York: Springer-Verlag.

De Leeuw, E.D and Collins, M. (1997). Data collection methods and survey quality: an overview. In: Lyberg, L., Biemer, P., Collins, M., de Leeuw, E., Dippo, C., Schwartz, N. and Trewin, D. (eds.), *Survey Measurement and Process Quality*. New York: Wiley.

De Leeuw, E.D., Hox, J.J. and Snijers, G. (1995). The effect of computer assisted interviewing on data quality: a review. *Journal of Market Research Society* **37**, 325–344.

Diaz, P., Mercier, C., Hachey, R., Caron, J. and Boyer, G. (1999). An evaluation of psychometric properties of the client's questionnaire of the Wisconsin Quality of Life Index–Canadian Version (CaW-QLI). *Quality of Life Research* **8**, 509–514.

Ellis, J.L. and Van den Wollenberg, A.L. (1993). Local homogeneity in latent trait models. A characterization of the homogeneous monotone IRT model. *Psychometrika* ***58***, 417–429.

Fayers, P.M., Hand, D.J., Bjordal, K. and Groenvold, M. (1997). Causal indicators in quality of life research. *Quality of Life Research* **6**, 393–406.

Fischer, G.H. and Molenaar, I.W., eds. (1995). *Rasch Models: Foundations, Recent Developments, and Applications*. New York: Springer-Verlag.

Fischer, G.H. (1995). Derivations of the Rasch model. In: Fischer, G.H. and Molenaar, I.W. (eds.), *Rasch Models: Foundations, Recent Developments, and Applications*. New York: Springer-Verlag.

Glas, C.A.W. and Verhelst, N.D. (1995). Testing the Rasch model. In: Fischer, G.H. and Molenaar, I.W. (eds.), *Rasch Models: Foundations, Recent Developments, and Applications*. New York: Springer-Verlag.

Grayson, D.A. (1988). Two-group classification in latent trait theory: scores with monotone likelihood ratio. *Psychometrika* **53**, 383–392.

Hawthorne, G., Richardson, J. and Osborne, R. (1999). The Assessment of Quality of Life (AQoL) instrument: a psychometric measure of health-related quality of life. *Quality of Life Research,* **8**, 209–224.

Hemker, B.T., Sijtsma K., Molenaar, I.W. and Junker, B.W. (1996). Polytomous IRT models and monotone likelihood ratio of the total score. *Psychometrika* **61**, 679–693.

Hemker, B.T., Sijtsma K., Molenaar, I.W. and Junker, B.W. (1997). Stochastic ordering using the latent trait and the sum score in polytomous IRT models. *Psychometrika* **62**, 331–347.

Junker, B.W. (2001). On the interplay between nonparametric and parametric IRT, with some thoughts about the future. In: Boomsma, A., van Duijn, M.A.J. and Snijders, T.A.B. (eds.), *Essays on Item Response Theory*. New York: Springer-Verlag.

Lindsay, B.G., Clogg, C.C. and Grego, J. (1991). Semiparametric estimation in the Rasch model and related exponential response models, including a simple latent class model for item analysis. *Journal of the American Statistical Association* **86**, 96–107.

Loevinger, J. (1948). The technique of homogeneous tests compared with some aspects of "scale analysis" and factor analysis. *Psychological Bulletin* **45**, 507–530.

Lord, F.M. and Novick, M.R. (1968). *Statistical Theories of Mental Test Scores*. Reading MA: Addison-Wesley.

Mokken, R.J. (1971). *A Theory and Procedure of Scale Analysis: With Applications in Political Research*. The Hague: Mouton, Berlin: De Gruyter.

Molenaar, I.W. (1992). Statistical Models for Educational Testing and Attitude Measurement. In: van der Heijden, P.G.M., Jansen, W. Francis, B. And Seeber, G.U.H. (eds.), *Statistical Modeling*. Amsterdam: Elsevier Science Publishers.

Molenaar, I.W. (1995). Some background for item response theory and the Rasch model. In: Fischer, G.H. and Molenaar, I.W. (eds.), *Rasch Models: Foundations, Recent Developments, and Applications*. New York: Springer-Verlag.

Molenaar, I.W. and Sijtsma, K. (2000). *User's manual MSP5 for Windows: A Program for Mokken Scale Analysis for Polytomous Items*. Version 5.0 [Software manual]. Groningen: ProGAMMA.

Neyman, J. and Scott, E.L. (1948). Consistent estimates based on partially consistent observations. *Econometrica* **16**, 1–32.

Ramsay, J.O. (1991). Kernel smoothing approaches to nonparametric item characteristic curve estimation. *Psychometrika* **56**, 611–630.

Rasch, G. (1960). *Probabilistic Models for Some Intelligence and Attainment Tests*. Copenhagen: The Danish Institute of Educational Research. [Expanded edition, 1980, Chicago: The University of Chicago Press].

Richman, W.L., Kiesler, S. Weisband, S. and Drasgow, F. (1999). A meta-analytic study of social desirability distortion in computer administered questionnaires, traditional questionnaires and interviews. *Journal of Applied Psychology* **84**, 754–775.

Ringdal, K., Ringdal, G.I., Kaasa, S., Bjordal, K., Wisløff, F., Sundstrøm, S. and Hjermstad, M.J. (1999). Assessing the consistency of psychometric properties of the HRQoL scales within the EORTC QLQ-C30 across populations by means of the Mokken scaling model. *Quality of Life Research* **8**, 25–43.

Sijtsma, K. (1998). Methodology review: nonparametric IRT approaches to the analysis of dichotomous item scores. *Applied Psychological Measurement* **22**, 3–32.

Sijtsma, K., and Van der Ark, L.A. (2001). Progress in NIRT analysis of polytomous item scores: dilemmas and practical solutions. In Boomsma, A., van Duijn, M.A.J. and Snijders, T.A.B. (eds.), *Essays on Item Response Theory* (pp. 297–318). New York: Springer-Verlag.

Stout, W.F. (1990). A new item response theory modeling approach with applications to unidimensionality assessment and ability estimation. *Psychometrika* **55**, 293–325.

Theunissen, N.C.M., Vogels, T.G.C., Koopman, H.M., Verrips, G.H.W., Zwinderman, K.A.H., Verloove-Vanhorick, S.P. and Wit, J.M. (1998). The proxy problem: child report versus parent report in health-related quality of life research. *Quality of Life Research* **7**, 387–397.

Tsutakawa, R.K. and Johnson, J.C. (1990). The effect of uncertainty of item parameter estimation on ability estimates. *Psychometrika* **55**, 371–390.

Van der Linden, W.J. and Hambleton, R.K., eds. (1997). *Handbook of Modern Item Response Theory*. New York: Springer Verlag.

Verhelst, N.D. and Glas, C.A.W. (1995). The one parameter logistic model. In: Fischer, G.H. and Molenaar, I.W. (eds.), *Rasch Models: Foundations, Recent Developments, and Applications*. New York: Springer-Verlag.

Wainer, H. (1990). *Computerized Adaptive Testing. A Primer*. Hillsdale NJ: Erlbaum.

Warm, T.A. (1989). Weighted likelihood estimation of ability in item response models. *Psychometrika* **54**, 427–450.

Zhang, J. and Stout, W.F. (1999a). Conditional covariance structure of generalized compensatory multidimensional items. *Psychometrika* **64**, 129–152.

Zhang, J., and Stout, W.F. (1999b). The theoretical DETECT index of dimensionality and its application to approximate simple structure. *Psychometrika* **64**, 213–249.

QUESTIONNAIRE RELIABILITY UNDER THE RASCH MODEL

AGNES HAMON AND MOUNIR MESBAH

Laboratory SABRES, University of South-Brittany

Quality of life studies must be concerned with the accuracy, or reliability (as it is usually called in psychometrics) of measurement. A reliability coefficient gives an evaluation of a questionnaire's ability to yield interpretable statements about the construct being measured. There are two classes of models for analyzing unidimensional scales: classical models and Item Response Theory (IRT) models. Classical models are based on a linear decomposition of the score, and reliability is estimated using Cronbach's alpha coefficient. IRT models focus on the relationship between the probability of a correct answer and a latent variable. The Rasch model is a special IRT model which having good measurement properties. In the context of the Rasch model, or IRT models in general, no reliability coefficient similar to Cronbach Alpha is clearly defined. Some authors have studied the Fisher information of the latent parameter, which provides a measure of accuracy of the estimator. In this chapter, we present how reliability is estimated for classical models, and we propose a reliability coefficient for the Rasch model. Simulated data and data derived from the communication subscale of the Sickness Impact Profile are used to illustrate the methods.

1. Introduction

The statistical validation of health-related quality-of-life (HRQoL) questionnaires involves techniques commonly used in a variety of fields. In educational science, specific questionnaires can be used to evaluate the impact of new teaching methodologies. In the social and behavioral sciences, interest may focus on diverse subjects such as political attitudes or consumer behavior. In medicine, psychiatric questionnaires are commonly used to measure depression. Recently, HRQoL scales have been developed and used in a range of contexts. These include comparing therapies in clinical trials, measuring health status in epidemiological studies, or comparing interventions in health policy studies.

Measurement of a variable requires an instrument. HRQoL is generally assessed by self-administered questionnaires consisting of a number of items (questions). Responses to these items are generally dichotomous (e.g., "yes" or "no", "agree" or "disagree") or ordinal (e.g., "not at all", "a little", "quite a bit" or "very much"). A HRQoL instrument must produce scalar scores (numbers) for each item (item measure). Items measuring the same underlying trait are grouped to produce a sub-dimensional score (subscale). Item scores and subscale scores constitute the measurements of the instrument. The purpose of this chapter is to focus on evaluating instrument reliability under the Rasch model. Reliability is a measurement

M. Mesbah et al. (eds.), Statistical Methods for Quality of Life Studies, 155–168.

property generally related to the classical psychometric theory. The Rasch model is the core of modern psychometric theory. We will consider only dichotomous items and unidimensional scales. The purpose of reliability evaluation is to identify poorly-performing items in a questionnaire.

Many standard HRQoL instruments are currently available. One of the most well-known is the Sickness Impact Profile (SIP). The SIP comprises 136 items distributed into 12 dimensions (Bergner *et al.*, 1976). The items of the SIP communication dimension appear in the Appendix.

The main goal of this work is to present a new reliability coefficient, similar to Cronbach's alpha, computed under Rasch model assumptions. In the next section, we briefly recall the principles of classical theory. We also explain how reliability is defined, estimated and used in practice. In Section 3, we focus on the Rasch model, beginning with a brief presentation of its assumptions and statistical properties. We then propose a new coefficient to estimate the reliability of the total score. We also present two other points of view: the Fisher information and the reliability of the estimates $\hat{\theta}$. In Section 4, simulations are presented to illustrate the new reliability coefficient in various situations and compare it with Cronbach's alpha. Using actual HRQoL data, we demonstrate satisfactory goodness of fit for the Rasch model and the reliability coefficient. Finally, we discuss other possibilities for estimating the reliability of a questionnaire and future work to better understand the properties of the new coefficient.

2. Classical Psychometric Theory

Let X_{ij} be the observed score (response) of a person i on item (question) j. Classical theory supposes that X_{ij} can be written

$$X_{ij} = \tau_{ij} + \epsilon_{ij},$$

where τ_{ij}, the "true score," and ϵ_{ij}, the "error score," are two unknown random variables generally assumed to be independent (or at least non-correlated).

2.1 The Parallel Model

The most popular classical model is a mixed one way model:

$$\tau_{ij} = \mu + a_i,$$

with the following five assumptions.

1. μ is a constant fixed effect.
2. a_i is a random effect with zero mean and standard error σ_a corresponding to the between-person variability (it produces the variance of the true item measure).
3. ϵ_{ij} is a random effect with zero mean and standard error σ_e corresponding to the additional measurement error.

4. The true item measure and the error are uncorrelated (i.e., $\operatorname{cov}(a_i, \epsilon_{ij}) = 0$).
5. For all $j = 1, \ldots, k$ and for $r \neq s$, (a_r, ϵ_{rj}) and (a_s, ϵ_{sj}) are independent.

These assumptions are typical in experimental design. This model defines relationships between different types of variables: the observed score X_{ij}, the true score τ_{ij} and the error ϵ_{ij}. We make the following remarks about these assumptions:

1. Each ϵ_{ij} is the measurement error for item j.
2. The "true" measure for person i, $\tau_i = \mu + a_i$, is independent of item j.
3. The measurement errors, ϵ_{ij}, are uncorrelated with the true measure τ_i.
4. X_{ij} is observed while τ_i is not.
5. It is easy to show that $E(X_{ij}) = \mu$, $\operatorname{var}(X_{ij}) = \sigma_a^2 + \sigma_e^2$, and $\operatorname{cov}(X_{ij}, X_{ij'}) = \sigma_a^2$

This model clearly applies to repeated biological measures, when the same measure is repeated steps with no systematic change (i.e., μ is a constant). In the case of HRQoL, we assume that all items measure the same quantity but at a different level or difficulty. Thus, a more realistic model for HRQoL is the parallel model, with the true score given by

$$\tau_{ij} = \mu_j + a_i.$$

This model allows the same covariance structure for the data but uses a slightly different mean structure. When $\mu_j = \mu$, it is called the strict parallel model.

2.2 Reliability of an Instrument

The classical test theory has a long history and the appropriate reliability coefficient depends on whether parallel forms are used or the test-retest approach is used (see Lord and Novick, 1968). In HRQoL studies, the most commonly used reliability measure is Cronbach's alpha (1951). This coefficient has many interpretations (see Cortina, 1998). In this section we focus on how it is deduced from the parallel model.

The reliability ρ of the instrument is defined as the ratio of two variances: the variance of the true (unobserved) measure and the variance of the observed measure. Under the parallel model (or the strictly parallel model), it can be shown that

$$\rho = \frac{\sigma_a^2}{\sigma_a^2 + \sigma_e^2}.$$

This quantity is also the constant correlation between any two items and is called the intra-class coefficient.

The reliability coefficient ρ can be interpreted as the correlation between the true measure and the observed measure. The k straight regression lines (X_{ij}, τ_{ij}), corresponding to the items $(j = 1, \ldots, k)$ are parallel and

$$\operatorname{corr}(X_{ij}, \tau_{ij}) = \rho^{1/2}.$$

Under the parallel model, the reliability of the sum of the k items is

$$\tilde{\rho} = \frac{k\rho}{(k-1)\rho + 1}.$$

This is known as the Spearman-Brown formula. Under the parallel model, the reliability tends to 1 as the number of items increases. Cronbach's alpha (α) is the maximum likelihood estimate of $\tilde{\rho}$ assuming normally-distributed error terms for the parallel model (Kristof, 1963). It is given by

$$\alpha = \frac{k}{k-1}\left[1 - \frac{\sum_{j=1}^{k} S_j^2}{S_{tot}^2}\right],$$

where

$$\begin{aligned} S_j^2 &= \frac{1}{n-1}\sum_{i=1}^{n}(x_{ij} - \bar{x}_j)^2 \\ S_{tot}^2 &= \frac{1}{nk-1}\sum_{i=1}^{n}\sum_{j=1}^{k}(x_{ij} - \bar{x})^2. \end{aligned}$$

A direct connection exists between α and the percent of variance of the first component in a principal components analysis (Moret *et al.*, 1993). There is a monotone relationship between $\tilde{\rho}$, which is estimated by α, and the first latent root λ_1, which is estimated by the corresponding value of the observed correlation matrix (and thus gives the percent of variance of the first principal component). As a result, α is often considered as a measure of unidimensionality.

Cronbach's alpha, α, can be used to find the most reliable subset of items (Curt *et al.*, 1997). The first step in this process is to use all items to compute α. In each subsequent step, one item is removed from the scale. The removed item is chosen so as to maximize the α for the remaining items. If we remove a poor item, the α coefficient will increase. If we remove a good item, the α coefficient must decrease. More precisely, under the parallel model, the Spearman-Brown formula shows that increasing the number of items increases the reliability of the total score, which is estimated by α. Thus, a decrease in the estimated curve following the addition of an item could lead us to suspect that the given item is a poor one (in term of goodness of fit of the model). If an instrument is already validated, the curve should increase when the number of items increases.

A supplementary way to assess the influence of an item on the goodness of fit of the parallel model is to examine the empirical correlation between the item and the number correct score (also known as the item-test correlation). Assuming the parallel model, these correlations must be high and equal to one another. A low correlation, differing from the remaining correlations, indicates a poor item. The major statistical software programs include routines for computing these statistics. Only a few specific software programs provide additional goodness of fit assessment.

3. Item Response Theory and the Rasch Model

Classical models handle quantitative item responses well, and they perform even better when responses are normally distributed. In practice, however, responses are rarely normally distributed. Modern psychometric theory takes into account the qualitative (dichotomous or polychotomous) nature of the item response. Instead of modeling the item score directly as in the classical theory, IRT relies on modeling the item response function (or characteristic curve; i.e., the probability of "taking a positive value" conditionally on the actual value of the latent trait). More precisely, classical methods are (generally mixed) linear models when modern methods are (often mixed) generalized linear models.

Let us consider a set of n people having answered a test of k dichotomous items. Let X_{ij} be the answer for subject i to item j, and let θ_i be the unobserved latent variable. The three assumptions, common to all unidimensional IRT models, are:

1. The latent variable θ_i is unidimensional (i.e., a scalar).
2. The variables X_{ij} are independent conditionally on θ_i. This property is called "local independence".
3. $P(X_{ij} = 1|\theta_i) = f(\theta_i, \gamma_j)$ where $\gamma_j \in \mathbb{R}^p$ is a vector of unknown item parameters and f is a monotone increasing function in θ (in most cases the logistic or probit link function).

A response of "1" corresponds to a high level of HRQoL, and a response of "0" corresponds to a low level of HRQoL. When θ_i is very large (towards $+\infty$), and thus when one considers an individual with a very good HRQoL level, the probability of answering 1 is very close to 1.

The local independence property is useful for deriving the likelihood. It links IRT models to the class of graphical models (Kreiner and Christensen, 2001). The marginal distribution of θ is often assumed to be Gaussian. The developer of a HRQoL instrument generally wishes to produce normally-distributed scores (obtained by estimation of the latent trait), thus the conditional Gaussian model (Lauritzen and Wermuth, 1988) could be efficiently used.

3.1 The Rasch Model

The Rasch model was first developed by the Danish mathematician Rasch (1960). It is also sometimes called the one parameter logistic model because of its formulation

$$\text{logit}\left(P\left(X_{ij} = 1|\theta_i\right)\right) = \theta_i - \beta_j \quad \text{or equivalently,} \quad P\left(X_{ij} = 1|\theta_i\right) = \frac{e^{\theta_i - \beta_j}}{1 + e^{\theta_i - \beta_j}},$$

where β_j is a scalar. The probability, when viewed as a function of θ, is called the item characteristic curve. It is $1/2$ when $\theta_i = \beta_j$, and it is decreasing for fixed θ_i. So a large values of β_j corresponds to a low probability of a correct response. The parameter β_j is thus called the item difficulty parameter. The central portions of these curves are nearly straight lines. Another interesting property is that the different curves corresponding to different items are parallel. In this sense, the Rasch model is also a parallel model.

The Rasch model distinguishes itself from the other IRT models by the following property: an individual's total score (i.e., the number of correct answers) is a sufficient statistic for the ability parameter. This is a characteristic property for the Rasch model, and it is the only IRT model with this property. Hence, when we use the total score as the measure produced by the instrument, and when responses are dichotomous, we must assume that the Rasch model is true.

Another interesting measurement property of the Rasch model is its specific objectivity. This property states that the comparison of any two persons v and w does not involve the instrument parameter. Again, this is true only for the Rasch model and not for any other link function (Fischer, 1995).

Three methods of estimation are commonly used: joint (or unconditional) maximum likelihood (JML), conditional maximum likelihood (CML), and marginal maximum likelihood (MML).

JML is the classical maximum likelihood method with θ_i and β_j considered as unknown fixed parameters. Using the local independence assumption and assuming independence between individuals, we can write the likelihood

$$L\left(x^1,\ldots,x^n;\theta_1,\ldots,\theta_n,\beta_1,\ldots,\beta_k\right)=\prod_{i=1}^{n}\prod_{j=1}^{k}\frac{\exp\left[x_{ij}\left(\theta_i-\beta_j\right)\right]}{1+\exp\left(\theta_i-\beta_j\right)},$$

where $x^i=(x_{i1},\ldots,x_{ik})$ is the response vector for person i. Letting $S_i=\sum_{j=1}^{k}x_{ij}$ and $T_j=\sum_{i=1}^{n}x_{ij}$, the log-likelihood can be written

$$\log L=\sum_{i=1}^{n}S_i\theta_i-\sum_{j=1}^{k}T_j\beta_j-\sum_{i,j}\log\left(1+e^{\theta_i-\beta_j}\right).$$

Taking derivatives with respect to θ_i and β_j, we find the following equations

$$\begin{cases} S_i=\sum_{j=1}^{k}\frac{e^{\theta_i-\beta_j}}{1+e^{\theta_i-\beta_j}} \\ T_j=\sum_{i=1}^{n}\frac{e^{\theta_i-\beta_j}}{1+e^{\theta_i-\beta_j}} \end{cases}$$

Unfortunately the estimates of θ_i and β_j thus obtained are asymptotically biased and inconsistent (Haberman, 1977) when $n\to\infty$ and k remains moderate.

The second method, CML, consists of maximizing the conditional likelihood given the sufficient statistics for the ability parameters. Under mild conditions, this method gives consistent and asymptotically normally distributed estimators of the item parameters (Andersen, 1970). Fischer (1981) derived a set of necessary and sufficient conditions for existence and uniqueness of the CML estimates.

The last method, MML, is directly related to the interpretation of the Rasch model as a mixed model with θ as a random effect with a distribution g having an unknown parameter ϕ. The likelihood is then

$$L\left(x^1,\ldots,x^n;\phi,\beta_1,\ldots,\beta_k\right)=\int\prod_{j=1}^{k}P\left(X_{ij}=x_{ij}|\theta_i,\beta_j\right)\times g\left(\theta_i,\phi\right)\,d\theta_i.$$

The problem with this method is that the integral is intractable, and maximum likelihood solutions are not straightforward. An EM algorithm may be used (Thissen, 1982). Considering θ as a missing variable, the complete likelihood is

$$l_c(x, \theta, \beta, \phi) = \prod_{i=1}^{n} \left\{ \prod_{j=1}^{k} \frac{\exp\left[x_{ij}(\theta_i - \beta_j)\right]}{1 + \exp(\theta_i - \beta_j)} \times g(\theta_i, \phi) \right\}.$$

The EM algorithm consists of two steps. Having current estimates $\left(\beta^{(p)}, \phi^{(p)}\right)$, the steps are:

E-Step: Compute the mean of the complete log-likelihood with respect to the distribution of the unobserved θ conditionally to the observations.

$$\begin{aligned} Q_p &= \mathrm{E}\left(\log l_c(x, \theta, \beta, \phi) \middle| x, \beta^{(p)}, \phi^{(p)}\right) \\ &= \int \log l_c(x, \theta, \beta, \phi) f\left(\theta \middle| x, \beta^{(p)}, \phi^{(p)}\right) \, d\theta \\ &= \sum_{i=1}^{n} \left\{ \int \log\left(g(\theta_i, \phi)\right) f^{(p)} + \sum_{j=1}^{k} \int \log\left(p\left(x_{ij} \left| \theta_i, \beta_j\right.\right)\right) f^{(p)} \, d\theta_i \right\} \end{aligned}$$

with $f^{(p)} = f\left(\theta_i \left| x_i, \beta^{(p)}, \phi^{(p)}\right.\right)$

M-Step: Update estimations by computing the point $\left(\beta^{(p+1)}, \phi^{(p+1)}\right)$ that maximizes Q_p

The E-step is difficult because there is no explicit form of the integral. A possible solution is to use Gauss-Hermite quadrature, to obtain a numerical approximation. Another solution is to implement a stochastic EM algorithm (Hamon and Iovleff, 2001). In this case, the E-step is replaced by a simulation step to impute the missing values of θ. One then performs an EM-step maximizing the complete log-likelihood.

3.2 Assessment of Reliability

In the previous section, we defined the reliability as a ratio of variances: the variance of the true score to the variance of the observed score. This can be done easily under a classical linear model, but it is not straight forward under a generalized linear model like the Rasch model. In current HRQoL research, the Rasch model is commonly used, and reliability is almost always evaluated using the alpha coefficient. In fact, assuming the mixed Rasch model, it is possible to define the true and observed scores as in classical theory. Then in the same manner, we can derive the reliability coefficient as the ratio of the variances of these two scores. More precisely, if we define the true score $T(\theta_i)$ as the conditional expected score for an individual with latent trait θ_i,

$$T(\theta_i) = \sum_{j=1}^{k} P(X_{ij} = 1 | \theta_i).$$

Then we have

$$\operatorname{var}(T(\theta_i)) = \int T(\theta_i)^2 g(\theta_i|\phi)\, d\theta_i - \left[\int T(\theta_i)\, g(\theta_i|\phi)\, d\theta_i\right]^2.$$

Using the general formula

$$\operatorname{var}(X) = \operatorname{var}(\mathrm{E}(X|Y) + \mathrm{E}(\operatorname{var}(X|Y)),$$

we have

$$\begin{aligned}\operatorname{var}\left(\sum X_{ij}\right) &= \operatorname{var}(T(\theta_i)) + \mathrm{E}(\operatorname{var}(T(\theta_i)|\theta_i))\\ &= \int T(\theta_i)^2 g(\theta_i|\phi)\, d\theta_i + \sum_{j=1}^{k} \int P(X_{ij} = 1|\theta_i)\,[1 - P(X_{ij} = 1|\theta_i)]\, g(\theta_i|\phi)\, d\theta_i,\end{aligned}$$

where ϕ could be any scalar or vector parameter. $g(\theta_i|\phi)$ is often specified as $N(\theta_i, \sigma^2)$, the normal distribution with variance σ^2.

As previously, we define the reliability of the total score $S_i = \sum_j X_{ij}$ by

$$\rho_S = \frac{\operatorname{var}(\mathrm{E}(S|\theta))}{\operatorname{var}(S)}.$$

We denote its estimate under the Rasch model by α_R. To compute this reliability, we must evaluate the following:

$$\sigma_T^2 = \operatorname{var}(T_i) = \int \left(\sum_{j=1}^{k} \frac{e^{\theta_i - \beta_j}}{1 + e^{\theta_i - \beta_j}}\right)^2 g(\theta_i|\phi) d\theta_i - \left[\int \sum_{j=1}^{k} \frac{e^{\theta_i - \beta_j}}{1 + e^{\theta_i - \beta_j}} g(\theta_i|\phi) d\theta_i\right]^2$$

For this purpose, Gauss-Hermite quadrature is very helpful.

In the IRT literature, no such reliability coefficient is clearly defined with links to the classical theory. The most common approach is to study the Fisher information for θ. Assume the item parameters are known. Individual measures of the latent trait can be obtained using the maximum likelihood estimator $\hat{\theta}_i$. A useful asymptotic result (Klauer, 1990) shows that if the sequence (β_j) is bounded, then when $k \to +\infty$, we have the following convergence in law:

$$\sqrt{I(\hat{\theta}_i(k), k)}\left(\hat{\theta}_i(k) - \theta_i\right) \longrightarrow N(0, 1).$$

Then, the Fisher information gives the precision of the measure of the latent trait θ_i. Under the Rasch model, the Fisher information is

$$I(\theta, k) = \sum_{j=1}^{k} \frac{\exp(\theta - \beta_j)}{(1 + \exp(\theta - \beta_j))^2}$$

If item difficulties are known (or previously estimated), the information function can be used to reduce the number of items without loosing precision. We note that the information is largest when the difficulty is equal to the latent value θ. So, if we choose items that can be adapted to the latent trait of every person, we would have the best questionnaire (in terms of the Fisher information). In educational sciences, this idea leads to the theory of adaptive testing (Lord ,1980), and more recently, computerized adaptive testing (CAT, Wainer, 1990). Adaptive testing requires a large set of items whose difficulty parameters are known. In the case of HRQoL, this situation is not yet met. The approach presented in this chapter is different because we want to estimate the reliability of a questionnaire when it is administered to one population. So here, we do not focus on individual precision (or local reliability) but on global precision (or global reliability).

Lord (1983) proposed to consider the difference between the true value of the latent parameter and its maximum likelihood estimate as the error of measurement. As in the classical theory, Lord defined this reliability coefficient as

$$\rho_L = 1 - \frac{\frac{1}{n}\sum_{i=1}^{n} \mathrm{E}\left[(\hat{\theta}_i - \theta_i)^2\right] - \mathrm{E}\left(\hat{\theta}_i - \theta_i\right)^2}{s^2_{\hat{\theta}}},$$

with $s^2_{\hat{\theta}} = s^2(\hat{\theta}_i) = \frac{1}{n-1}\sum_{i=1}^{n}\left(\hat{\theta}_i - \overline{\hat{\theta}}\right)^2$. The line above $\hat{\theta}$ denotes the average of all $\hat{\theta}_i$. We note that the numerator is the variance of the error, and the denominator is the observed variance. Using asymptotic convergence of the maximum likelihood estimators when $k \to \infty$, and assuming that all β_j are known, Lord proved that the previous coefficient can be approximated by

$$\rho_L = 1 - \frac{\frac{1}{n}\sum_{i=1}^{n} \frac{1}{I(\theta,k)}}{s^2_{\hat{\theta}}} + o(k^{-1}).$$

We estimate the reliability coefficient by replacing the latent parameters by their maximum likelihood estimates. We note that this coefficient is also related to the Fisher information. The main difference with the information function approach is that the Lord coefficient gives just one number and not a function. A similar coefficient based on the Fisher information was also proposed by Fischer and Molenaar (1995).

If the number of items is small, the approximation is not valid, and the coefficient ρ_L can be negative. The main drawback of the Lord coefficient is that it evaluates the reliability of the maximum likelihood estimate of θ and not of the total score, which is generally used by HRQoL researchers. Moreover, the use of this coefficient, and the Fisher information, require knowledge of the values of the difficulty parameters. This is seldom the case in HRQoL research.

4. Illustrations

4.1 Simulations

We performed simulations to compare Cronbach's coefficient and the Rasch coefficient. We used 3 sets of items, given in Table 1. For the first test, the difficulty parameters are uniformly distributed in the interval $(-2, 2)$. For the second test, the last item is very difficult (i.e., $\beta_9 = 4$) and the first one is very easy ($\beta_1 = -4$). For the third test, all of the difficulties of the first test are incremented by $+1$. These distributions are chosen because they represent various situations that can occur in practice. For each test we performed 200 simulations with $n = 100$ individuals. We used the Rasch model assumption to simulate the answers. The latent distribution is Gaussian with mean 0 and standard deviations of 0.5, 1 and 1.5.

Table 1. Difficulty parameters used in the simulations

	Difficulty Parameters								
	β_1	β_2	β_3	β_4	β_5	β_6	β_7	β_8	β_9
Test 1	–2	–1.5	–1	–0.5	0	0.5	1	1.5	2
Test 2	–4	–1.5	–1	–0.5	0	0.5	1	1.5	4
Test 3	–1	–0.5	0	0.5	1	1.5	2	2.5	3

Table 2 shows the mean reliability estimates of Cronbach's α and the approximated true Rasch reliability coefficient, α_R. For this approximation, we used the true values of β and σ and computed α_R using Gauss-Hermite approximation.

Table 2. The average α coefficient and the approximated α_R based on 200 simulations for each test case

Standard Deviation of the Latent Trait (σ)		Test 1	Test 2	Test 3
0.5	α	0.28	0.23	0.25
	α_R	0.28	0.26	0.27
1	α	0.59	0.54	0.56
	α_R	0.60	0.57	0.58
1.5	α	0.74	0.70	0.73
	α_R	0.76	0.73	0.75

The results show that when the latent trait variance decreases, the approximated and estimated reliability also decrease. This indicates that the reliability of a questionnaire is not an absolute value but a value that depends also on the spread of the latent variable. The results also show that when the latent trait variance is fixed, there is not much variation in the reliability across the different questionnaires. Extreme items decreases the reliability, however. With these simulations, we see that the influence of the difficulty parameters, and thus of the items, is small.

These results also show that the α estimates are very near to the α_R estimates, but the Cronbach coefficient is always less than the reliability estimated under the Rasch model. This is because the Cronbach coefficient is an estimate of a lower bound of the reliability (Ten Berge and Zegers, 1978). The biggest difference between the estimates occurred for the second set of difficulty parameters, where one item had a very high difficulty. The classical Cronbach alpha seems nevertheless to remain a good reliability coefficient under Rasch model assumptions. Unfortunately it is not straightforward to prove this result more generally or to determine conditions that assure the approximation is valid.

4.2 Example: the Communication Scale of the SIP

In this section, we illustrate the reliability estimation using responses from 483 patients with depression who completed the SIP questionnaire. The approach illustrated here is different from the one presented at the end of the Section 2.2. In Section 2.2, the items were chosen using a criterion related to the reliability estimation. Now, we retain the set of items that gives a good fit to the Rasch model. Then, we estimate the reliability. Therefore, before estimating the reliability coefficient, we must first test whether the data follow the Rasch model. Secondly, we must estimate the difficulty parameter (using the MML method). We used the mixed Rasch model. We assumed that the distribution of the latent trait is Gaussian ($\theta \sim N(\mu, \sigma^2)$). We used two goodness of fit tests. The first (denoted R_0) is detailed by Glas and Verhelst (1995). This χ^2-type test is based on a comparison of the observed scores and the expected scores under the null hypothesis (that the latent trait is Gaussian). The second test, proposed by Glas (1988), is denoted R_1. It is also a χ^2-type test, and it compares the observed number of individuals who achieved a score s and who correctly answered item j to the expected number under the null hypothesis (that the Rasch model is true).

Table 3 shows the estimated item difficulty parameters (in the first 9 rows) for two cases. In the first case, all items were considered. In the second case, item 7 was removed to improve the p-value of the goodness of fit test R_1 (denoted Prob(R_1)). The difference between the observed and expected numbers of good answers is the largest for item 7, suggesting a lack of fit for this item.

In both cases, the most difficult item was number 2 ("I communicate mostly by gestures"). We also give the estimated mean and standard deviation of the latent Gaussian distribution (here the identifiability condition is that the sum of the difficulties is zero). Finally, the two last rows of Table 3 give the estimated reliability coefficient. To estimate α_R, we replaced the values of the parameters in the Gauss-Hermite approximation by their respective estimates.

The estimated standard deviation is approximately 1.5. The reliability estimated by alpha or $\hat{\alpha}_R$ is nearly equal to the value found in the simulations. We note that the alpha coefficient gives a good estimate of the reliability even when the assumptions of the Rasch model hold. The conclusion of this example is that if we remove the more apparent deviant item (item 7), we find a decrease in reliability, so we choose to keep the complete scale. In some cases, removing an item can improve the fit and increase the reliability. In this situation, the question of keeping such an item must be evaluated (and not only on the basis of the reliability or goodness of fit but also by examining its content or formulation).

Table 3. Reliability analysis of the communication scale of the Sickness Impact Profile ($n = 483$)

Item Number	9 Items	8 Items
1	–1.23	–1.23
2	1.39	1.32
3	1.28	1.22
4	–0.03	–0.06
5	–0.78	–0.79
6	0.06	0.02
7	–0.24	–
8	0.83	0.78
9	–1.28	–1.27
$\hat{\mu}$	–1.13	–1.12
$\hat{\sigma}^2$	1.52	1.43
Prob(Z_1)	0.931	0.818
Prob(R_1)	0.309	0.681
α	0.742	0.698
$\hat{\alpha}_R$	0.761	0.716

5. Discussion

In this chapter we have shown how it is possible to define the reliability of the total score under the specific assumptions of the Rasch model. The simulations we presented show that the alpha coefficient is a robust estimator of the reliability. Other studies to evaluate the finite sample properties, like the mean square error, would be very interesting to complete the present work. Our simulations showed that there is an important influence of the standard deviation of the latent trait on the reliability coefficient α_R and a small influence of the difficulties. The influence of the number of items is not evaluated here. It would be interesting to investigate how the number of items could have an impact on the differences between alpha and the approximated α_R. In this chapter, we focused on the Rasch model because it is an important IRT model and a powerful tool for designing and validating a HRQoL questionnaire. We note that there are nonparametric alternatives to the Rasch model (for a good introduction see Mokken, 1996). In this context Sijstma and Molenaar (1987) have proposed an estimation of the reliability coefficient which is now implemented in the software MSP5 (Molenaar and Sijstma, 2000). It would be interesting to compare the estimates obtained in the nonparametric and parametric frameworks. We restricted our study of reliability to the case of dichotomous items; the relatively easy extension to polytomous items would be very useful.

ACKNOWLEDGMENTS

The authors thank Ivo Molenaar, Bernard F. Cole and an anonymous reviewer for numerous helpful comments.

REFERENCES

Andersen, E.B. (1970). Asymptotic properties of conditional maximum likelihood estimators. *Journal of the Royal Statistical Society, Series B* **32**, 283–301.

Bergner, M., Bobbit, R.A., Pollard, W.E., Martin, D.P. and Gilson, B.S. (1976). The Sickness Impact Profile: validation of a health status measure. *Medical Care* **14**, 57–67.

Cortina, J.M. (1998). What is coefficient Alpha? An examination of theory and applications. *Journal of Applied Psychology* **78**, 98–104.

Curt, F., Mesbah, M., Lellouch, J. and Dellatolas, G. (1997). Handedness scale: how many and which items? *Laterality* **2**, 137–154.

Fischer, G.H. (1981). On the existence and uniqueness of maximum-likelihood estimates of the Rasch model. *Psychometrika* **46**, 59–77.

Fischer, G.H. (1995). Derivations of the Rasch model. In: Fischer, G.H. and Molenaar, I.W. (eds.), *Rasch Models, Foundations, Recent Developments, and Applications*, New-York: Springer-Verlag.

Fischer, G.H. and Molenaar, I.W. (1995). *Rasch Models, Foundations, Recent Developments, and Applications*, New-York: Springer-Verlag.

Glas, C.A.W. (1988). The derivation of some tests for the Rasch model from the multinomial distribution. *Psychometrika* **53**, 525–546.

Haberman, S.J. (1977). Maximum likelihood estimates in exponential response models. *Annals of Statistics* **5**, 815–841.

Hamon, A. and Iovleff, S. (2001). Estimation in a longitudinal Rasch model via three stochastic EM algorithms. *Technical report, Laboratoire SABRES, Université de Bretagne Sud.*

Klauer, K.C. (1990). Asymptotic properties of the ML estimator of the ability parameter when item parameters are known. *Methodika* **4**, 23–26.

Kreiner, S. and Christensen, K.B. (2001). Graphical Rasch models. In Mesbah, M., Cole, B.F. and Lee, M.L.T. (eds.), *Statistical Methods for Quality of Life Studies: Design, Measurements and Analysis*, Amsterdam: Kluwer.

Kristof, W. (1963). The Statistical theory of stepped-up reliability coefficients when a test has been divided into several equivalent parts. *Psychometrika* **28**, 221–238.

Lauritzen, S.L. and Wermuth, N. (1989). Graphical models for associations between variables, some of which are qualitative and some quantitative. *Annals of Statistics* **17**, 31–54.

Lord, F.M. (1980). *Applications of Item Response Theory to Practical Testing Problems,* Hillsdale, NJ: Lawrence Erlbaum.

Lord, F.M. (1983). Unbiased estimators of ability parameters, of their variance, and of their parallel-forms reliability, *Psychometrika* **48**, 233–245.

Lord, F.M. and Novick, M.R. (1968). *Statistical Theories of Mental Test Scores*, Reading, MA: Addison-Wesley.

Mokken, R.J. (1996). Nonparametric models for dichotomous responses. In: van der Linden, W. and Hambleton, R.K. (eds.), *Handbook of Modern Item Response Theory*, New-York: Springer-Verlag.

Moret, L., Mesbah, M., Chwalow, J. and Lellouch, J. (1993). Internal validation of a measurement scale: relation between principal component analysis, Cronbach's alpha coefficient and intra-class correlation coefficient. *Revue d'Epidépidémiologie et de Santé Publique* **41**, 179–186.

Molenaar, I.W. and Sijtsma, K. (2000). MSP, a program for Mokken scale analysis for polytomous items. *iec ProGAMMA,* Groningen, The Netherlands.

Nunnally, J.C. and Bernstein I.H. (1994). *Psychometric Theory, 3rd Edition*, New-York: McGraw-Hill.

Rasch G. (1993). *Probabilistic Models for some Intelligence and Attainment tests.* Chicago: MESA Press.

Sijtsma, K. and Molenaar, I.W. (1987). Reliability of test scores in noparametric item response theory. *Psychometrika* **52**, 79–97.

Ten Berge, J.M.F. and Zegers, F.E. (1978). A series of lower bounds to the reliability of a test. *Psychometrika* **43**, 575–579.

Thissen, D. (1982). Marginal maximum likelihood estimation for the one-parameter logistic model. *Psychometrika* **47**, 175–186.

Tjur, T. (1982). A Connection between Rasch's item analysis model and a multiplicative Poisson model. *Scandinavian Journal of Statistics*, **9**, 23–30.

Wainer, H., Dorans, N.J., Flaugher, R., Green, B.F., Mislevy, R.J., Steinberg, L. and Thissen, D., Eds. (1990). *Computerized Adaptive Testing: A Primer.* Hillsdale, NJ: Lawrence Erlbaum.

APPENDIX

Below are listed the 9 items of the communication dimension of the Sickness Impact Profile. The response to each item is either "agree" or "disagree."

1. I am having trouble writing or typing
2. I communicate mostly by gestures, for example, moving head, pointing, sign language
3. My speech is understood only by e few people who know me well
4. I often lose control of my voice when I talk, for example, my voice gets louder or softer, trembles, changes unexpectedly
5. I don't write except to sign my name
6. I carry on a conversation only when very close to the other person or looking at him
7. I have difficulty speaking, for example, get stuck, stutter, stammer, slur my words
8. I am understood with difficulty
9. I do not speak clearly when I am under stress

ITEM RESPONSE THEORY (IRT): APPLICATIONS IN QUALITY OF LIFE MEASUREMENT, ANALYSIS AND INTERPRETATION

DAVID CELLA, CHIH-HUNG CHANG AND ALLEN W. HEINEMANN

Northwestern University

This article discusses basic concept of quality of life (QOL) measurement and item response theory (IRT). In a way complementary to that of traditional methods, IRT models can be applied to analyze and interpret QOL data collected in various settings. Growing interest in precise QOL measurement in research and clinical settings demands the development of psychometrically sound and clinically meaningful measurement tools. This in turn contributes to the appropriate use of QOL data that are collected. Advances in IRT, also referred to as modern test theory, make it possible for one to more critically evaluate questionnaire performance at its initial development and subsequent refinement and validation. It also offers better methodology to make interpretation of QOL data and comparisons between different populations or occasions more meaningful by converting ordinal observations into linear measures. Empirical results from different studies are provided to assist in the understanding of different IRT models and their applications. It is feasible and promising to integrate IRT models and advanced computer technology to develop a computerized adaptive testing platform to deliver tailored test to arrive at more precise QOL measurement. Administration of more targeted test items according to patient's level of health via CAT with real-time scoring and reporting is not just possibility but a reality. This can facilitate better use of QOL information between patients and physicians, and ultimately improve patient care.

1. Introduction

Health care in the United States is in transition. Fundamental to outcomes management is the notion that high quality outcomes assessment and monitoring will enable providers to evaluate directly from patients the value of a given treatment. Perceiving this as an opportunity, many health care organizations have taken an interest in adding patient-based outcomes assessment, such as quality of life (QOL) measurement, to their existing efforts in quality management or quality improvement. Thus, providers need precise, efficient outcomes data acquisition.

Designing timely and effective treatments to prevent or treat physical and psychosocial concerns of patients with cancer has been a challenge, in part because of deficiencies in the acquisition and use of patient-reported QOL in clinical settings. Earlier emphasis upon instrument development and quality assurance of data collection in clinical trials has recently expanded to include emphasis on data analysis and interpretation. While there is a growing interest in QOL monitoring outside of controlled clinical trials, including clinical practice, there is a continuing need for practical, user-friendly, and psychometrically sound data acquisition technology. The optimal QOL evaluation program is one which is well-integrated with other clinical and laboratory data, and

M. Mesbah et al. (eds.), Statistical Methods for Quality of Life Studies, 169–185.

connected to a reporting mechanism that allows for self-correction of the treatment system.

The effective use of well-organized QOL information for patient care requires easily recorded data that can be presented in a manner that enhances clinical decision making. One barrier faced by physicians is the need to have QOL information summarized in an interpretable fashion available during the office visit. Data collected in paper-and-pencil (P&P) format during the office visit is not scored or summarized at the time when it is needed to inform decision-making, and therefore is not as useful to the physician or patient. The majority of QOL questionnaires are designed to be administered via P&P format, which limits their usefulness in clinical decision-making.

If QOL data are to be useful in clinical settings, they must be accurate, responsive to meaningful change and interpretable. Advances of computer technology and modern test theory now make it possible to administer and score QOL questionnaires within a single system. Unlike the labor-intensive P&P data collection method, computerized QOL assessments provide an efficient way to collect and present QOL information for patients and physicians.

1.1 The Over-Supply of QOL Questionnaires

There is an abundant supply of QOL questionnaires available to investigate outcomes of treatment for chronic illnesses, including cancer, HIV/AIDS and other chronic conditions such as stroke [1–3]. Indeed, our group has been among the leaders in the development of QOL questionnaires and methods that are widely used in oncology [4–12], HIV/AIDS [13,14], multiple sclerosis [15] and post-stroke rehabilitation [16–18]. It has become increasingly unlikely that a single "gold standard" will emerge. In fact, the diverse instruments that have evolved are valuable in that they provide the user with choices based upon specific characteristics of a given disease site or QOL domain of interest. However, the plethora of QOL questionnaires also carries risk of "confusing the marketplace" with different questions, rating scales, and aggregate scores. Indeed, despite wide availability of QOL instruments, few providers use them in practice. Why is this? Genuinely interested users of these data resist committing to patient-based assessment because it is too expensive, complicated or confusing to master [19–22]. A practical concern is the requirement that assessment be brief, immediately available, and easily interpreted. Physicians consider the *quality* of their patients' lives to be as important as *quantity* [19–21,23], and yet little attention is paid to patient-rated QOL data *per se* [20,21,24]. One major problem is that QOL measures are diverse in scaling properties and require sophistication to understand and appropriately interpret. There are other barriers to the integration of QOL data into practice [20–22,24–27]. These barriers include: (1) misunderstanding of QOL, including the myth that it cannot be measured reliably; (2) a tendency to disregard subjective patient data in favor of objective data; and (3) time, effort and cost required to accomplish valid assessment. A solution to these barriers exists: equating five commonly used QOL questionnaires in both cancer and HIV/AIDS patients. This solution provides a common language for QOL that can facilitate widespread application of QOL measurement.

1.2 What is Needed?

Clinicians frequently request the minimum-required number of questions to obtain a desirable level of precision. They want clinically relevant, responsive questions that can be aggregated and available during the same medical encounter. Our work has sought to simplify and standardize patient-based outcomes data monitoring via computer in a way that is valid, clinically useful, practical, psychometrically sound and robust. This work required a comprehensive bank of QOL questions relevant and sensitive to the concerns of people with chronic illness, and a computer-based administration platform. Computerized Adaptive Testing (CAT) is used in educational testing and professional certification. It uses probabilistic measurement models (either Rasch or item response theory measurement) to guide selection of subsequent questions from a large bank, based upon previous responses. This maximizes measurement precision with a limited number of questions. CAT application in medicine is a recently advocated innovation [28–30].

2. Quality of Life Measurement

Although the quality of patient care has traditionally been measured with such objective outcomes as survival and tumor response, there is a growing recognition of the importance of subjective patient-rated outcomes. Quality of life (QOL) evaluation differs from classical physical indicator rating (e.g., survival and toxicity) in two important ways: (1) it incorporates more aspects of function (e.g., mood, affect, social well-being) than those which have typically been attributed to treatment; and (2) it focuses on the patient's perspective. QOL evaluation entails a multidimensional quantification of health and well-being, as reported by the patient. Major QOL dimensions are physical well-being (disease symptoms, treatment side effects), emotional well-being (coping, distress, enjoyment), social well-being (social activity/support, relationship quality, family well-being), and functional well-being (activities of daily living, role performance).

The measurement of QOL is becoming more common in clinical trials and treatment decision making. QOL measurement is used to reflect the extent to which one's usual or expected physical, emotional, and social well-being are affected by a medical condition or its treatment [31]. Cella and Webster [32] report that "the desire for QOL assessment in clinical practice has outstripped current capability to provide valid, streamlined, and cost-effective assessment methods."

Although QOL evaluation has matured dramatically over the past 20 years, the unmet need is in the area of practical, user-friendly data acquisition technology that captures clinically meaningful, responsive data about patient health status. Also needed is a psychometrically robust, precise indicator of patient-rated QOL that is interpretable by clinicians, useful for cost-effectiveness considerations and applicable to treatment decision-making. The integration of contemporary test theory and computer technology fills a pressing need in health care outcomes management by creating a survey platform to make real-time QOL information acquisition and retrieval a reality.

3. Item Response Theory (IRT) and its Applications

IRT methods and classical methods work compatibly with one another, often providing both overlapping and unique information. Unlike traditional ("classical") psychometric methods, IRT models mathematically describe the relationship between the persons being measured and items used to measure persons on the same unidimensional underlying continuum, which allows us to establish an underlying dimension on a continuum, along which respondents and items can be jointly placed, ordered and compared. This allows us to examine the content and degree of magnitude (severity) of questions along the continuum, and thereby better understand and define what is being measured. Another attractive feature of IRT models is that the item parameter estimates are relatively more independent of the sample from which the analyses were done. Likewise, person-ability measures are relatively independent of the particular choice of items used from the population of items that were calibrated. In classical test methods, analyses are sample dependent. Therefore, when using classical methods, any given instrument must typically be "re-validated" in new populations, as psychometric data from one sample cannot easily be generalized to another.

3.1 Item Response Theory (IRT)

IRT models employ mathematical equations to determine the characteristics (e.g., "difficulty") of test questions and to estimate the level, or "ability" of people on the underlying dimension being measured [33,34]. It posits an underlying, unobserved trait on which the items are hierarchically arrayed from the easiest to the hardest. The three most popular unidimensional IRT models are the one-, two-, and three-parameter logistic (PL) models, so named because of the number of item parameters each incorporates. The 1PL models focus on item difficulty as the sole parameter of interest, the 2PL models add item discrimination to item difficulty, and the 3PL models incorporate a third guessing parameter. All models are appropriate for dichotomous response items. The one-parameter is also referred to as the Rasch model, after its developer, Georg Rasch [35]. Extensions of dichotomous IRT models to handle polytomous response data have been developed. Masters and Wright [36] reviewed extensions of the Rasch model, including the partial credit model, rating scale model, binomial trials, and Poisson count model. Thissen and Steinberg [37] also reviewed a larger collection of models developed to deal with categorical data and provided a framework of classifying them. More recently developed multidimensional IRT models also exist [38]. Unlike other IRT models, the Rasch measurement model specifies that the questions to be included in a measure discriminate equally with the other questions in the set. If the data do not fit this requirement, the differentially discriminating items misfit. This is identifiable from fit statistics provided by the analysis program. For example, using Rasch measurement software, e.g, WINSTEPS [39], one can analyze multiple rating scales within instruments. Other factors that might systematically contribute to measurement (e.g., interrater differences) can be analyzed in a multifaceted analysis using *Facets* [39,40]. Rather than eliminate items that do not discriminate equally, the 2PL models estimate item discrimination and include that information in determining the relative value of different items at the same level of difficulty.

This chapter concerns itself primarily with illustrating opportunities made available with IRT methods. To illustrate some of the applications of IRT in health status, we drew data from two psychometric studies funded by the national Cancer Institute (US). The first study, referred to as "BIOQOL" (Bilingual Intercultural Oncology Quality of Life), collected English language and Spanish language QOL data on 1,615 people with cancer.

The primary purpose of the second study, referred to as "Q-Score," was to equate several commonly-used QOL questionnaires in oncology and HIV disease, for the purpose of deriving a single, common metric. A total of 1,720 patients were recruited. The five instruments are the Medical Outcomes Study Short Form-36 (SF-36), European Organization for Research and Treatment of Cancer Core Quality of Life Questionnaire (EORTC QLQ-C30), Cancer Rehabilitation Evaluation System-Short Form (CARES-SF), Functional Assessment of Cancer Therapy-General (FACT-G), and the Spitzer Quality of Life Index (QLI).

3.2 Comparing One Parameter Logistic (1PL) Versus Two Parameter Logistic (2PL) Models

From the Q-Score data we analyzed the 10 physical functioning items (PF-10) from the Medical Outcomes Study SF-36 to illustrate the potential comparability and complementarity of the approaches. The WINSTEPS program [39] was used for 1PL rating scale analysis and the PARSCALE program [41] was used for 2PL generalized partial credit model analysis. The item location (difficulty) hierarchies obtained from the 2 models are identical (see Table 1). The correlation between infit mean square (MNSQ) and slope is –0.892. The possible misfitting items (PF10 and PF1) have the lowest slope (or discrimination) parameters. We also investigated the relationships between person measures obtained from the two models with original SF-36 physical functioning scoring. The correlations are very high; PF10 original scoring correlates 0.979 with 1PL Rasch measure and 0.988 with 2PL measure. The relationship between person measures

Table 1. Comparison of one- versus two-parameter logistic model analysis of 10-item Physical Functioning subscale of the SF-36

	1PL Model			2PL model	
Item	Location	Infit MNSQ*	Outfit MNSQ*	Slope	Location
PF10	–3.61	1.34	3.08	1.104	–1.963
PF9	–1.79	0.87	0.65	1.901	–1.049
PF5	–1.20	0.87	0.72	1.690	–0.878
PF6	–0.28	1.19	1.33	1.154	–0.613
PF3	–0.09	0.92	0.82	1.440	–0.466
PF8	0.08	0.81	0.66	2.194	–0.313
PF2	0.76	1.04	0.91	1.423	–0.118
PF4	0.79	0.88	0.81	1.686	–0.088
PF7	1.51	0.95	0.84	1.815	0.158
PF1	3.84	1.32	3.74	1.111	1.108

*The infit mean square is (MNSQ) an information-weighted fit statistic, which is particularly sensitive to unexpected responses to items near the person's trait level. The outfit MNSQ is an outlier-sensitive statistic that is particularly sensitive to unexpected responses by persons on items far from the person's trait level. Fit statistics have an expected value of 1.0, and range from 0 to infinity. Values substantially above 1 indicate noise in the data or a "misfitting" item; values substantially below 1 indicate redundancy or an "overfitting" item.

obtained by two IRT models is 0.995, indicating both models yields almost identical ordering of patients in measuring physical functioning. We conclude that these approaches yield comparable results and have good potential for providing complementary rather than conflicting data.

3.3 Standardized Scores

We believe communication among health professionals about patient QOL will be enhanced if generalizable, interpretable scores can be derived from common questionnaires. In order to derive standardized scores (ranging from 0–100) for each FACT subscale (Physical Well-Being, Social/Family Well-Being, Emotional Well-Being, and Functional Well-Being) and total score, 27 FACT-G items were analyzed using the Rasch rating scale model [42]. The data were drawn from a heterogeneous group of cancer and HIV patients. The quality of life measures for the separate FACT-G scales were calibrated with the BIGSTEPS computer program [39]. The scaled measures, originally expressed in log-transformed units (called "logits"), were then transformed linearly, to a 0–100 scale (called "standardized scores"). We set "0" = worst quality of life and "100" = best quality of life. The values on both scales (logits or standardized scores) are interval. Standardized scores can therefore now easily be derived from raw scores by using the conversion tables provided in the scoring section of the manual, and illustrated here in Table 2. Work on validating the standardized scores and their usefulness in research and clinical trials is continuing.

3.4 Cross-Instrument Equivalence/Equating

By calibrating scores of one questionnaire to another, QOL can be estimated using a common metric across questionnaires. This common metric, "Q-score," allows one to be indifferent to questionnaire used, because the score can be transformed into the common metric for ease of interpretation, and equivalent scores among instruments can be established. This was done by calibrating all 140 items from the five QOL instrument mentioned earlier and creating a common metric (hierarchy of item difficulties). Patients' QOL measures for each instrument were then re-estimated separately using anchored item and step measures obtained from the joint calibration. Person measures were then linked from the five separate calibrations. We then created score conversion tables similar to that shown in Table 3. These tables allow a user to administer any of the five instruments and derive a total logit score that can be converted to a comparable logit score for any of the other questionnaires. It is also possible to convert raw scores from different settings into corresponding Q-scores for comparison. This innovation helps to advance QOL research by supporting the use of a number of well validated QOL measures, to increase communication about QOL among physicians and researchers who use different measures for different purposes, and ultimately to enhance patient QOL by helping doctors understand and use QOL concepts.

3.5 Cross-Group and Cross-Cultural Equivalence

Although the definition of a construct such as QOL may differ from culture to culture, the questionnaire designed to measure QOL must capture a common underlying construct. In order to make quantitative comparisons cross-culturally, it is essential to establish cross-cultural equivalence of translated questionnaires to evaluate such comparisons.

We have employed a methodology based on IRT for examining, anchoring and fixing conceptual issues across languages, so data collected can be meaningfully compared. The extent to which items in a questionnaire perform similarly across different reference groups is of critical interest when determining whether a given questionnaire can be used as an unbiased basis for comparing groups. Having determined individual item difficulty (location) which for Rasch analysis is independent of the sample, we can then identify items displaying differential item functioning (DIF) [43]. The principal of conjoint additivity provides this property. The most important indicator of DIF is *not* whether

Table 2A. Raw Score to Standardized Score Conversion Table for FACT-G Subscales

	Standardized Score			
Raw Score on Each Scale	Physical Well-Being	Social/Family Well-Being	Emotional Well-Being	Functional Well-Being
0	0	0	0	0
1	9	11	9	9
2	19	20	18	18
3	24	25	23	24
4	28	29	28	28
5	32	32	31	32
6	34	34	34	34
7	37	36	36	37
8	39	38	38	39
9	41	40	41	41
10	43	41	43	43
11	45	43	45	45
12	47	44	47	47
13	49	46	49	49
14	50	47	51	50
15	52	49	53	52
16	54	50	55	54
17	56	52	58	56
18	58	53	60	57
19	60	55	64	59
20	62	57	67	61
21	64	59	72	64
22	66	61	79	66
23	69	64	89	69
24	72	67	100	72
25	76	71		76
26	82	77		82
27	91	88		91
28	100	100		100

Table 2B. Raw Score to Standardized Score Conversion Table for FACT-G Total

Raw Score	Stand. Score	Raw Score	Stand. Score	Raw Score	Stand. Score	Raw Score	Stand. Score
0	0	28	41	56	49	84	58
1	8	29	41	57	50	85	59
2	16	30	42	58	50	86	59
3	20	31	42	59	50	87	59
4	23	32	42	60	50	88	60
5	25	33	43	61	51	89	60
6	27	34	43	62	51	90	61
7	28	35	43	63	51	91	62
8	29	36	44	64	52	92	62
9	31	37	44	65	52	93	63
10	32	38	44	66	52	94	63
11	32	39	45	67	52	95	64
12	33	40	45	68	53	96	65
13	34	41	45	69	53	97	66
14	35	42	45	70	53	98	67
15	35	43	46	71	54	99	68
16	36	44	46	72	54	100	69
17	36	45	46	73	54	101	70
18	37	46	47	74	54	102	72
19	37	47	47	75	55	103	74
20	38	48	47	76	55	104	76
21	38	49	47	77	55	105	79
22	39	50	48	78	56	106	84
23	39	51	48	79	56	107	92
24	40	52	48	80	57	108	100
25	40	53	48	81	57		
26	40	54	49	82	57		
27	41	55	49	83	58		

Table 3. Segment of a Raw Score Equation Table for Overall QOL

Measure	Instrument				Q-Score (0-100)
	CARES-SF	EORTC QLO-C30	FACT-G	SF36	
–1.14	27	–	–	–	34
–1.12	28	–	21	–	34
–1.10	–	52	–	56	35
1.03	137	98	97	–	54
1.05	–	–	–	121	55
1.07	138	–	–	–	55

items systematically differentiate relevant subgroups, but whether they do so in an unmodeled (i.e., unpredicted) way. Unmodeled differences reflect differential interaction between some items and some persons, which in turn confuses interpretation of results. Items which differentiate groups in unexpected ways can be identified and investigated to determine the likely source of DIF. This process is done for each bivariate comparison between two patient groups (e.g., African American vs. Caucasian). DIF detection procedures are described below and actions to be taken in each procedure are also noted.

1. After all data are collected, calibrations of item responses is completed *separately* for the two groups (e.g., African American vs. Caucasian).
2. The calibrated item difficulties from the separate analysis of each sample is centered and plotted against each other (e.g., Spanish on the *y*-axis and English on the *x*-axis).
3. An identity line is drawn through the origin of each plot with a slope of one.
4. Statistical control (95% confidence interval) lines are drawn around the identity line to guide interpretation, and the plots are examined to see if any items fall outside the control lines, thereby reflecting possible bias.
5. Items identified as possibly biased (displaying DIF) are reviewed plot-by-plot to obtain direction on interpreting the plots and determining the appropriate disposition of the item, given the content and the context of the misfitting item.

The end product of these analyses and plots is an understanding of the extent to which questions in a scale are unbiased across the two groups compared. The sample result shown in Figure 1 indicates that the FACT-G Physical Well-Being (PWB) subscale works very similarly among African-American versus European American (Caucasian), with all items falling within 0.5 logit of the identity line. However, due to the relatively large sample size, three of the seven items fall outside of the 95% confidence interval, suggesting mild DIF. Of these three items, one ("I feel ill") was <u>more</u> likely to be endorsed by African-Americans at the same level of QOL, whereas two ("I have a lack of energy," "I am bothered by side effects of treatment") were <u>less</u> likely to be endorsed by African-Americans at the same level of QOL. Differences in mean FACT scores between these two patient groups can then be evaluated as to whether these potentially "biased" items are retained or deleted prior to pooling data or comparing groups. One can then be more confident that differences found between groups are not attributable to biased assessment, but rather to true differences.

3.6 Defining Primary Dimensions of QOL

QOL is multi-dimensional. One practical problem is that HRQOL measures have diverse scaling properties and require a high degree of familiarity and prior experience to understand and interpret. By equating five commonly-used HRQOL questionnaires in both cancer and HIV/AIDS patients, the Q-Score project [44,45] is an effort to foster use of a common language for HRQOL. We employed mixed Rasch measurement models in the same analysis, including the dichotomous Rasch model [35], Andrich's rating scale model [46–48] for questionnaires with a common rating scale (i.e., response choices) across all items, and Masters' partial credit model [42], for questionnaires in which the response choices vary across items in a questionnaire.

Figure 1. Sample Differential Item Functioning (DIF) plot comparing item locations for African American versus Caucasian patients for the Physical Well Being scale. Item difficulties are shown with 95% confidence bands (dashed lines)

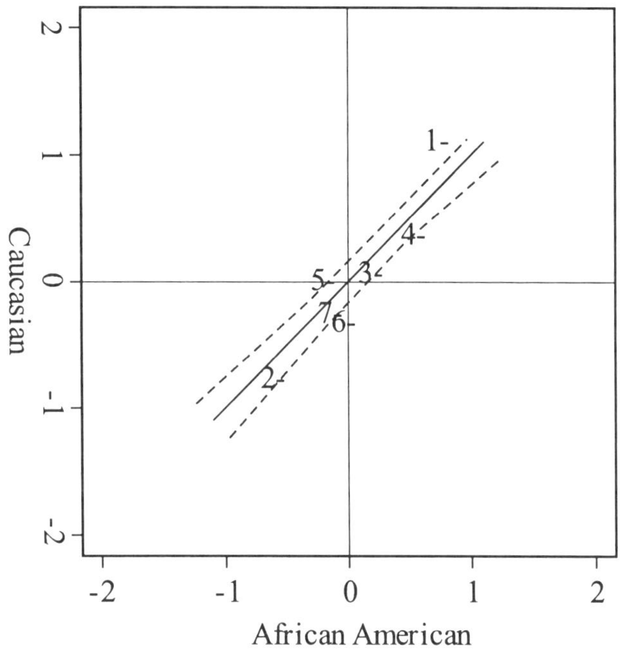

We calibrated all items together so as to define one core construct. Joint calibration is a useful way to investigate improvements in scale definition, even when one anticipates ultimately dividing items into sub-dimensions [49–51]. The reliability of this single HRQOL construct was above 0.90, implying that all HRQOL instruments tapped a single construct. Then, we conducted a principal components analysis of the data residuals from this common core [52]. We found two clear subsets of items. The first factor was similar to the Physical Well-Being (PWB) dimension in the two-factor solution described above. Specifically, 75 items were extracted, including 69 of the 72 PWB items from the exploratory factor analysis (96% overlap). The second residual factor was similar to the Mental Well-Being (MWB) factor from the exploratory analysis, extracting 65 items, with 55 of the 57 MWB items from the exploratory factor analysis (97% overlap). Identical overlap (96% PWB; 97% MWB) in assignment to physical versus mental dimension occurred when all items (including those with loadings <0.30) were assigned to a factor based solely upon magnitude of loading. Thus, we are confident that it is important to distinguish two sub-dimensions of QOL, PWB and MWB. When data were randomly split into halves (n = 856 each) and analyzed with Rasch residual factor analysis, the item compositions for each of the two factors remained stable, with four exceptions. Two items ("I find that my clothes do not fit." and "My partner spends too much time taking care of me.") in random sample 1 were classified as PWB items but were classified as MWB items in the combined sample. Two items ("Have you had trouble sleeping?" and "Has your physical condition or medical treatment caused you financial problem?") in sample 2 were identified as PWB items but were identified as MWB items in the whole sample. Further work is needed here to define these dimensions clearly enough to assure that the data collected in future samples will adequately fit the measurement model. In addition, newer multidimensional IRT models, as they become more practical in their application, may shed important light on the multidimensionality of QOL [53].

3.7 Item Banking and Computerized Adaptive Testing (CAT)

Clinicians frequently request short instruments to minimize patient fatigue. They want clinically relevant, responsive questions that can be aggregated and available during the same medical encounter. Fulfilling this request requires a comprehensive bank of QOL questions that are relevant and sensitive to specific patient concerns and a computer-based administration platform. Computerized Adaptive Testing (CAT) is used routinely in educational testing and professional certification. It uses probabilistic measurement models (item response theory; IRT) to guide selection of subsequent questions from a large bank. This technique maximizes measurement precision with a minimum number of questions. Medical application of CAT is a recent innovation that allows simplification and standardization of patient-based outcomes data monitoring via a computer in a way that is valid, clinically useful, practical, and psychometrically sound.

What is an item bank and how is it useful? More than a collection of items; an *item bank* is comprised of carefully calibrated questions that help define and quantify a common theme and thus help evaluate an operational definition of a concept [54–58]. A bank is as good as its coverage of the entire continuum of the latent trait being measured. The items in the bank are concrete manifestations of positions along the continuum that represent differing amounts of that trait. The bank could contain all items that could be written to measure a trait.

A well-constructed QOL item bank provides the basis for designing the best possible set of questions (a "test") for a particular application. A well-calibrated item bank makes it possible to compare the QOL of patients who complete different sets of questions in the bank. Not only does this allow for tailored, "adaptive" testing (see later), it also allows one to compare the QOL of patients across studies which have used different questionnaires. Patients complete a subset of items that are appropriate to their level of QOL. And because all items drawn from the bank are calibrated onto one common metric, we can compare QOL status between diverse groups of patients, even when there are no common items. Finally, a well-organized item bank with wide ranging item difficulties also enables researchers and clinicians to select items to construct a wide variety of tests, depending on the target population and the purpose of the assessment. Theoretically, the items selected should be immaterial to the measurement. The most important parameter is item difficulty. At a given difficulty level, an item should provide the same increment of information. In the specific context of QOL (or one of its dimensions), the content of questions at comparable difficulty levels may vary in clinical relevance. By using item bank information, the user is able to select that item, within a given difficulty level, according to its clinical relevance. Specific items can thus be selected from among those in the bank to maximize precision of the estimate and clinical relevance of the questions.

What is CAT? Computerized Adaptive Testing is a process of test administration in which items are selected on the basis of the examinee's responses to previously administered items [59]. This process utilizes an algorithm to estimate person *level* ("ability"), to choose the next best item and to administer the test with certain test specifications such as content coverage and length. In fact, the capacity to measure all examinees on the same continuum, even if they have not been presented any items in common, provides a test that is individually tailored to each examinee. CAT uses microcomputer technology and a psychometric framework such as *Rasch measurement*. CAT targets the "difficulty" of questions to the "level" of the patient. With item banking, each patient need only answer a sample of items in order to obtain a measure that accurately estimates what would have been obtained had the entire set of items been administered. Adaptive tests are greatly facilitated by a computer because of the computational requirements of the algorithm and the logistics of item and data management [60].

Why CAT? CAT has been used successfully in educational, licensing and achievement testing [61–63], personality assessment [64–66] and military personnel selection [67]. *A measurement model such as Rasch measurement is crucial to implementing CAT because it guides efficient question selection.* The opportunity to apply CAT does not exist within traditional test theory [68–70]. CAT can reduce test length without loss of precision [60,66,71–76]. A CAT platform for QOL outcome assessment has at least six advantages: Compared to paper-and-pencil tests, CAT technology (1) requires fewer questions to arrive at an accurate estimate; (2) allows patients to receive immediate feedback on their QOL status; (3) allows users to compare their QOL to one another on a common metric, as defined and measured by the IRT models; and (4) dynamically tailors the test to the trait level of the individual patient. In principle, then, (5) CAT reduces floor and ceiling effects. Reducing floor and ceiling effects not only yield measures that allow accurate selection and classification decisions, but reduce patient boredom or frustration; and (6) since CAT automates question administration, data recording, scoring and reporting, human clerical error is eliminated. It remains to be determined whether implementation of CAT in clinical practice or clinical research is as feasible as it is appealing.

4. Summary

Quality of life assessment urgently needs practical, user-friendly data acquisition technology that captures clinically-meaningful and responsive data. Also needed is a psychometrically robust, precise indicator of patient-rated quality of life which is interpretable by clinicians, useful for cost-effectiveness considerations and applicable to treatment decision-making.

Contemporary psychometric approaches (item response theory) advance the development and validation of reliable, valid and robust quality of life instruments and the computer technology make real-time questionnaire administration and reporting possible. The integration of modern test theory and computer technology facilitates better health care outcomes management by making real-time QOL and outcomes information acquisition and retrieval a reality.

Internet and wireless technologies allow, for instance, a physician to use a wireless Personal Digital Assistant (PDA) to collect QOL data at the point of service and immediately develop a treatment plan based on immediate feedback. Alternatively, the physician can access the same application and data via Internet on any type of computer, dramatically reducing system deployment and maintenance costs. Questionnaire administration can be interactive by selecting questions based on responses to previous questions.

REFERENCES

1. Berzon R.A., Donnelly, M.A., Simpson, R.L., Jr., Simeon, G.P. and Tilson, H.H. (1995). Quality of bibliography and indexes: 1994 update. *Quality of Life Research* **4**, 547–569.
2. Erickson, P. (1998). *On-line Guide to Quality of Life Assessment (OLGA).* http://olga-qol.com.
3. Spilker, B., ed. (1996). *Quality of Life and Pharmacoeconomics in Clinical Trials, (Second Edition).* Philadelphia: Lippincott-Raven Publishers.
4. Brady, M.J., Cella, D.F., Mo, F., Bonomi, A.E., Tulsky, D.S., Lloyd, S.R., Deasy. S., Cobleigh, M. and Shiomoto, G. (1997). Reliability and validity of the Functional Assessment of Cancer Therapy – Breast (FACT-B) quality of life instrument. *Journal of Clinical Oncology* **15**, 974–986.
5. Cella, D.F. (1997). *Manual of the Functional Assessment of Chronic Illness Therapy (FACIT Scales – Version 4.* Chicago: Center on Outcomes Research and Education (CORE), Evanston Northwestern Healthcare and Northwestern University.
6. Cella, D.F. and Bonomi, A.E. (1996). The Functional Assessment of Cancer Therapy (FACT) and Functional Assessment of HIV Infection (FAHI) quality of life measurement system. In: Spilker, B. (ed.), *Quality of Life and Pharmacoeconomics in Clinical Trials (Second Edition).* Philadelphia: Lippincott-Raven Publishers.
7. Cella, D.F., Tulsky, D.S., Gray, G., Sarafian, B., Lloyd, S., Linn, E., Bonomi, A., Silberman, M., Yellen, S.B., Winicour, P., Brannon, J., Eckberg, K., Purl, S., Blendowski, C., Goodman, M., Barnicle, M., Stewart, I., McHale, M., Bonomi, P., Kaplan, E., Taylor, S., Thomas, C. and Harris, J. (1993) The Functional Assessment of Cancer Therapy (FACT) scale: development and validation of the general measure. *Journal of Clinical Oncology* **11**, 570–579.
8. Cella, D.F., Bonomi, A.E., Lloyd, S.R., Tulsky, D.S., Kaplan, E. and Bonomi, P. (1995). Reliability and validity of the Functional Assessment of Cancer Therapy-Lung (FACT-L) quality of life instrument. *Lung Cancer* **12**, 199–220.
9. D'Antonio, L.L., Zimmerman, G.J., Cella, D.F. and Long, S.A. (1996). Quality of life and functional status measures in patients with head and neck cancer. *Archives of Otolaryngology–Head & Neck Surgery* **122**, 482–487.
10. Esper, P., Mo, F., Chodak, G., Sinner, M., Pienta, K. and Cella, D. (1997). Measuring quality of life in men with prostate cancer using the Functional Assessment of Cancer Therapy – Prostate (FACT-P) instrument. *Urology* **50**, 920–928.

11. McQuellon, R.P., Russell, G.B., Cella, D.F., Craven, B.L., Brady, M., Bonomi, A.E. and Hurd, D.D. (1997). Quality of life measurement in bone marrow transplantation: development of the Functional Assessment of Cancer Therapy – Bone Marrow Transplant (FACT-BMT) scale. *Bone Marrow Transplantation* **19**, 357–368.
12. Ward, W.L., Hahn, E.A., Mo, F., Hernandez, L., Tulsky, D.S. and Cella, D. (1999). Reliability and validity of the Functional Assessment of Cancer Therapy – Colorectal (FACT-C) quality of life instrument. *Quality of Life Research* **8**, 181–195.
13. Peterman, A.H., Cella, D.F., Mo, F. and McCain, N. (1997). Psychometric validation of the revised Functional Assessment of Human Immunodeficiency Virus Infection (FAHI) quality of life instrument. *Quality of Life Research* **6**, 572–584.
14. Cella, D.F., McCain, N.L., Peterman, A.H., Mo, F. and Wolen, D. (1996). Development and validation of the Functional Assessment of Human Immunodeficiency Virus Infection (FAHI) quality of life instrument. *Quality of Life Research* **5**, 450–463.
15. Cella, D.F., Dineen, K., Arnason, B., Reder, A., Webster, K.A., Karabatsos, G., Chang, C., Lloyd, S., Mo, F., Stewart, J. and Stefoski, D. (1996). Validation of the Functional Assessment of Multiple Sclerosis quality of life instrument. *Neurology* **47**, 129–139.
16. Heinemann, A.W., Hamilton, B.B., Linacre, J.M., Wright, B.D. and Granger, C. (1995). Functional status and therapeutic intensity during inpatient rehabilitation. *American Journal of Physical Medicine and Rehabilitation* **74**, 315–325.
17. Linacre, J.M., Heinemann, A.W., Wright, B.D., Granger, C.V. and Hamilton, B.B. (1994). The structure and stability of the functional independence measure. *Archives of Physical Medicine and Rehabilitation* **75**, 127–132.
18. Segal, M.E., Heinemann, A.W., Schall, R.R. and Wright, B.D. (1997). Rasch analysis of a brief physical ability scale for long-term outcomes of stroke. *Physical Medicine and Rehabilitation: State of the Art Reviews* **11**, 385–396.
19. Fallowfield, D., Ratcliffe, D. and Souhami, R. (1997). Clinicians? attitudes to clinical trials of cancer therapy. *European Journal of Cancer* **33**, 2221–2229.
20. Morris, J., Perez, D. and McNoe, B. (1998). The use of quality of life data in clinical practice. *Quality of Life Research* **7**, 85–91.
21. Taylor, K.M., Feldstein, M.L., Skeel, R.T., Pandya, K.J., Ng, P. and Carbone, P.P. (1994). Fundamental dilemmas of the randomized clinical trial process: results of a survey of the 1,737 ECOG investigators. *Journal of Clinical Oncology* **12**, 1796–1805.
22. Wasson, J., Keller, A., Rubenstein, L., Hays, R., Nelson. E. and Johnson, D. (1992). Benefits and obstacles of health status assessment in ambulatory settings. *Medical Care* **30**, MS42–49.
23. Gough, I.R. and Dalgleish, L.I. (1991). What value is given to quality of life assessment by health professionals considering response to palliative chemotherapy for advanced cancer? *Cancer* **68**, 220–225.
24. Taylor, K.M., DePetrillo, D., Macdonald, K., Awrey, J., Nicolson, J., Ng, P. and the Clinical Advisory Committee. (1993). Quality of Life (QOL) information: how do/would oncologists use it? *Proceedings of ASCO* **12**, 1573.
25. Bergner, M. (1989). Quality of life, health status and clinical research. *Medical Care* **27**, S148–156.

26. Deyo, R.A. and Patrick, D.L. (1989) Barriers to the use of health status measures in clinical investigation, patient care and policy research. *Medical Care* **27** (Suppl), 254–S268.
27. Nelson, E.C. and Berwick, D.M. (1989). The measurement of health status in clinical practice. *Medical Care* **27** (Suppl 3), 77–90.
28. Chang, C.-H. and Cella, D.F. (1997). Equating health-related quality of life instruments in applied oncology settings. *Physical Medicine and Rehabilitation: State of the Art Reviews* **11**, 397–406.
29. McHorney, C.A. (1997). Generic health measurement: past accomplishments and a measurement paradigm for the 21st century. *Annals of Internal Medicine* **127**, 743–750.
30. Revicki, D.A. and Cella, D.F. (1997). Health status assessment for the twenty-first century: item response theory, item banking and computer adaptive testing. *Quality of Life Research* **6**, 595–600.
31. Cella, D.F. (1995). Measuring quality of life in palliative care. *Seminars in Oncology* **22** (Suppl 3), 73–81.
32. Cella, D. and Webster, K. (1997). Linking outcomes management to quality-of-life measurement. *Oncology* **11**, 232–235.
33. Lord, F.M. (1980). *Applications of Item Response Theory to Practical Testing Problems*. Hillsdale, NJ: Erlbaum L.
34. Lord, F.M. and Novick, M.R. (1968). *Statistical Theories of Mental Test Scores.* Reading, MA: Addison-Wesley.
35. Rasch, G. (1960). *Probabilistic Models for Some Intelligence and Attainment Tests.* Copenhagen: Danish Institute for Educational Research.
36. Masters, G.N. and Wright, B.D. (1984). The essential process of a family of measurement models. *Psychometrika* **49**, 529–544.
37. Thissen, D. and Steinberg, L. (1984) Taxonomy of item response models. *Psychometrika* **51**, 567–578.
38. van der Linden, W.J. and Hambleton, R.K., eds. (1997). *Handbook of Modern Item Response Theory*. New York: Springer-Verlag.
39. Wright, B.D. and Linacre, J.M. (1997). *A User's Guide to BIGSTEPS Rasch Model Computer Program, Version 2.7.* Chicago: Mesa Press.
40. Linacre, J.M. and Wright, B.D. (1997). *Facets: Many-Faceted Rasch Analysis.* Chicago: MESA Press.
41. Muraki, E. and Bock, R.D. (1993). *PARSCALE: Parameter scaling of rating data (Version 3.5).* Chicago: Scientific Software International, Inc.
42. Wright, B.D. and Masters, G.N. (1982) *Rating Scale Analysis: Rasch Measurement.* Chicago: Mesa Press.
43. Holland, P.W. and Wainer, H., eds. (1993). *Differential Item Functioning*. Hillsdale, NJ: Lawrence Erlbaum Associates.
44. Cella, D.F. and Chang, C.-H. (1997). Establishing equivalence measures from different health-related quality of life instruments. *Quality of Life Research* **6**, 631.
45. Chang, C.-H. and Cella, D.F. (1997). Equating health-related quality of life instruments in applied oncology settings. *Physical Medicine and Rehabilitation: State of the Art Reviews* **11**, 397–406.

46. Andrich, D. (1978). Application of a psychometric rating model to ordered categories which are scored with successive integers. *Applied Psychological Measurement* **2**, 581–594.
47. Andrich, D. (1978). Scaling attitude items constructed and scored in the Likert tradition. *Educational and Psychological Measurement* **38**, 665–680.
48. Andrich, D. (1978). A rating formulation for ordered response categories. *Psychometrika* **43**, 561–573.
49. Chang, C.-H. (1998). Confirming test structure and measurement characteristics. *Rasch Measurement* Transaction **12**, 622–623.
50. Gehlert, S. and Chang, C.-H. (1998). Psychometric properties of the Multidimensional Health Locus of Control scales in measuring patients with epilepsy. *Journal of Outcome Measurement* **2**, 173–190.
51. Prieto, L., Alonso, J., Lamarca, R. and Wright, B.D. (1998). Rasch measurement for reducing the items of the Nottingham Health Profile. *Journal of Outcome Measurement* **2**, 285–301.
52. Linacre, J.M. (1998). Detecting multidimensionality: which residual data-type works best? *Journal of Outcome Measurement* **2**, 266–283.
53. Kelderman, H. and Rijkes, C.P.M. (1994). Loglinear multidimensional IRT models for polytomously scored items. *Psychometrika* **59**, 149–176.
54. Choppin, B. (1968). An item bank using sample-free calibration. *Nature* **219**, 870–872.
55. Choppin, B. (1976). Recent developments in item banking. In: de Gruijter, D.N.M. and van der Kamp, L.J.T. (eds.), *Advances in Psychological and Educational Measurement*. New York: John Wiley.
56. Choppin, B. (1978). *Item banking and the monitoring of achievement [Research in Progress, Series No. 1]*. Slough, England: National Foundation for Educational Research.
57. Choppin, B. (1979). Testing the questions; the Rasch model and item banking. *MESA Research Memorandum No. 49*. Chicago: University of Chicago, MESA Psychometric Laboratory.
58. Choppin, B. (1981). Educational measurement and the item bank model. In: Lacey, C. and Lawton, D. (eds.), *Issues in Evaluation and Accountability*. London: Methuen.
59. Weiss, D.J. and Kingsbury, G.G. (1984). Application of computerized adaptive testing to educational problems. *Journal of Educational Measurement*, **21**, 361–375.
60. Bergstrom, B.A. and Lunz, M.E. (1992). Confidence in pass/fail decisions for computer adaptive and paper and pencil examinations. *Evaluation and the Health Professions* **15**, 453–464.
61. Bunderson, V.C., Inouye, D.K. and Olsen, J.B. (1986). The four generations of computerized educational measurement. In: Linn, R.L. (ed.), *Educational Measurement*. New York: Macmillan Publishing.
62. Lautenschlager, G.J. and Flaherty, V.L. (1990). Computer administration of questions: more desirable or more social desirability? *Journal of Applied Psychology* **75**, 310–314.
63. Reckase, M.D. (1989). Adaptive testing: the evolution of a good idea. *Educational Measurement: Issues and Practice* **8**, 3.

64. Butcher, J.N. (1987). *Computerized Psychological Assessment: A Practitioner's Guide*. New York: Basic Books.
65. Waller, N.G. and Reise, S.P. (1989). Computerized adaptive personality assessment: An illustration with the absorption scale. *Journal of Personality and Social Psychology* **57**, 1051–1058.
66. Weiss, D.J. (1985). Adaptive testing by computer. *Journal of Consulting and Clinical Psychology* **53**, 774–789.
67. Sand, W.A., Waters, B.K., and McBride, J.R., eds. (1997). *Computer adaptive testing: From inquiry to operation*. Washington, DC: American Psychological Association.
68. Fisher, W.P., Jr. (1997). Equating the MOS SF36 and the LSU HIS Physical Functioning Scales. *Journal of Outcome Measurement* **1**, 329–362.
69. Fisher, W.P., Jr. (1997). Physical disability construct convergence across instruments: towards a universal metric. *Journal of Outcome Measurement* **1**, 87–113.
70. Fisher, W.P., Jr. (1998). A research program for accountable and patient-centered health outcome measures. *Journal of Outcome Measurement* **2**, 222–239.
71. Green, B.F., Bock, R.D., Humphreys, L.G., Linn, R.B. and Reckase, M.D. (1984). Technical guidelines for assessing computerized adaptive tests. *Journal of Educational Measurement* **21**, 347–360.
72. McKinley, R.L. and Reckase, M.D. (1980). Computer applications to ability testing. *Association for Educational Data Systems Journal* **13**, 193–203.
73. McKinley, R.L. and Reckase, M.D. (1984). Implementing an adaptive testing program in an instructional program environment. Paper presented at the meeting of the American Educational Research Association, New Orleans, LA.
74. Urry, V.W. (1977). Tailored testing: a successful application of latent trait theory. *Journal of Educational Measurement* **14**, 181–196.
75. Olsen, J.B., Maynes, D.D., Slawson, D. and Ho, K. (1986). Comparison and equating of paper-administered, computer-administered and computerized adaptive test of achievement. Paper presented at the meeting of the American Educational Research Association, San Francisco, CA.
76. Weiss, D.J. (1983). *New Horizons in Testing: Latent Trait Test Theory and Computerized Adaptive Testing*. New York: Academic Press.

GRAPHICAL RASCH MODELS

SVEND KREINER[1] AND KARL BANG CHRISTENSEN[2]

[1]*University of Copenhagen and* [2]*National Institute of Occupational Health, Denmark*

This paper defines a class of multivariate models combining features of Rasch type models with features of graphical interaction models into a common framework for analysis of criterion related construct validity and differential item functioning. Item analysis by Graphical Rasch models is illustrated with reanalysis of a summary Health scale counting numbers of experienced symptoms within the last six months.

1. Introduction

Index scales summarizing information from item responses are often used to analyze the association between outcomes on Health related QOL items and other variables. Analyses of validity and quality of such scales using a psychometric model often address the properties of the summary scales relative to clinical applications. The validity of the index scales for statistical purposes is rarely considered. Kreiner (1993) discussed a Health scale counting the number of different symptoms experienced within a period of half a year. The scale appears to be criterion valid and construct valid, and item analysis accepts the Rasch (1960) model as an adequate description of item responses. The subsequent analysis of the relationship between the number of symptoms and exogenous variables found no evidence of a relationship between age and the number of symptoms. An analysis of the relationship between separate items and age suggests that the items consist of two groups, one consisting of symptoms that appear more frequently with age and another consisting of symptoms that appear less frequently with age. The conclusion of this more careful analysis is that age is a factor of importance for Health. Even though the summary scale was strongly correlated with Self Reported Health and even though the item responses seemed to fit the Rasch model it turned out that the scale was inappropriate for the analysis of the association between age and health. Analysis of Differential Item Functioning (DIF) can identify this type of problem. Because standard techniques only treat the potential sources of DIF as stratification factors defining groups that may be compared with respect to item responses this type of analysis will not always be able to pinpoint the exact nature of DIF. A more powerful analysis requires that items, latent variables and exogenous variables are integrated into one common modeling framework within which both the reasons for and the consequences of differential item functioning may be addressed.

This paper suggests one such framework using the graphical models first described by Darroch, Lauritzen and Speed (1980). A model fitting this framework will be referred to as a graphical Rasch model (GRM). Section 2 defines the model and discusses the difference between the assumptions of the Rasch model and the assumptions of the graphical Rasch model. Section 3 discusses the implication for item analysis by the

M. Mesbah et al. (eds.), Statistical Methods for Quality of Life Studies, 187–203.

graphical Rasch models focusing analysis of DIF and of local dependence. Section 4 discusses the implications of the Graphical Rasch model for analysis of association among raw scores, latent variables and exogenous variables. The focus here will be on the implications in terms of collapsibility and the possible problems created by violations of the assumptions of the GRM. Finally section 5 illustrates the methods with a reanalysis of the symptom scale discussed above.

2. Definition: The Graphical Rasch Model.

2.1 Graphical Models

Let $X_1,\ldots,X_k$ be a set of random variables organized into a recursive set of blocks

$$(X_1,\ldots,X_a) \Leftarrow (X_{a+1},\ldots,X_b) \Leftarrow (X_{b+1},\ldots,X_c) \Leftarrow \ldots \Leftarrow (X_{j+1},\ldots,X_k).$$

This recursive structure is often assumed to represent temporal and/or causal structure. When focus is on a single variable or a subset of variables we refer to variables in the same block as current variables and to variables in earlier blocks as prior variables. A model defined by the product of conditional distributions of variables in separate blocks given the sets of prior variables is called recursive. A chain graph model is a block recursive model defined by conditional independence of pairs of variables given all other current or prior variables. A graphical model may be illustrated by interaction graphs where variables are represented by nodes connected by edges (among variables in the same block) and arrows (among variables in different blocks) omitting edges and arrows between conditionally independent variables. We refer to Whittaker (1990), Edwards (2000), Lauritzen (1996) and Cox and Wermuth (1996) where graphical models are discussed at some length.

Unconnected variables of undirected interaction graphs are conditional independent given sets of variables that separate the variables in the graph. This result is referred to as the separation theorem, (Whittaker, 1990). This means that any path between the two variables along the edges of the graph has to visit at least one of the variables of the separating set. For directed graphs representing chain graph models a similar result applies, permitting all kinds of paths between prior explanatory variables whether or not these are connected. In Figure 1 below items are separated by the latent variable. It therefore follows that items are pairwise conditionally independent given the latent variable. Other examples of separation in graphical models will be discussed in the following sections.

Nothing has been said about the nature of the variables of graphical models or the way they are distributed apart from the assumptions on conditional independence. Such assumptions are in most case too weak to define useful statistical models. If all variables are categorical graphical models are hierarchical loglinear models defined by generating sets corresponding to the so-called cliques of the graphs (Darroch, Lauritzen and Speed, 1980). Graphical models are therefore in most cases models where higher order interaction parameters are assumed to be present. Assuming that associations among variables are homogeneous across different levels of some variables leads to the full class of hierarchical loglinear models. If some or all variables are continuous some kind of assumptions concerning the distribution of these variables have to be imposed on the models. For the moment the only practical assumption is that the conditional distribution of a set of continuous variables given all current or prior categorical variables is a multivariate normal distribution.

One of the advantages of graphical models is that collapsibility properties of the models may be read directly off the interaction graphs. A multidimensional model is collapsible unto a smaller marginal model if some of the properties of the complete model may be recovered in the marginal model. One may distinguish between parametric collapsibility where some of the parameters of the complete model, e.g. parameters describing the association between two variables, survives unchanged after collapsing and stronger kinds of collapsibility where not only parameters, but also estimates and certain test statistics relating to these parameters are the same for the complete and the marginal models. Kreiner (1998) discusses the relationship between collapsibility and separation and decomposition of graphical models.

The GRM defined in Section 2.3 below is a graphical model enhanced by another type of assumption concerning the distribution of items. The assumption implies that the model is characterized not by one but by two different interaction graphs.

2.2 Rasch Models

The Rasch model (RM) assumes that item responses depend on a univariate latent variable and that:

1. Items are conditionally independent given the latent variable (local independence),
2. The raw score is a sufficient statistic for the person parameter (the main feature of the Rasch type models) in the conditional distribution of items given the latent variable,
3. The conditional distribution of items given the latent variable is the same, whichever way the persons are sampled (one of several consequences of Rasch's definition of specific objectivity, Rasch, 1977).

Assumption 1 contains an explicit reference to conditional independence, the basic concept underlying graphical models. Assumptions 2 and 3 can however also be interpreted in terms of conditional independence.

These assumptions leads for dichotomous items to the classical Rasch (1960) model where item responses, $Y_1,\ldots,Y_k$ depend on item parameters, φ_i, and person parameter θ:

$$P(Y_i = 1) = \frac{\theta\phi_i}{1+\theta\phi_i}.$$

In the setup discussed here, θ will however be regarded as a latent variable. As definitions of sufficiency usually assume that parameters are unknown constants we therefore have to paraphrase assumption 2 in terms of Bayesian sufficiency as suggested by Kolmogoroff (1942). The definition of Bayesian sufficiency hinges on the following result discussed by Arnold (1988):

> Let X be a vector of observed variables while θ is an unknown random vector and $S(X)$ is a statistic defined as function of X. θ is conditionally independent of X given $S(X)$ if and only if $S(X)$ is a sufficient statistic for θ in the conditional distribution of X given θ.

This result suggests that Bayesian sufficiency is a question of conditional independence: $S(X)$ is a Bayesian sufficient statistic if the conditional (posterior) distribution of θ given X only depends on X through $S(X)$, that is if θ and X are conditionally independent given S.

The equivalence of sufficiency in the frequentist sense of the word and Bayesian sufficiency as defined above implies that assumption 2 should be replaced with the assumption that items and the latent variable are conditionally independent given the latent variable.

Specific objectivity according to Rasch implies that distributions of item responses and estimates of item parameters should only depend on the values of the latent variables and not on the way persons are sampled as long as they are sampled from within the specific frame of reference where objectivity is assumed to be feasible. Item characteristic curves describing the probabilities of specific responses as functions of person parameters should therefore be the same whether or not the sample only includes men, women, old, young or consists of in fact of persons from any sub-population for which an exogenous variable has a specific value. Or in other words: Item characteristic curves must not depend on values of any variable that can be defined within the frame of reference of the measurement-items and exogenous variables must be conditionally independent. In addition to this objectivity also requires that items are interchangeable in the sense that any subscale defined by a subset of items also adhere to the Rasch models and that Baysian sufficiency therefore applies for all subsets of items.

It has been shown that local independence and sufficiency characterize the dichotomous RM under very general constraints, Andersen (1977). Restated in terms of Bayesian sufficiency for latent variables we therefore see that the RM for dichotomous items is characterized by certain assumptions on conditional independence. The RM for dichotomous items is therefore related to graphical models in a natural way as a model defined by conditional independence. This has been one of the main motivations for the definition of the GRM models below.

2.3 *Graphical Rasch Models*

Consider a set of (dichotomous or polytomous) items, $Y_1,\ldots,Y_k$, a summary raw score, $S = \Sigma Y_i$, a latent variable, θ, a set of criterion variables, $C_1,\ldots,C_c$, and a set of exogenous variables, $X_1,\ldots,X_m$. We use the following notation

$$Y = (Y_1,\ldots,Y_k)$$

$$Y^{(i)} = (Y_1,\ldots,Y_{i-1},Y_{i+1},\ldots,Y_k)$$

$$Y^{(ij)} = (Y_1,\ldots,Y_{i-1},Y_{i+1},\ldots,Y_{j-1},Y_{j+1},\ldots,Y_k).$$

In the same way X, $X^{(i)}$ and $X^{(ij)}$ denote sets of exogenous variables from which none, one or two has been removed. Criterion variables are included to provide a general setting for both item analysis and criterion validity. Apart from this consideration criterion variables are regarded as exogenous variables. Unless otherwise specifically stated any reference to exogenous variables may refer to both criterion variables and/or proper exogenous variables.

A graphical Rasch model (GRM) is defined by the assumptions of conditional independence given by formulas (1) to (4) below (illustrated in Figures 1 and 2 for four items). The assumptions of conditional independence and absence of DIF are

$$Y_i \perp Y_j \mid \theta, Y^{(ij)}, X \quad (1)$$

$$Y_i \perp X_j \mid \theta, Y^{(j)}, X^{(j)} \quad (2)$$

for all items and exogenous variables. Items are assumed to be pairwise conditionally independent given the latent variable, and all other items, and all exogenous variables. These assumptions are stronger than established definitions. Criterion validity within the GRM is a stronger requirement than criterion validity based on assumptions on marginal relationships, because not only marginal, but also non-vanishing partial correlation between scales and criterion variables is required. Conditioning on all other variables of the model should not result in conditional independence between the latent variable and a criterion variable. Figure 1 illustrates assumptions (1) and (2). Bold arrows indicate associations that are specifically assumed to exist, while ordinary arrows/edges represent potential associations among variables.

We are not only interested in the set of items but also in the possibilities of using the raw score as a measure of the latent variable. To justify the use of the score in such a way we introduce the assumptions

$$Y \perp \theta \mid S, X \quad (3)$$

$$Y \perp X_j \mid S, \theta, X^{(j)}. \quad (4)$$

If Y is regarded as one variable, (3) and (4) define the graphical model illustrated in Figure 2. A consequence of the graphical structure is that the joint distribution of all the variables may be partitioned into a product of the conditional distribution of items given the latent variable and the joint distribution of the latent variable and exogenous variables:

$$P(Y_1,\ldots,Y_k \mid \theta)\, P(\theta,X).$$

Figure 1. Local independence and absence of DIF in a model with two criterion variables (Crit1 and Crit2) and three exogenous variables (Exo1, Exo2 and Exo3).

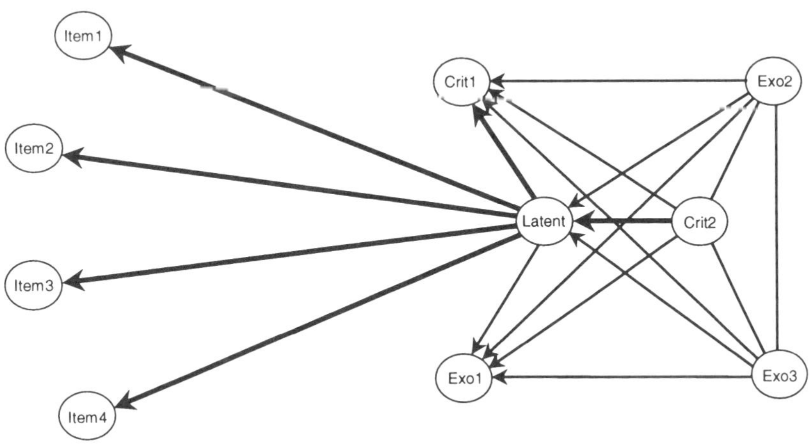

Figure 2. Interaction graph implying Bayesian sufficiency. The items are treated as one variable.

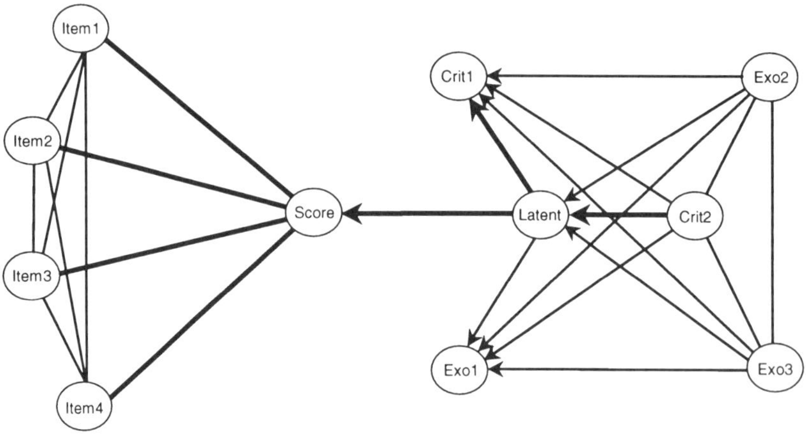

The measurement model may be further decomposed into the conditional distribution of items given the raw score and the conditional distribution of the raw score given θ:

$$P(Y_1,\ldots,Y_k \mid S)\ P(S \mid \theta)\ P(\theta,X). \tag{5}$$

It follows from (5) that inference about the association between θ and the exogenous variables may be performed in the marginal (S,θ,X) distribution. In other words, the model is collapsible over the items. The GRM in this way provides the justification for using the raw score instead of the complete set of item responses for the analysis.

The GRM is defined in terms of conditional independence. Additional assumptions about the conditional distribution of item responses given the latent variable are needed for a complete specification of the model. A large family of Rasch models for polytomous items, including the partial credit model of Masters (1982) and the rating scale model of Andrich (1978), all share the property of sufficiency and exchangeability of items with the dichotomous RM. This family consists of distributions for which the conditional distribution of an item given the latent variable is a power series distribution

$$P(Y_i = y|\theta) = \frac{\theta^y \gamma_{iy}}{\sum_z \theta^z \gamma_{iz}}, \tag{6}$$

where γ_{ix} are item parameters depending on item scores. Constraints are needed to identify the parameters, and additional constraints may be imposed to simplify the models. The rating scale model thus assumes that item parameters may be expressed as a function of an one dimensional item parameter and a common score parameter for all items:

$$\gamma_{iy} = \varphi_i^y \gamma_y.$$

In the remaining part of this paper we assume that the measurement component of the Graphical Rasch models is defined by the power series distribution (6).

2.4 Differential Item Functioning

The separation property of GRM implies that the requirement of no DIF is satisfied no matter if the latent variable or the raw score is used as a stratifying control variable, i.e.

$$Y_i \perp X_j \mid \theta \tag{7}$$

$$Y_i \perp X_j \mid S \tag{8}$$

both (7) and (8) have been used as the criteria of no item bias. The separation properties of GRM insist that both criteria must be satisfied and furthermore that the definition of no DIF can be extended to requirements of conditional independence of subsets of items and subsets of exogenous variables. That is,

$$(Y_1,\ldots,Y_j) \perp (X_a,\ldots,X_b) \mid \theta$$

$$(Y_1,\ldots,Y_j) \perp (X_a,\ldots,X_b) \mid S. \tag{9}$$

It is not unusual that analysis of DIF suggests that certain items seem to be biased for more than one exogenous variable. In this situation it is difficult to understand the reason for the DIF and thus to decide how to deal with it. GRM is a framework within which it is fairly straightforward to deal with this, because it possible to distinguish between genuine and spurious DIF. Assume for instance that item Y_i seems to be biased for several exogenous variables, $X_1,\ldots,X_a$ in the sense that (7) and (8) are rejected for all these variables. If the hypotheses

$$Y_i \perp X_j \mid \theta, X_1,\ldots X_{j-1},X_{j+1},\ldots,X_a \tag{10}$$

$$Y_i \perp X_j \mid S, X_1,\ldots X_{j-1},X_{j+1},\ldots,X_a \tag{11}$$

are acceptable the bias of item Y_i with respect to X_j should be regarded as spurious item bias. This distinction between spurious and genuine item bias allows a definition of the *origin* of item bias as the complete set of exogenous variables for which item bias is genuine.

2.5 Graphical and Loglinear Rasch Models

Glas and Verhelst (1995) discuss different directions to be followed when evidence against the RM has been disclosed. If the motive is to construct a pure Rasch scale, ill-fitting items must be removed. This section describes an alternative approach based on GRM models that in several cases has proven viable.

The GRM is based on four different types of assumptions: existence of a univariate latent variable, a Bayesian sufficient raw score, locally independent items, and absence of DIF. The two first assumptions are the basic substantial assumptions on which the idea of a summary index scale is founded. The two remaining assumptions are technical and relate to the selection or creation of items. It is important to recognize that evidence against a GRM in some cases only means that technical assumptions have been violated. The set of items and the scoring may be substantially sound in the sense that there actually is an univariate latent variable responsible for the variation among items with a Bayesian sufficient raw score for which (3) applies even though (1), (2) and/or (4) is fallacious. In this case, one should first try to model the item bias or local dependence of which evidence has been disclosed before removing items or rejecting the hypothesis of a univariate latent variable.

The assumptions of local independence and no item bias may be relaxed by introduction of a loglinear structure among items and exogenous variables in the conditional distribution of items given then latent and exogenous variables, (θ,X).

The joint conditional distribution of item responses given (θ,X) is a distribution across a multidimensional contingency table. This means that the model can be parametricized as a loglinear model. The model may in the completely general case be a saturated model with parameters depending on the observed values of both θ and X. For the model with locally independent responses, no item bias, and distributions given by (6) the joint distribution of items given specific values of θ and X is a particular simple loglinear model with main effect parameters depending on θ.

$$\begin{aligned}\ln[\mathrm{P}(Y_1 = y_1, \ldots, Y_k = y_k|\theta, X)] &= \ln\left(\frac{\prod_i \theta^{y_i}\gamma_{iy_i}}{\prod_i \sum_z \theta^z \gamma_{iz}}\right) \\ &= \ln\left(\frac{\theta^{\sum_i y_i}\prod_i \gamma_{iy_i}}{\prod_i \sum_z \theta^z \gamma_{iz}}\right) \\ &= \alpha_0 + \sum_i \alpha_{iy_i} + \beta \sum_i y_i \\ &= \alpha_0 + \sum_i (\alpha_{iy_i} + \beta y_i),\end{aligned} \tag{12}$$

where $\alpha_{iy} = \ln(\gamma_{iy})$ and $\beta = \ln(\theta)$.

The model (12) contains no higher order interactions among items and exogenous variables. Adding interaction terms to (12) that do not depend on θ yields a so-called loglinear Rasch model (Kelderman, 1984, 1995). Including interactions between item 1 and item 2 and between item 3 and the first exogenous variables in (12) thus defines a model

$$\ln[\mathrm{P}(Y_1, \ldots, Y_k|\theta, X)] = \alpha_0 + \sum_i (\alpha_{iy_i} + \beta y_i) + \lambda^{1,2}_{y_1 y_2} + \kappa^{3,1}_{y_3 x_1} \tag{13}$$

incorporating local dependence and DIF without sacrificing the idea of a unidimensional latent variable and a sufficient raw score.

Notice first, that removing items Y_1 to Y_3 from the model defined by (13) leads to a model for an uncontaminated set of items satisfying all the assumptions of GRM. If Y_3 is reintroduced, a model is defined where the set of items fits the GRM for different levels of X_1 and where item contrasts (differences between item parameters) between the other items are the same for all X_1 levels. The only difference between the models for different levels of X_1 is the contrasts between Y_3 and the other items. This situation is referred to as uniform item bias by Hanson (1998) and Whitmore and Schumacker (1999).

The situation complicates if the first two items are reintroduced. The λ parameters of (13) define a model where the two first items are no longer locally independent because these two items are not conditionally independent. (13) assumes that the latent variable does not influence the size of the λ parameters in exactly the same way as it did not influence the item bias parameters discussed above. In accordance with the definition of uniform item bias we will refer to this situation as a case of uniform local dependency.

Model (12) may be augmented with any number of interaction parameters describing uniform local dependency and item bias. As long as the latent variable has no effect on the interactions between items and exogenous variables the raw score will still be a sufficient statistic for the latent variable and conditioning with the raw score will still separate item parameters from the distribution of the latent variable in exactly the same way as for the classical Rasch models. The analysis of the association between the latent and exogenous variables complicates however as discussed in the next section of this paper.

The family of loglinear Rasch models fits easily within the GRM framework leading to a family of Graphical and loglinear Rasch models (GLLRM). The complete family of models discussed here can be summarized in the following way, where the term "graphical" refers to the structure connecting the measurement model to the exogenous variables while the "loglinear" terms refer to the specific item structure within the measurement component.

Rasch models describing the dependence of item responses on the latent variable. There are no exogenous variables in this family of models. Items are assumed to be locally independent.

Graphical Rasch models are models with both items and exogenous variables. Items are assumed to be unbiased and locally independent. The model decomposes into a measurement component – a Rasch model – and a graphical model describing associations between the latent variable and the exogenous variables.

Loglinear and graphical Rasch models are models permitting uniform local dependence and uniform item bias. That is, association among items and exogenous variables that do not depend on the latent variable. Decomposition properties may be somewhat more complicated than for graphical Rasch models, but the raw score is still a Bayesian sufficient statistic.

3. Item Analysis by Graphical and Loglinear Rasch Models

3.1 Testing the adequacy of the Graphical Rasch model

The techniques connected with conditional inference in the Rasch model carries over to the GRM because the model decomposes into two parts. The first part consists of the measurement model describing the dependence of items on the latent variable while the second part is the association model of the joint distribution of the latent variable and the exogenous variables. Collapsing over all exogenous variables lead to a marginal Rasch model characterized by local independent items and a sufficient raw score. Conditional maximum likelihood estimates of the item parameters are still consistent and evidence against the Rasch model disclosed by Andersen's (1973) conditional likelihood ratio tests comparing estimates of item parameters in different score groups is also evidence against a graphical Rasch model.

Marginal inference in the RM is based on the assumption that the latent variable follows a specific distribution. The univariate normal distribution is a very popular choice. Within the framework defined by GRM the distribution of the latent variable has to be specified as a *conditional* distribution of θ given the set of current and prior exogenous variables. The standard techniques for marginal inference implemented in several computer packages therefore do not automatically apply for the GRM.

3.2. Analysis of Differential Item Functioning

The Graphical Rasch model reconciles two basically different approaches to conditional analysis of DIF: The Mantel-Haenszel test discussed in Holland and Wainer (1993) tests the hypotheses (8) of conditional independence in $2 \times 2 \times M$ contingency tables, showing the conditional relationship between an item and an exogenous variable given the score. The Andersen (1973) test comparing conditional likelihood ratio estimates of item parameters in different groups is a test of the hypothesis given by (9). Both (8) and (9) are necessary consequences of the GRM. Both procedures are therefore valid attempts to disqualify the models.

The Mantel-Haenszel test is restricted to binary items and binary exogenous variable. The hypotheses given by (8) apply however also for ordinal items and exogenous variables with more than two levels. A more general approach to tests for conditional independence of ordinal items and ordinal exogenous variables would be to use a partial gamma coefficient instead of the odds-ratio statistic used by the Mantel-Haenszel procedure. We refer to Agresti (1984) for a discussion of test statistics for ordinal data and to Kreiner (1987) who describes Monte Carlo techniques for exact conditional tests using partial gamma coefficients. The partial gamma coefficient for binary items and binary exogenous variables degenerates to a test statistic which is an estimate of a one-to-one function of the same partial odds ratio value estimated by the Mantel-Hanszel statistic.

The above mentioned standard techniques for analysis of differential item functioning can without problems be extended to analysis of the origins of item bias as defined by (10) and (11). Mantel-Haenszel techniques and partial gamma coefficients apply equally well for tests of conditional independence in multidimensional contingency tables of any dimension. A conditional likelihood ratio tests that an exogenous variable is not an origin of item bias requires that conditional likelihood ratio test comparing item parameter estimates in subpopulations defined by the exogenous variable are in several different strata and later added together into one summary likelihood ratio statistic.

3.3 Analysis of Local Dependency

The fact that any subset of items defines a Bayesian sufficient subscore of items suggests a whole range of tests for local dependence. To see this consider two different items, Y_i and Y_j and a score, T, defined by a subset of item including one but not both items as illustrated in Figure 3 showing the independence graph of a model with a subscore excluding a single item. It is an immediate consequence of the separation theorem of graphical models that the two items has to be conditionally independent given T.

The result is quite general: Let Y and X be the vectors of items and exogenous variables of a graphical Rasch model. It the follows for all pairs of items, Y_i and Y_j and all subscores, T, including one but not both items that

$$Y_i \perp Y_j \mid T. \tag{14}$$

Note that (14) does not depend on the exogenous variables and therefore applies for all kinds of Rasch type models where the set of exogenous variables is empty.

Figure 3. Independence graph for a subscore defined by a graphical Rasch model

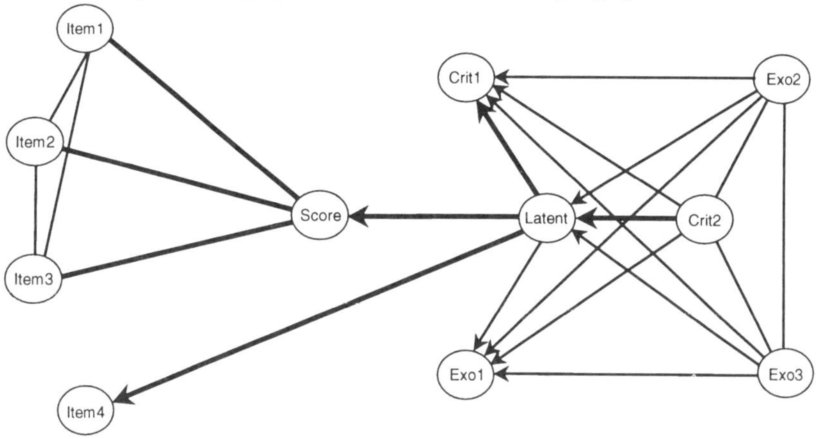

Tjur (1982) showed for the RM for dichotomous items that any items Y_1 and Y_2 will be conditionally independent given the sum of one of these items with a third item, $Y_1 \perp Y_2 \mid Y_1 + Y_2$. (14) generalizes this result to conditional independence of polytomous items given any subscore including one of the two items. We will therefore refer to violation of (14) as violation of Tjur conditions depending only on the Bayesian sufficiency of subscores. We also notice that analysis of local dependency based on (14) in technical terms is equivalent to analysis of different item functioning because subtraction of an item from a summary score as in Figure 3 redefines the item as an exogenous variable. It follows therefore not only that a test of (14) is equivalent to the test of item bias suggested by (10), but also that all other approaches to analysis and modeling of item bias may be used for analysis and modeling of local dependency.

3.4 Item Analysis by Loglinear Rasch Models

Evidence that certain items do not fit within a GRM framework may suggest that these items should be rejected before the raw score is calculated. While it is true that a pure Rasch scale in many ways lead to a fairly simple statistical analysis of association, removing items will reduce the reliability of the scale and therefore also result in reduced power of the statistical analysis. Items should therefore only be removed as a last resort when all other attempts to deal with the problems indicated by the evidence against the Rasch models have failed. Before items are removed one should examine whether or not uniform item bias or uniform local dependency seems to be the reason for the lack of fit of the Rasch model. If this turns out to be the case loglinear modeling of item bias and local dependency is feasible and may be a better solution than simply removing contaminated items.

One advantage of the loglinear Rasch models is that conditional inference still applies. Conditioning with respect to the raw score effectively separates the latent nuisance variable from item parameters and the item bias parameters. Estimates of this extended set of item parameters are consistent and conditional likelihood ratio tests apply in exactly the same way as for standard Rasch models. The loglinear Rasch model framework in this way leads to

(1) Tests of homogeneity of the extended set of item parameters across different score groups or across sub groups defined by exogenous variables.
(2) Conditional likelihood ratio tests of vanishing parameters for item bias and local dependency.
(3) Loglinear modeling of item bias by standard strategies for model search among loglinear models based on conditional likelihood ratio tests, identifying not only origins of item bias but also sources of apparent local dependency.

4. Analysis of Association by GRM

Items are assumed to be discrete. The summary score will therefore also be a discrete variable with a finite number of possible outcomes. Collapsibility properties inferred by decomposition of graphical models imply that results of an analysis of the association between the score and the exogenous variables will be the same as the results from an analysis of the association between the complete set of items and the exogenous variables. In other words: If the assumptions underlying the graphical models are satisfied then data reduction by replacement of the complete set of item responses with the summary scores is justified.

When uniform DIF and/or local dependency is present the index scale may still be a useful summary measure, but collapsibility properties will be more complicated. The situation is illustrated in Figure 4 showing a graphical and loglinear Rasch model with uniform local dependence between two items and one uniformly biased item. To simplify the structure some assumptions of conditional independence among exogenous variables have been added to the model. For the same reason the model has been collapsed over the latent variable even though no assumption has been made at this point whether or not the analysis of association should address the manifest or the latent structure.

The model represented by Figure 4 is strictly speaking not a ordinary graphical model because the loglinear structure of the measurement component implies that certain higher order interaction parameters vanish. There can for instance be no 3-way interaction between the score, Item 4 and Exo 1. Collapsibility properties may nevertheless be read off the interaction graph as for any standard graphical model.

Notice first that the local dependency of items 1 and 2 has no influence on the way the model collapses for an analysis of the association between the score and the exogenous variables. Local dependency will of course influence the estimates of the item parameters and therefore also the parameters of the conditional distribution of the score given the latent variable, but there is no way in which local dependency can influence the interaction parameters describing the effect of the exogenous variables.

The item bias will on the other hand confound the analysis of the effect of the exogenous variables if it is not taken into account during the analysis. Assume that the purpose of the study is to analyze the effect of the exogenous variables, Exo1 and Exo3, on the raw score. For this purpose the model collapses in two different ways one of which may actually be regarded as somewhat surprising.

The model given by Figure 4 is collapsible onto the marginal model of the score, Item 4, the two criterion variables and Exo1 with respect to the interaction between Exo1 and the score. The Score-by-Exo1 interaction can therefore be analyzed conditionally given Item4, Crit1 and Crit2. As Item 4 is part of the definition of the raw score this

Figure 4. An interaction graph for a graphical loglinear Rasch model collapsed unto the manifest variables. The bold edge between Item 1 and Item 2 indicates that these items are assumed to be uniformly locally dependent. The edge between Item 4 and Exo 1 represents uniform item bias of Item 4 with Exo 1 as the origin of differential item functioning.

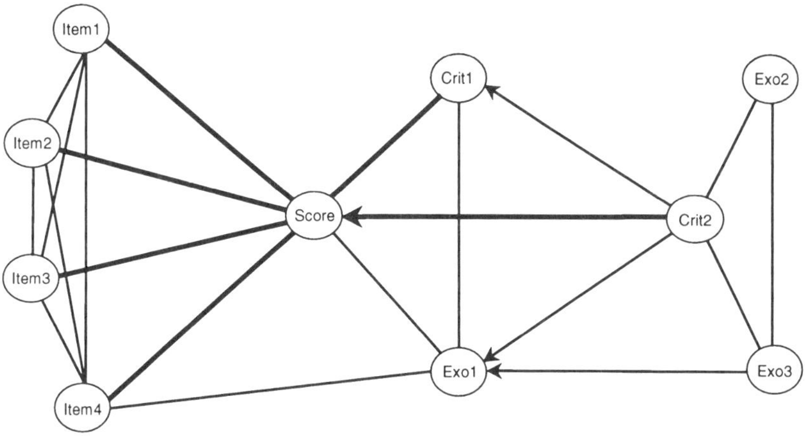

means that the analysis of the association between the score and Exo1 reduces to an analysis of the conditional distribution of the sub score, S_4 = S-Item 4 given Item 4, Crit1 and Crit2. For this specific purpose the differential functioning of Item 4 means that the item should be removed from the score. This does not imply however, that Item 4 should be completely disregarded during then analysis. For the analysis of the association between the score and Exo3 the model given by Figure 4 is however also collapses onto the marginal model of the Score, Exo1, Exo3 and Crit2. Crit2 and the Score-by-Exo3 interaction parameters should be estimated conditionally given Exo1 and Crit1 and a test of vanishing Score-by-Exo3 interaction parameters should be a test of conditional independence of the score and Exo3 given Exo1 and. This means that the complete score can be used for an analysis of the association between the score and Exo3 even though one of the items is biased as long as the origin of item bias is included in the analysis as well.

5. An Example

We illustrate the item analysis by graphical loglinear Rasch models by reanalysis of data from a population study of self-care and health related behavior in Denmark. A previous analysis (Kreiner, 1993) examined the criterion related construct validity of a symptom scale summarizing responses to questions concerning twelve different symptoms. The analysis disclosed evidence DIF with respect to age, suggesting that the symptom scale covered two different Health dimensions, the first of which was positively and the second negatively related to Age. Table 1 shows the items of the two different subscales:

Even though Rasch models seemed to be adequate for the two subscales the question remained whether a two-dimensional latent construct was justified. First, no substantial arguments were forwarded supporting the distinction between two different symptom

Table 1. Symptoms included in two symptom indices

Items that were positively related to age	Items that were negative related to age
Cough	Nose and throat
Muscle Pain	Fever
Eyes	Stomach
Dizziness, fainting	Indigestion
Back pain	Rash
Chest pain	Mouth and gums

Table 2. Conditional LR tests of homogenous item and DIF parameters. Test are shown for both the GRM with no DIF and no local dependence and for the GLLRM of Figure 5

Groups defined by	GRM	GLLRM
Score groups 1, 2, 3+	$\chi^2 = 31.4$, df = 22, p = 0.09	$\chi^2 = 58.0$, df = 44, p = 0.08
Sex	$\chi^2 = 11.6$, df = 11, p = 0.40	$\chi^2 = 13.7$, df = 20, p = 0.85
SRH	$\chi^2 = 36.9$, df = 33, p = 0.29	$\chi^2 = 32.5$, df = 38, p = 0.72
Age	$\chi^2 = 50.8$, df = 22, p = 0.0004	$\chi^2 = 38.8$, df = 26, p = 0.051

Figure 5. Independence graph of loglinear graphical Rasch model for symptom items

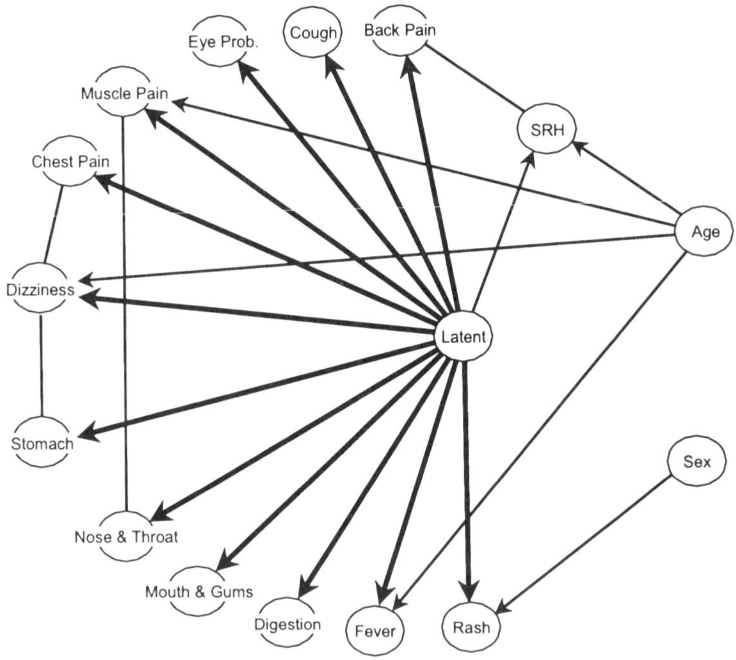

dimensions and second strong evidence of item bias only existed for muscle pain and fever. Second, no attempt was made to formulate a complete model covering the complete inference frame of items, latent variables and exogenous variables. The data was therefore reanalyzed to investigate the degree to which departures from the Rasch model for the complete set of items could be explained by the presence of uniform differential item functioning and/or uniform local dependency. Figure 5 shows the interaction graph for the most parsimonious GLLRM with two exogenous variables (sex and age) and one criterion variable (self-reported health) fitting the data. Tests of fit by conditional likelihood ratio tests comparing item and DIF parameters in subgroups defined by score groups and exogenous variables are shown in Table 2.

The model indicates that one latent susceptibility variable gives an adequate description of responses to the symptom items if local dependency and DIF is taken into account. Age is the origin of item bias for three items two of which (muscle pain and dizziness) occur more frequently with increasing age while the third, fever, occurs with decreasing frequency with increasing age. Some evidence of DIF against sex and self reported health (SRH) was also disclosed. We notice that the association between SRH and back pain was found to be stronger than one would expect if they had been conditionally independent given the latent variable.

It was suggested by Kreiner (1993) that symptom depended on two related but different latent dimensions. If this had been correct one would have expected to find evidence of positive local dependency between items from one and the same dimension and negative local dependency between items from different dimensions. The fact that very little evidence of local dependency was disclosed in the current analysis with one latent dimension supports the impression that the prior conclusion was incorrect. It is worth noting also that evidence of positive local dependency was found only for dizziness and chest pain and that all remaining suggestions of local dependency indicate negative local dependency between some (apparently competing) symptoms.

Age and sex are both origins of DIF, but neither variable seems to be directly related to the latent variable. There is an effect of age and sex on specific symptoms, but no effect of these variables on susceptibility as such: Partial γ coefficients controlling for exogenous variables and biased items were equal to -0.14 ($p = 0.082$) for age and equal to $+0.10$ ($p = 0.204$) for sex. Finally criterion validity is established by a strongly significant positive partial correlation ($\gamma = 0.31$, $p < 0.0005$) between the symptom index and SRH.

6. Discussion

The main purpose of this paper has been to define an integrated association and measurement model that justifies the use of a summary scale instead of a high dimensional vector of item responses. The GRM and GLLRM are two such models. Many of the important features of Rasch models transfer to the GRM and one might with some justification argue that the GRM are nothing but a common sense representation of much practice related to use of the Rasch models. The main advantage of building such models lies however not only in the way that the assumptions on which the use of Rasch scales for analysis of association are founded is clarified and additional test are suggested. GRM and GLLRM are also important because they shed light on the role of some basic concepts. The fact for instance that local dependency is a minor problem and that differential item functioning is of no consequence for certain applications of the index scales can not be seen or hardly discussed without a complete model defining the complete inference frame for the intended analysis.

REFERENCES

Agresti, A. (1984). *Analysis of Ordinal Categorical Data*. New York: Wiley.

Andersen, E.B. (1973). A goodness of fit test for the Rasch model. *Psychometrika* **38**, 123–140.

Andersen, E.B. (1977). Sufficient statistics and latent trait models. *Psychometrika* **42**, 69–81.

Andrich, D. (1978). A rating formulation for ordered response categories. *Psychometrika* **43**, 561–573.

Arnold, S.F. (1988). Sufficient Statistics. In: Kotz, S. and Johnson, N.L. (eds.), *Encyclopedia of Statistical Sciences*. New York: Wiley.

Cox, D.R. and Wermuth, N. (1996). *Multivariate Dependencies: Models, Analysis and Interpretation*. London: Chapman and Hall.

Darroch, J.N., Lauritzen, S.L. and Speed, T. (1980). Markov fields and log-linear interaction models for contingency tables. *Annals of Statistics* **8**, 522–539.

Edwards, D. (2000). *Introduction to Graphical Modelling. 2nd Edition*. New York: Springer-Verlag.

Glas, C.A.W and Verhelst, N.D. (1995). Testing the Rasch Model. In: Fischer, G.H. and Molenaar, I.W. (eds.), *Rasch Models: Foundations, Recent Developments and Applications*. New York: Springer-Verlag.

Hanson, B.A. (1998). Uniform DIF and DIF defined by differences in item response functions. *Journal of Educational and Behavioral Statistics* **23**, 244–253.

Holland, P.W. and Wainer, H., eds. (1993). *Differential Item Functioning*. Hillsdale: Lawrence Erlbaum Associates.

Kelderman, H. (1984). Loglinear Rasch model tests. *Psychometrika* **49**, 223–245.

Kelderman, H. (1995). The polytomous Rasch model within the class of generalized linear symmetry models. In: Fischer, G.H. and Molenaar, I.W. (eds.), *Rasch Models: Foundations, Recent Developments and Applications*. New York: Springer-Verlag

Kolmogoroff, A.N. (1942). Definitions of center of dispersion and measure of accuracy from a finite number of observations. *Izv. Akad. Nauk. SSSR Ser. Mat.* **6**, 3–32. (Russian).

Kreiner, S. (1987). Analysis of multidimensional contingency tables by exact conditional tests: techniques and strategies. *Scandinavian Journal of Statistics* **14**, 97–112.

Kreiner, S. (1993). Validation of index scales for analysis of survey data: The Symptom Index. In: Dean, K. (ed.), *Population Health Research*. London: Sage Publications.

Kreiner, S. (1998). Interaction model. In: Armitage, P. and Colton, T. (eds.), *Encyclopedia of Biostatistics*. Chichester: Wiley.

Lauritzen, S.L. (1996). *Graphical Models*. London: Clarendon Press.

Masters, G.N. (1982). A Rasch model for partial credit scoring. *Psychometrika* **47**, 149–174.

Rasch, G. (1960). *Probabilistic Models for Some Intelligence and Attainment Tests*. Copenhagen: The Danish Institute of Educational Research.

Rasch, G. (1977). On specific objectivity. An attempt at formalizing the request for generality and validity of scientific statements. In: Blegvad, M. (ed.), *The Danish Yearbook of Philosophy*. Copenhagen: Munksgaard.

Tjur, T. (1982). A connection between Rasch's item analysis model and a multiplicative Poisson model. *Scandinavian Journal of Statistics* **9**, 23–30.

Whitmore, M.L and Schumacker, R.E. (1999). A comparison of logistic regression and analysis of variance differential item functioning detection methods. *Educational and Psychological Measurement* **59**, 910–927.

Whittaker, J. (1990). *Graphical Models in Applied Multivariate Statistics.* Chichester: Wiley.

Chapter 4

Joint Analysis of Quality of Life and Survival

SEMI-MARKOV MODELS FOR QUALITY OF LIFE DATA WITH CENSORING

NATACHA HEUTTE[1] AND CATHERINE HUBER-CAROL[1,2]

[1] *Université René Descartes and* [2] *U472 INSERM*

We present a semi-parametric, semi-Markov, multi-state model for quality of life data measured in continuous time with right censoring. The model is based on the same principles as the Cox proportional hazards model. The states are defined by categorizing a quality of life score as measured using a standard instrument. Death is considered as a separate state in the model. Transitions between the states represent changes in quality of life (or death) and follow a competing risk framework. We describe the model and derive relevant estimators. We illustrate the methodology using data from a cancer clinical trial comparing quality of life for two treatment regimens.

1. Introduction

When two drugs have equivalent efficiency, it is useful to compare the quality of life they provide to the patients. For this purpose, we propose a method based on a multi-state model (Keiding, Klein and Horowitz, 2000) with competing risks. Each state is defined by a range of quality of life scores as measured using a standard instrument. Death is considered as a separate state. Transitions between the states represent changes in quality of life or the occurrence of death. We assume that the corresponding process is semi-Markov (Pyke, 1961; Cocozza-Thivent, 1997) with a finite number m of states. We take states $1, \cdots, m_1$ to be transient and states $m_1 + 1, \cdots, m$ to be absorbing. To account for the possible effect of covariates, we present a semi-Markov model in continuous time, which assumes a multiplicative model for each waiting time and is analogous to the semi-parametric Cox model (Cox, 1972; Anderson *et al.*, 1992; Dabrowska, Horowitz and Sun, 1994; Kalbfleisch and Prentice, 1980). The covariates may be qualitative or quantitative. They may be time-dependent provided that the time considered is restricted to the current state.

One may consider the time spent in a specific state as a competing risk problem (Tsiatis, 1975), where the states that can be possibly entered are in competition with one another. We define state $m + 1$ as the censored state which occurs when a transition is right censored. Under relevant assumptions about the corresponding hazards, we may consider separately the different waiting times and apply Cox's partial likelihood to each of them. This allows us to easily estimate the impact of the covariates and the probability law of the waiting time in state i before a transition to state j. We test the impact of the covariates using likelihood ratio

M. Mesbah et al. (eds.), Statistical Methods for Quality of Life Studies, 207–218.

tests and estimate the transition probability from state i to state j as a function of the time spent in state i. We apply this method to a study of the quality of life in a cancer clinical trial.

2. Description of the Data

The aim of the trial was to compare two drugs A and B in terms of quality of life. To protect confidentiality, we do not reveal details of the trial, and therefore, we refer to the two treatments simply as A and B. Drug A ($N = 109$) was the reference or control group, and drug B ($N = 106$) was the experimental group. To identify the treatment groups, we use an indicator variable ξ which is equal to 0 for drug A and 1 for drug B. Quality of life was measured at different timepoints during study follow-up using the QLQ-C30 instrument (Aaronson *et al.*, 1996). Original scores ranged from 1 to 7, with higher values denoting better quality of life. For simplicity and due to the relatively small sample size, we reduced the number of quality of life states to 3 in this analysis. State 1 is bad quality of life, state 2 is neutral quality of life, and state 3 is good quality of life. State 4 is death, and we define state 5 as the censored state. Thus we have $m_1 = 3$ transient states, one absorbing state and the special censored state.

Every patient in the study has a history that can be described as follows:

$$H = \{J_0, X_1, J_1, X_2, J_2, \ldots, X_{s-1}, J_{s-1}, X_s, J_s\},$$

where J_i is the state visited after the i-th transition ($1 \leq J_i \leq m_1$ for $i < s$, $m_1 < J_s \leq m+1$, and $m = 4$), $m_1 = 3$ is the number of transient states, and X_i is the sojourn time for state J_{i-1}. The number of visited states s may differ among the the patients.

The methodology we propose accounts for patients whose history is censored. The right censored patients are in state $J_s = m + 1$. The observed transition numbers in this study are shown in Table 1. The number of transitions from state 1 to state 3 is small, only 4 patients, and among those, 2 were in the drug A group. We therefore assume that for these patients, there was a transition through state 2 before state 3 was reached. Accordingly, we replaced the direct transition from state 1 to state 3 by a transition from state 1 to state 2 followed by a transition from state 2 to state 3. We estimate the sojourn time in state 2, $E(X|\xi)$ by $\bar{X}_{23}$, the mean duration of time spent in state 2 before entering state 3. For the patients who received drug A, $\bar{X}_{23} = 30.2$ days, and for drug B, $\bar{X}_{23} = 36.4$ days.

Table 1. Number of observed transitions

Drug A						Drug B					
States	1	2	3	4	5	States	1	2	3	4	5
1	0	17	2	20	6	1	0	13	2	22	1
2	18	0	19	21	7	2	15	0	21	30	5
3	13	22	0	32	23	3	11	30	0	26	22

Figure 1 shows the possible transitions between the different states. The patients enter into the study with a specific quality of life, bad (state 1), neutral (state 2) or good (state 3). The only covariate used here is the treatment group; however, the model could easily accommodate additional covariates. In general covariates may be qualitative or quantitative. They may be time-dependent, but in this case, the dependence must be based only on the time spent in the current state. These conditions are necessary to fulfill the semi-Markov assumption.

Figure 1. Multi-state model: quality of life in a cancer clinical trial ($1 \equiv$ bad, $2 \equiv$ neutral, $3 \equiv$ good, $4 \equiv$ death

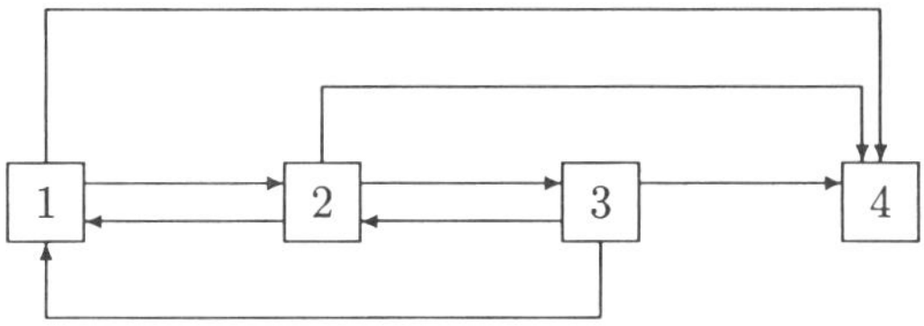

3. Model

We assume that the distribution of the sojourn time X in state i before a transition to state j may depend not only on state i but on the next state j ($\neq i$). This implies that we assume a semi-Markov model for our multi-state data.

For each patient, we observe a process $(J, X) = \{(J_s, X_s) : 0 \leq s\}$. We assume this process is semi-Markov. A semi-Markov process is a stochastic process whose state space is denumerable and whose sequence of visited states is a Markov chain. Conditionally on the Markov chain J, the sojourn times form a sequence $X = \{X_s, 0 \leq s\}$ of independent random variables with probability laws depending on the current state as well as on the next visited state. Precisely, (J, X) is a renewal process if the distribution of the sojourn times satisfies:

$$P(J_n = j, X_n \leq x | J_0, X_1, \ldots, J_{n-1}, X_{n-1}) = P(J_n = j, X_n \leq x | J_{n-1})$$

This process can be viewed as a Markov chain for which the time scale has become random. We define the sojourn times laws through the following hazard functions, conditional on the two adjacent states:

$$\lambda_{|ij,\xi}(t) = \lim_{\Delta t \to 0} \frac{P(t \leq X_{n+1} < t + \Delta t | X_{n+1} \geq t, J_n = i, J_{n+1} = j, \xi)}{\Delta t}.$$

Let $J(i)$ be the set of states that can be reached from state i. We can sketch the competing assumption as follows. If we consider independent random variables $W_{i1}, \ldots, W_{im}$ where $i = 1, \ldots, m_1$, having survival functions $G_{|i1,\xi}(t), \ldots, G_{|im,\xi}(t)$, respectively, the sojourn time X_{n+1} in state $J_n = i$ before a transition to state J_{n+1} is:

$$X_{n+1} = \min_{l \in J(i)} W_{il},$$

and $J_{n+1} = j$ if and only if $W_{ij} < W_{il}\ \forall l \in J(i), l \neq j$.

$W_{il}, l \in J(i)$ are potential sojourn times in state i before a transition to state l, the smallest of which determines the current sojourn time and the next state. The likelihood may be derived using the independence assumption.

We now write the likelihood of our model. The likelihood contribution of a transition between $J_n = i$ and $J_{n+1} = j$, with no censoring, after a sojourn time in state i equal to x is:

$$\begin{aligned}
&P(J_{n+1} = j|J_n = i, \xi)\frac{\partial}{\partial u}\left[-P(X_{n+1} > u|J_n = i, J_{n+1} = j, \xi)\right]\Big|_{u=x} \\
&= P\left(\bigcap_{\substack{l \neq j \\ l \in J(i)}} \{W_{il} > x\} \cap \{x \leq W_{ij} < x + dx\} \middle| \xi\right) \\
&= \prod_{\substack{l=1 \\ l \neq j}}^{m} P(W_{il} > x|\xi) dP(W_{ij} = x|\xi) \\
&= -\prod_{\substack{l=1 \\ l \neq j}}^{m} G_{|il,\xi}(x)\frac{\partial G_{|ij,\xi}(x)}{\partial x}
\end{aligned}$$

The likelihood contribution, of a censored sojourn time in state i equal to x is:

$$\begin{aligned}
&\sum_{l=1}^{m} P(J_{n+1} = l|J_n = i, \xi)P(X_{n+1} > x|J_n = i, J_{n+1} = l, \xi) \\
&= P\left(\bigcap_{l \in J(i)} \{W_{il} > x\} \middle| \xi\right) \\
&= \prod_{l=1}^{m} P(W_{il} > x|\xi) \\
&= \prod_{l=1}^{m} G_{|il,\xi}(x).
\end{aligned}$$

Let $j^h_{s^h}$ be the last observed state for patient h ranging from 1 to 5; δ^h is equal to 0 when censoring occurs. In others words $j^h_{s^h} = 5$, and 1 otherwise. Then the likelihood L is:

$$\begin{aligned}
L &= \prod_{h=1}^{N}\prod_{n=0}^{s^h-2} \lambda_{|j^h_n j^h_{n+1},\xi}(x^h_{n+1})\left[\prod_{\substack{l=1 \\ l \neq j^h_n}}^{m} G_{|j^h_n l,\xi}(x^h_{n+1})\right] \\
&\times \left[\lambda_{|j^h_{s^h-1} j^h_{s^h}}(x^h_{s^h}) \prod_{\substack{l=1 \\ l \neq j^h_{s^h-1}}}^{m} G_{|j^h_{s^h-1} l,\xi}(x^h_{s^h})\right]^{\delta^h} \\
&\times \left[\prod_{l=1}^{m} G_{|j^h_{s^h-1} l,\xi}(x^h_{s^h})\right]^{(1-\delta^h)}
\end{aligned}$$

Thus, the likelihood L is a product for each transition from state i to state j of terms such as:

$$L_{ij} = \prod_{h=1}^{N} \prod_{n=0}^{s^h-1} \left\{ [\lambda_{|ij,\xi}(x_{n+1}^h) G_{|ij,\xi}(x_{n+1}^h)]^{1\{j_n^h=i, j_{n+1}^h=j, j\neq m+1\}} \right. \\ \left. \times [G_{|ij,\xi}(x_{n+1}^h)]^{1\{j_n^h=i, j_{n+1}^h\neq j\}} [G_{|ij,\xi}(x_{s^h}^h)]^{1\{j_{s^h-1}^h=i, j_{s^h}^h=m+1\}} \right\} \quad (1)$$

and

$$L = \prod_{\substack{i=1,\cdots,m_1 \\ j\in J(i)}} L_{ij}$$

For each transition from state i to state j, we assume a Cox regression, and we consider that each transition from state i to any state $j' \neq j$ as a censored transition. Then, (1) is the total likelihood corresponding to the Cox model. The parameters β_{ij} and $G^0_{|ij}$ are estimated by the standard Cox method with covariates, using the partial likelihood:

$$V_{ij} = \prod_{h=1}^{N} \prod_{n=0}^{s^h-1} \left\{ \frac{[\exp(\beta_{ij}\xi^h)]^{1\{j_n^h=i, j_{n+1}^h=j\}}}{\sum_{u=1}^{N} \sum_{s=0}^{s^u-1} [\exp(\beta_{ij}\xi^u)]^{1\{j_s^u=i, x_{n+1}^h \leq x_{s+1}^u\}}} \right\}$$

We have, in the denominator, all the patients present in state i, at risk to have a transition to state j at time x_{n+1}^h. In other words, the denominator represents the patients who have not yet had a transition to state j or who are not yet censored. To obtain the estimates of β_{ij}, we maximize this expression.

The estimated parameters from the cancer clinical trial are given in Table 2. Figure 2 shows the probability of being in the bad quality of life state over time, and Figure 3 shows the probability of being in the good quality of life state. Only the coefficient $\hat{\beta}_{14}$ is significantly different to zero. This transition is from the state of bad quality of life to death.

Table 2. Estimates of regression parameters β_{ij}

Transition	$\hat{\beta}_{ij}$	$SE(\hat{\beta}_{ij})$	p-value
(1,2)	0.185	0.347	0.6
(1,4)	1.010	0.331	0.002
(2,1)	-0.207	0.350	0.6
(2,3)	0.013	0.302	1.0
(2,4)	0.463	0.286	0.1
(3,1)	-0.087	0.410	0.8
(3,2)	0.388	0.281	0.2
(3,4)	-0.107	0.265	0.7

Having fitted the transition intensities, we want to estimate $P_{ij;\xi}(t)$, the probability that a patient is in state j at time t given he was initially in state i with a

Figure 2. Probability of being in the bad quality of life state given being initially in the neutral state: $\hat{P}_{21,\xi}(t)$ with 95% confidence limits

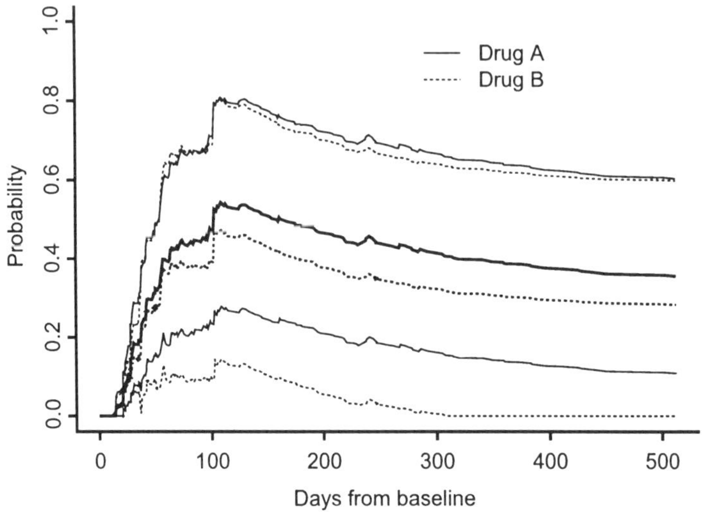

covariate value equal to ξ, $i \in \{1, \ldots, m_1\}, j \in \{1, \ldots, m\}$. We compute this probability when we have a hierarchical model. In a hierarchical model, if you can reach state j from state i, you cannot reach state i from state j. It is always possible to transform a model into a hierarchical model. Let

$$S_{i|\xi}(t) = \exp\left\{-\int_0^t \sum_j \lambda_{|ij;\xi}(u)du\right\}$$

be the survival function of the sojourn time in state i given ξ. Then, for a direct transition from state i to state j, we have:

$$\begin{aligned} P_{ij;\xi}(t) &= P(X_{n+1} = s, J_{n+1} = j, X_{n+2} \geq t - s | J_n = i, \xi) \\ &= \int_0^t S_{i|\xi}(s^-)\lambda_{|ij,\xi}(s)S_{j|\xi}(t-s)ds \quad 0 < s < t \end{aligned}$$

Remark: if state j is an absorbing state, the expression of $P_{ij;\xi}(t)$ becomes simpler because $S_{j|\xi}(t-s) = 1$.

Let $N_{ij}(t)$ be the number of direct transitions from state i to state j in $[0, t]$ and $Y_{i;\xi}(s)$ the number of sojourn times in state i exceeding s with covariable equal to ξ. We estimate $P_{ij;\xi}(t)$ by:

$$\hat{P}_{ij;\xi}(t) = \int_0^t \hat{S}_{i|\xi}(s^-)\frac{I\{Y_{i;\xi}(s) > 0\}}{Y_{i;\xi}(s)}\hat{S}_{j|\xi}(t-s)dN_{ij}(s)$$

Figure 3. Probability of being in the good quality of life state given being initially in the bad state: $\hat{P}_{13,\xi}(t)$ with 95% confidence limits

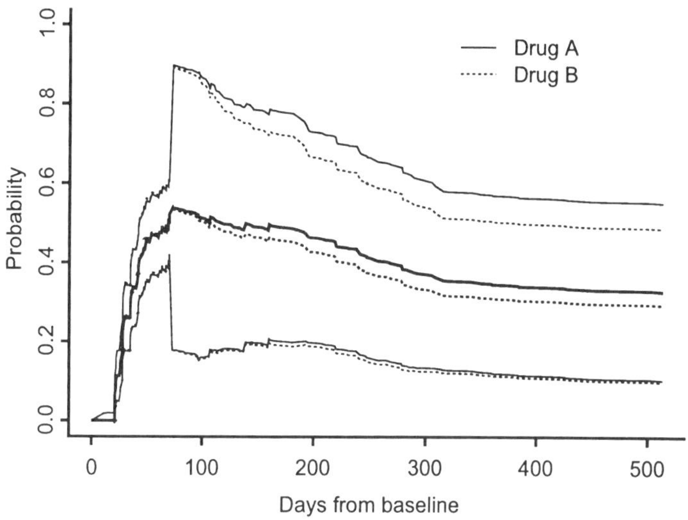

Let $\hat{A}_{|ij,\xi}$ be the estimated cumulative transition rate from state i to state j given ξ and (i,j):

$$\hat{A}_{|ij,\xi}(t) = \hat{A}^0_{|ij,\xi}(t)\exp(\hat{\beta}_{ij}\xi) \text{ for } i \neq j$$

and

$$\hat{A}_{|ii,\xi}(t) = -\sum_{j:i\neq j} \hat{A}_{|ij,\xi}(t) \text{ for } i \in \{1,\cdots,m_1\}.$$

We estimate this cumulative transition rate through the Nelson-Aalen estimator. As $\hat{A}_{|ij,\xi}$ is a step function, we can rewrite $\hat{P}_{ij;\xi}(t)$ as:

$$\hat{P}_{ij;\xi}(t) = \sum_{0<s<t} \hat{S}_{i;\xi}(s^-)d\hat{A}_{|ij;\xi}(s)\hat{S}_{j;\xi}(t-s)$$

with $\hat{S}_{i;\xi}(t) = \prod_{0<u<t}\{1-\sum_j d\hat{A}_{|ij;\xi}(u)\}$ (i.e., the Kaplan-Meier estimator).

We now generalize this estimator to a transition from state i to state j going through p successive states: we suppose that a patient moves now through p different states, staying in each state a random sojourn time before jumping in another state:

$$i \xrightarrow{s_1} l \xrightarrow{s_2} k \xrightarrow{s_3} \cdots \xrightarrow{s_{p-1}} j$$

The probability $P_{ij;\xi}(t)$ associated to this path π is:

$$P^{\pi}_{ij;\xi}(t) =$$
$$\int_{\sum_{l=1}^{p} s_l = t} S_{i|\xi}(s_1^-)\lambda_{|il,\xi}(s_1)S_{l|\xi}(s_2^-)\lambda_{|lk,\xi}(s_2)\cdots$$

$$S_{j|\xi}\left(t - \sum_{u=1}^{p-1} s_u\right) ds_1 ds_2 \cdots ds_{p-1}$$

Let $t_k = \sum_{l=1}^{k} s_l$. The estimated transition probabilities are given by:

$$\hat{P}^{\pi}_{ij;\xi}(t) = \sum_{0<t_1<t_2\cdots<t_n<t} \hat{S}_{i;\xi}(t_1^-)d\hat{A}_{|il;\xi}(t_1)\hat{S}_{l;\xi}([t_2-t_1]^-)d\hat{A}_{|lk;\xi}(t_2-t_1)\cdots\hat{S}_{j;\xi}(t-t_n)$$

Let $C(i,j)$ be the set of all possible paths from state i to state j. Then $\hat{P}_{ij;\xi}(t) = \sum_{\pi\in C(i,j)} \hat{P}^{\pi}_{ij;\xi}(t)$.

Voelkel and Crowley (1984) show how to obtain large sample properties of this estimator To obtain the variance of this estimator, we use a bootstrap procedure. The variance was obtained using 500 iterations. Figure 4 shows the estimated survival curve for each type of transition according to treatment group. The probability of being in state of bad quality of life given initially being in the neutral state is shown in Figure 4C, and the probability of being in state of good quality of life given initially being in the neutral state is shown in Figure 4G.

Figure 4. Transition-specific survival curves with 95% confidence limits

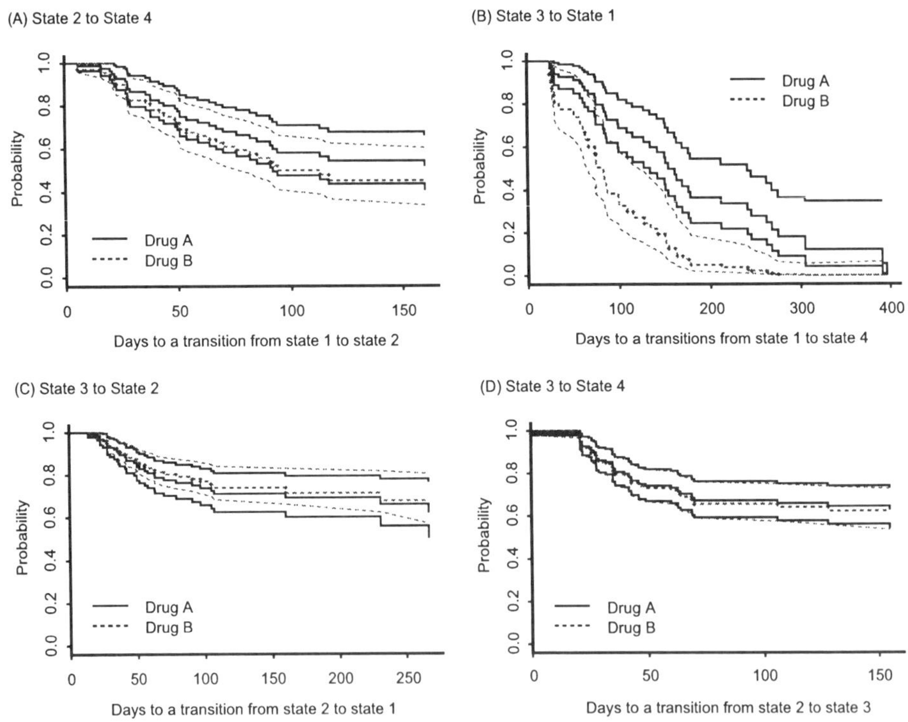

Figure 4 continued

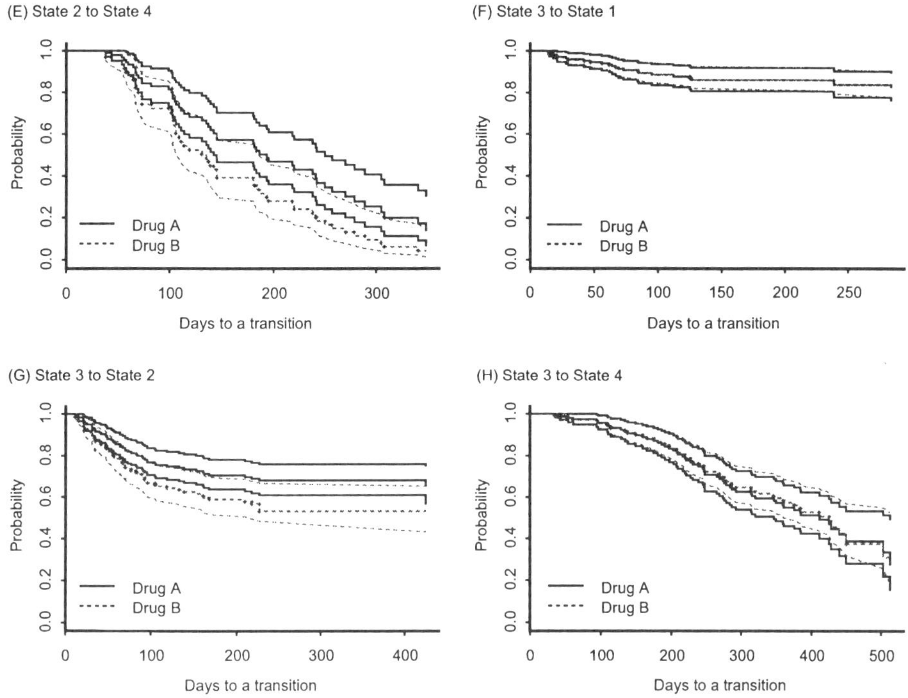

5. Conclusion

For the various survival curves (Figure 4 and Figure 5) and for the estimated regression parameters (Table 2), we observe that there is no difference between the two drugs with respect to quality of life. On the other hand, we observe a difference in efficiency between the two drugs for patients who have a bad quality of life. If we look at the probability of being in a state of bad quality of life initially being in the neutral state and the probability of being in a state of good quality of life given t initially being in the bad state, we note that there is no difference between the two drugs.

We have assumed a Cox model for each hazard function. We could also model each hazard function with a parametric model or another semi-parametric model. We have presented in this paper a method to compare the quality of life of patients who are treated by two different drugs. Cole, Gelber and Goldhirsch (1993) and Cole, Gelber and Anderson (1994) proposed other methods based on Cox regression and accelerated failure time regression for multi-state models.

Acknowledgements

We thank Professor M. Mesbah who gave us the data which are used for the example. We thank also Professor N. Keiding for his precious advise.

References

Aaronson, N.K., Cull, A.M., Kaasa, S. and Sprangers, M.A.G. (1996). The European Organisation for Research and Treatment of Cancer (EORTC) modular approach to quality of life assessment in oncology: an update. In: Spiker, B. (ed.), *Quality of Life and Pharmacoeconomics in Clinical Trials, 2nd Edition.* New York: Raven Press, pp. 179–189.

Andersen, P.K., Borgan, O., Gill, R.D. and Keiding, N. (1992). *Statistical Models Based on Counting Processes*, New York: Springer-Verlag.

Cocozza-Thivent, C. (1997). *Processus stochastiques et fiabilité des systèmes.* Berlin: Springer-Verlag.

Cole, B.F, Gelber, R.D. and Goldhirsch, A. (1993). Cox regression models for quality adjusted survival analysis. *Statistics in Medicine* **12**, 975–987.

Cole, B.F., Gelber, R.D. and Anderson, K.M. (1994). Parametric approaches to quality-adjusted survival analysis. *Biometrics* **50**, 621–631.

Cox, D.R. (1972). Regression models and life-tables. *Journal of the Royal Statistical Society, Series B* **34**, 269–276.

Dabrowska, D., Horowitz, G. and Sun, M. (1994). Cox regression in a Markov renewal model: an application to the analysis of bone marrow transplant data. *Journal of American Statistical Association* **89**, 867–877.

Keiding, N., Klein, J.P. and Horowitz, M.M. (2000). Multistate models and outcome prediction in bone marrow transplantation. *Research Report 00/1, Department of Biostatistics, University of Copenhagen.*

Kalbfleisch, J.D. and Prentice, R.L. (1980). *The Statistical Analysis of Failure Time Data*, New York: Wiley.

Pyke, R. (1961). Markov renewal processes: definitions and preliminary properties. *Annals of Mathematical Statistics* **32**, 1231–1342.

Tsiatis, A. (1975). A nonidentifiability aspect of the problem of competing risks. *Proceedings of the National Acadamy of Sciences* **72**, 20–22.

Voelkel, J. and Crowley, J. (1984). Nonparametric inference for a class of semi-markov processes with censored observations. *The Annals of Statistics* **12**, 142–160.

Appendix

In this appendix, we give the asymptotic properties when n covariates are present. Let $Y_i^k(t)$ be the indicators of presence of patient k in state i at time t. The functions Y_i^k are left continuous. Let τ be the maximal duration of observation. Let $N_{ijk}(x)$ be the number of transitions from state i to state j that have occurred before time x on patient k. We observe n independent point processes on $[0, \tau]$ with respective counts N_{ijk}. Then, we can write the partial log-likelihood as:

$$\mathcal{L}_{ij} = \sum_{k=1}^{M} \int_0^{\tau} \beta_{ij}\xi^k dN_{ijk}(x) - \int_0^{\tau} \log\left(\sum_{k=1}^{M} Y_i^k(x)\exp(\beta_{ij}\xi^k)\right) dN_{ij}(x)$$

We consider that vectors ξ are column vectors. For given β_{ij} and x, let:

$$S_{ij}^{(0)}(\beta_{ij}, x) = \sum_{k=1}^{M} e^{\beta_{ij}\xi} Y_i^k(x),$$

$S_{ij}^{(1)}(\beta_{ij}, x)$ be a column vector of dimension k:

$$S_{ij}^{(1)}(\beta_{ij}, x) = \sum_{k=1}^{M} e^{\beta_{ij}\xi} Y_i^k(x)\xi,$$

and let $S_{ij}^{(2)}(\beta_{ij}, x)$, $V_{ij}(\beta_{ij}, x)$ and $J_{ij}(\beta_{ij})$ be $n \times n$ matrices given by:

$$\begin{aligned} S_{ij}^{(2)}(\beta_{ij}, x) &= \sum_{k=1}^{M} e^{\beta_{ij}\xi} Y_i^k(x)\xi\xi^t, \\ V_{ij}(\beta_{ij}, x) &= \frac{S_{ij}^{(2)}(\beta_{ij}, x)}{S_{ij}^{(0)}(\beta_{ij}, x)} - \frac{S_{ij}^{(1)}(\beta_{ij}, x) S_{ij}^{(1)}(\beta_{ij}, x)^t}{[S_{ij}^{(0)}(\beta_{ij}, x)]^2}, \\ J_{ij}(\beta_{ij}) &= \int_0^{\tau} V_{ij}(\beta_{ij}, x) dN_{ij}(x). \end{aligned}$$

Assumptions: We assume that there exists a neighborhood ν of β_{ij}, $s_{ij}^{(0)}$, a column vector $s_{ij}^{(1)}$ and a matrix $s_{ij}^{(2)}$ defined on $\nu \times [0, \tau]$ such that for all $u = 0, 1, 2$:

1. $\sup_{\beta_{ij}\in\nu, t\le\tau} \|\frac{1}{n} S_{ij}^{(u)}(\beta_{ij}, t) - s_{ij}^{(u)}(\beta_{ij}, t)\| \xrightarrow[n\to\infty]{P} 0.$

2. $s_{ij}^{(u)}(.)$ is a continuous function of $\beta_{ij} \in \nu$, uniformly in $t \subset \tau$ and bounded on $\nu \otimes [0, \tau]$.

3. There exists $a > 0$ such that function $t \to s_{ij}^{(0)}(\beta_{ij}, t)$ is bounded on $[a, \tau]$.

4. For $\beta_{ij} \in \nu, t \le \tau$:
   $s_{ij}^{(1)}(\beta_{ij}, t) = \partial \frac{s_{ij}^{(0)}(\beta_{ij}, t)}{\beta_{ij}}$, $s_{ij}^{(2)}(\beta_{ij}, t) = \partial^2 \frac{s_{ij}^{(0)}(\beta_{ij}, t)}{\beta_{ij}^2}$.

5. Let $v_{ij} = \frac{s_{ij}^{(2)}}{s_{ij}^{(0)}} - \frac{s_{ij}^{(1)}(s_{ij}^{(1)})^t}{(s_{ij}^{(0)})^2}$, the matrix $\Sigma_{ij} = \int_0^{\tau} v_{ij}(\beta_{ij}, t) s_{ij}^{(0)}(\beta_{ij}, t)\lambda_{j|i,\xi}(t)dt$ is positive definite.

6. There exists $\delta > 0$ such as $\frac{1}{\sqrt{n}} \sup_{\substack{0\le v\le t \\ 1\le k\le n}} |\xi Y_i^k(t) I_{\{\beta_{ij}\xi > -\delta|\xi|\}}| \xrightarrow[n\to\infty]{P} 0.$

Theorem: Under the previous assumptions,

$$\begin{aligned}\hat{\beta}_{ij} &\xrightarrow{P} \beta_{ij},\\ \sqrt{M}(\hat{\beta}_{ij}-\beta_{ij}) &\xrightarrow{\mathcal{L}} \mathcal{N}(0,\Sigma_{ij}^{-1}),\\ \frac{1}{M}J_{ij}(\hat{\beta}_{ij}) &\xrightarrow{P} \Sigma_{ij}.\end{aligned}$$

For all $x_1,\cdots,x_u$ in $[0,\tau]$ let

$$\begin{aligned}C_{ij}(k,\cdot) &= \int_0^{x_k}\frac{\lambda_{j|i}^0(u)}{s_{ij}^{(0)}(\beta_{ij},u)}s_{ij}^{(1)}(\beta_{ij},u)du,\\ \Gamma_{ij}(k,l) &= \int_0^{x_k\wedge x_l}\frac{\lambda_{j|i}^0(u)}{s_{ij}^{(0)}(\beta_{ij},u)}du,\\ K_{ij} &= \Gamma_{ij}+C_{ij}\Sigma_{ij}^{-1}C_{ij}^t,\end{aligned}$$

then

$$\sqrt{M}[\hat{A}_{ij}^0(x_1)-A_{ij}^0(x_1),\cdots,\hat{A}_{ij}^0(x_u)-A_{ij}^0(x_u)]\xrightarrow{\mathcal{L}}\mathcal{N}(0,K_{ij}),$$

and

$$\hat{K}_{ij}(k,l)\xrightarrow{P}K_{ij}(k,l),$$

where

$$\hat{K}_{ij}(k,l)= n\left(\int_0^{x_k\wedge x_l}\frac{1}{[S_{ij}^{(0)}(\hat{\beta}_{ij},u)]^2}dN_{ij}(u) + \int_0^{x}\frac{[S_{ij}^{(1)}(\hat{\beta}_{ij},u)]^t}{[S_{ij}^{(0)}(\hat{\beta}_{ij},u)]^2}dN_{ij}(u)J(\hat{\beta}_{ij})^{-1}\int_0^{v_l}\frac{S_{ij}^{(1)}(\hat{\beta}_{ij},u)}{[S_{ij}^{(0)}(\hat{\beta}_{ij},u)]^2}dN_{ij}(u)\right).$$

More generally:

$$\sqrt{M}[\hat{\beta}_{ij}-\beta_{ij},\hat{A}_{ij}^0(x_1)-A_{ij}^0(x_1),\cdots,\hat{A}_{ij}^0(x_u)-A_{ij}^0(x_u)]\xrightarrow{\mathcal{L}}\mathcal{N}(0,K_{ij}^1),$$

with

$$K_{ij}^1=\begin{pmatrix}\Sigma_{ij}^{-1} & -\Sigma_{ij}^{-1}C_{ij}^t\\ -C_{ij}\Sigma_{ij}^{-1} & K_{ij}\end{pmatrix}$$

and for all l

$$-MJ_{ij}(\hat{\beta}_{ij})^{-1}\int_0^{v_l}\frac{(S_{ij}^{(1)}(\hat{\beta}_{ij},u)}{[S_{ij}^{(0)}(\hat{\beta}_{ij},u)]^2}dN_{ij}(u)\xrightarrow{P}-\Sigma_{ij}C_{ij}^t(\cdot,l).$$

A MODEL RELATING QUALITY OF LIFE TO LATENT HEALTH STATUS AND SURVIVAL

MEI-LING TING LEE[1,2] AND G. ALEX WHITMORE[3]

[1] *Channing Laboratory, Brigham & Women's Hospital*
[2] *Harvard University,* [3] *McGill University*

QOL assessments measure a subject's state of health and well-being in a global sense or with reference to particular domains of function, symptoms and living. In this chapter, we define a QOL process for a subject as a continuous-time stochastic process that is periodically assessed by means of a survey instrument. The QOL process is assumed to have three components: a survival component that is correlated with the survival time of the subject, a palliative component that reflects a subject's comfort, freedom from pain and other aspects of well-being that are not correlated with survival, and a noise component that represents a combination of measurement errors and extraneous effects. We present a statistical model that can be used to distinguish between the survival component and the combined palliative and noise components. Our model also provides a way of incorporating markers of health status in the analysis and evaluating their importance. The model assumes that health status and related health markers follow a joint stochastic process. The markers are assumed to be observable whereas the health status process is assumed to be latent or unobservable. The primary endpoint, which we take to be death, is assumed to be triggered when this latent process first crosses a failure threshold level. Inferences for the model are based on censored survival data and marker measurements. Covariates, such as treatment variables, risk factors and other baseline variables, are related to the model parameters through generalized linear regression functions. We interpret the model as a joint process for QOL, latent health status and, possibly, markers of health status. The portion of the QOL process that is correlated with the latent health status process forms the survival component of QOL. The proposed model provides a rich conceptual framework for the study of QOL issues and offers a flexible and tractable methodology for associated statistical inferences. The model and methods are illustrated by a small case demonstration.

1. Introduction

A substantial literature has accumulated on the subject of quality of life (QOL) assessment in connection with health care and medical treatment programs, as illustrated by some of our cited references. A QOL assessment may measure a subject's state of health and well-being with reference to a particular domain of physical, emotional, social and cognitive function, a domain of symptoms, or some other domain of living. It may also be a single global measure of overall well-being. A typical QOL study involves an assessment instrument, covering one or more assessment domains, applied to a sample of subjects from a relevant population.

M. Mesbah et al. (eds.), Statistical Methods for Quality of Life Studies, 219–230.

The assessment might be done once for a subject, or in a longitudinal series from the commencement of a study until the end of follow-up or the occurrence of a primary endpoint, such as death.

In our conceptual framework, QOL is a continuous-time stochastic process for a subject that we shall refer to as the *QOL process.* This process is not monitored continuously but, instead, is periodically assessed by means of a survey instrument. The QOL process is assumed to consist of three components. The key idea underlying these components is the recognition that QOL is partly determined by aspects of health that influence survival time, partly by aspects that involve the simple alleviation of pain and suffering and, finally, partly by the inevitable presence of noise or inherent variability. We define the three components as follows.

1. *Survival component.* This component is related to the force of mortality that acts on the individual subject. This force describes the combined causes that lead inevitably to an individual's death. The survival component of QOL is the one that is correlated with the survival time of the subject.

2. *Palliative component.* This component reflects a subject's comfort, freedom from pain and other aspects of well-being that are not correlated with survival *per se.* It is mainly this component that sets QOL methodology apart from other measurement methods for medical and health outcomes.

3. *Noise component.* This component is a combination of measurement errors and extraneous effects that are found in all survey contexts.

In statistical terms, these three components are mutually uncorrelated or orthogonal and add together to make up the QOL process and, hence, the QOL assessments derived from the process.

In this chapter, we present a statistical model that can be used to distinguish between the survival component and the combined palliative and noise components. We wish to distinguish the components of QOL for two reasons. First, the relative magnitudes of the three components elicited by a QOL assessment instrument have implications for the scientific reliability and use of the instrument. The choice of instrument will depend on its ability to differentiate among the three components. Medical treatment can be curative and palliative in varying degrees. The tradeoff being made between these components needs to be assessed. Second, a QOL assessment instrument may only partially capture information about health status and survival. Markers for health status and survival may be available that can supplement the QOL process. Our model provides a way of incorporating markers in the analysis and evaluating their importance.

As a framework for studying health status and survival, we adopt the model described in Lee, DeGruttola and Schoenfeld (2000), which itself is an extension of one described in Whitmore, Crowder and Lawless (1998). We use the model structure of Lee *et al.* but, initially, do not use their distributional assumptions. In brief, their model assumes that health status and related health markers follow a joint stochastic process. The health markers are assumed to be observable. In contrast, the health status process is assumed to be latent or unobservable. The primary endpoint, which we take to be death, is assumed to be triggered when this latent process first crosses a failure threshold level. Inferences for the model are based on censored survival data and marker measurements. Covariates, such as treatment variables, risk factors and other baseline variables, are related to the model parameters through generalized linear regression functions.

In this chapter, we build on a suggestion by Cox (1999) and interpret the Lee *et al.* model as a joint process for latent health status, QOL and, possibly, markers of health status. The part of the QOL process that is correlated with the latent health status process forms the survival component of QOL, as defined earlier. Inferences about model parameters are based on censored survival data, longitudinal QOL assessment data, and measurements for marker processes. The proposed model provides a rich conceptual framework for the study of QOL issues and offers a flexible and tractable methodology for associated statistical inferences.

2. Model

Consider a two-dimensional continuous-time stochastic process $\{H(t), Q(t)\}$ for $t \geq 0$, with initial values $\{H(0), Q(0)\}$. Process $\{H(t)\}$ represents a latent *health status process* for a subject while $\{Q(t)\}$ represents an observed *QOL process* that is correlated with the health status process $\{H(t)\}$ and partly tracks its progress. It is the process $\{Q(t)\}$ that consists of survival, palliative and noise components. The survival component of $\{Q(t)\}$ is the one that is correlated with the health status process $\{H(t)\}$. For the moment, we assume that only one QOL process is under consideration, ignoring QOL assessments for multiple domains or health status markers that may be of interest. We extend the model to incorporate these other elements later.

We assume that both processes $\{H(t)\}$ and $\{Q(t)\}$ have stationary independent increments. Thus, the vector $\{H(t), Q(t)\}$ has a bivariate distribution, of unspecified form, with mean vector $\{H(0), Q(0)\} + t\mu$, where $\mu = (\mu_H, \mu_Q)$, and covariance matrix $t\Sigma$, where

$$\Sigma = \begin{pmatrix} \sigma_{HH} & \sigma_{HQ} \\ \sigma_{QH} & \sigma_{QQ} \end{pmatrix}.$$

The subject's initial health status is at some positive level $h_0 = H(0) > 0$. The value h_0 is unknown and must be estimated. We set the failure threshold at zero on the health status scale so the closer $H(t)$ is to zero, the more ill is the subject. Failure (death) occurs when the subject's health status reaches zero for the first time. We denote the first passage time from the initial health status h_0 to the failure threshold at zero (i.e., the survival time) by the random variable S. The initial QOL level $q_0 = Q(0)$ will be known and will be used as a baseline covariate. Figure 1 illustrates a sample path of the joint process from its initial level to failure.

The extent to which the QOL process tracks latent health status depends on the strength of its correlation ρ with the health status process. By definition, the correlation parameter for these two processes is defined by $\rho = \sigma_{HQ}/(\sigma_{HH}\sigma_{QQ})^{1/2}$. The closer $|\rho|$ is to 1, the more closely movements in the QOL process track or

Figure 1. Correlated QOL and health status processes with failure threshold

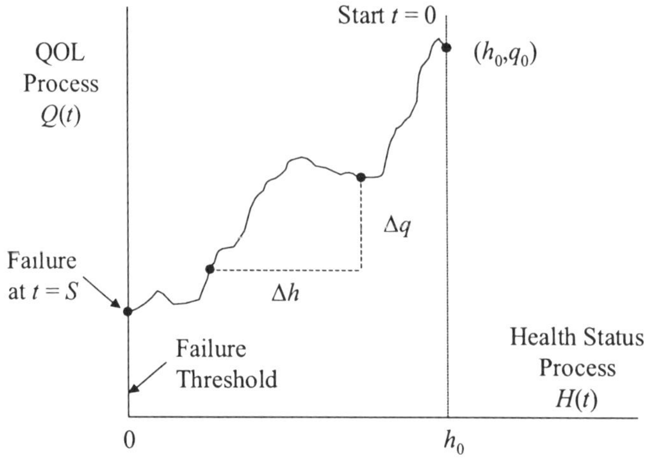

mimic movements in the latent health status process. The parameter μ_H describes the mean change per unit time in health status. A negative value for μ_H indicates that the subject's health status is tending toward failure. The variance parameter σ_{HH} describes the variability per unit time in health status. The parameter μ_Q describes the mean change per unit time in the QOL process. The parameter σ_{QQ} is the variance per unit time of the QOL process. Finally, the covariance parameter σ_{HQ} measures the extent to which changes in the QOL and health status processes covary.

In our model, a regression of the QOL process on the health status process yields an estimate of the survival component of QOL. The correlation of the QOL and health status processes measures the strength of their linear relationship. By definition, the part of the QOL process that is uncorrelated with health status represents the combined effects of the palliative and noise components. The regression of the QOL process on the health status process accounts for ρ^2 of the variability in QOL. The residual fraction of variability, given by $1 - \rho^2$, reflects the palliative and noise components of QOL.

In our conceptual framework, covariates are fixed characteristics of the subject. Examples include treatment indicators, baseline characteristics (such as age and initial QOL level) and subject characteristics (such as gender and ethnicity). Effects of covariates are easily incorporated in the parameters. Letting $\mathbf{z}$ represent a covariate vector, we connect each parameter to a linear combination of covariates using general link functions as follows.

$$h_0 = g_0(\mathbf{z}\boldsymbol{\beta}_0), \quad \mu_H = g_H(\mathbf{z}\boldsymbol{\beta}_H), \quad \mu_Q = g_Q(\mathbf{z}\boldsymbol{\beta}_Q)$$

$$\rho = g_\rho(\mathbf{z}\boldsymbol{\beta}_\rho), \quad \sigma_{QQ} = g_{QQ}(\mathbf{z}\boldsymbol{\beta}_{QQ})$$

The forms of the link functions are chosen as appropriate for each application. At the least, however, the forms must preserve the requirements for h_0 and σ_{QQ} to be positive and for $|\rho|$ to be less than one.

3. Data Structure and Parametric Estimation

As the health status process is assumed to be latent, inferences about the health status of subjects must be based on observations on the QOL process and censored survival data, possibly supplemented with information on associated marker processes. No direct observation is made of the latent health status process, although one can infer that the H process has reached the failure threshold level at the moment a subject fails and that H has not reached that level at any time in the interval $(0, t)$ if the subject has survived to time t.

We assume that there are n subjects in the study, indexed by $i = 1, \ldots, n$. In the most general setup, longitudinal QOL assessments will be available. The observation times for subject i will be denoted by $t_{ij}, j = 1, \ldots, m_i$, where $t_{i,0} = 0$. The number of observations m_i may be as small as 1. We consider this situation in our subsequent case example. For a failing subject, $t_{i,m_i} = s_i$, where s_i is the subject's survival (failure) time and, for a surviving subject, $t_{i,m_i} = c_i$, where c_i is an independent censoring time. The set of QOL increments observed for each subject i are denoted by $\Delta q_{ij} = Q_i(t_{ij}) - Q_i(t_{i,j-1}), j = 1, \ldots, m_i$ (see Figure 1). The corresponding time increments are $\Delta t_{ij} = t_{ij} - t_{i,j-1}, j = 1, \ldots, m_i$. The initial QOL level for subject i is denoted by q_{i0}.

Parameter estimation may proceed in two basic ways, with or without an explicit distributional model. Lee and Whitmore (2000b) describe an estimation methodology that is distribution free, relying only on the first two moments of the joint distribution of $\{H(t), Q(t)\}$. In contrast, an explicit distributional form might be given to the joint process $\{H(t), Q(t)\}$ and then either a frequentist or Bayesian estimation method employed. Candidate distributions for the process might vary widely. Lee *et al.* (2000) and Whitmore *et al.* (1998) consider a bivariate Wiener process and then use maximum likelihood estimation. We assume that the chosen joint process has stationary independent increments, as required earlier.

In both the distribution-free and distribution-based approaches, the solution of the estimation problem with general longitudinal data is computationally intensive. The computational burden arises because both approaches require data augmentation in which the latent health status increments $\Delta h_{ij} = H_i(t_{ij}) - H_i(t_{i,j-1})$ are treated as unknown data points that must be estimated (see Figure 1). For the case where $m_i = 1$ for all subjects i (i.e., one QOL increment derived from initial and ending QOL assessments), the computational routines (with covariates) described in Lee *et al.* (2000) and Lee and Whitmore (2000b) are easily implemented. The subsequent case example uses the routine in Lee *et al.* (2000).

We note for future reference that the health status process $\{H(t)\}$ has an arbitrary scale because it is latent. We choose to scale $H(t)$ by setting $\sigma_{HH} = 1$. Thus, the measurement units of the unknown h_0 and the parameters μ_H and σ_{HQ} are established accordingly.

4. QOL Domain Assessments and Supplemental Markers

QOL applications may involve simultaneous assessments being made on several QOL domains. Each of these individual domain assessments can be considered separately as the single QOL process in the preceding model and the analysis would proceed in the same fashion for each domain, as it also would for a global QOL assessment. On the other hand, there may be an interest in forming a composite QOL measure by combining the domain assessments so that the composite measure has the largest possible survival component in the sense of being as highly correlated with the latent health status process as possible. More precisely, let $Q_{(1)}(t), \ldots, Q_{(d)}(t)$ denote d QOL domain assessments, where $q_{(k)0} = Q_{(k)}(0)$ is the initial QOL domain reading for $k = 1, \ldots, d$. We require $Q_{(k)}(t), k = 1, \ldots, d$, and $H(t)$ to form a $d+1$ dimensional continuous-time joint process, having stationary independent increments. We form a linear combination of the QOL domain measures that is most highly correlated with the latent health status process. We refer to this optimal linear combination of processes as the *composite QOL index* and denote it by

$$Q(t) = \sum_{k=1}^{d} \gamma_k Q_{(k)}(t),$$

where $\gamma_k, k = 1, \ldots, d$, denote regression parameters to be estimated. The regression parameter estimates will be chosen jointly with estimates of the other process parameters in such a way as to maximize the estimated correlation coefficient $\hat{\rho}$ between the composite QOL process and the health status process. For this estimation, we calculate the QOL composite increments from the individual QOL domain assessment increments as follows.

$$\Delta q_{ij} = \sum_{k=1}^{d} \gamma_k \Delta q_{(k)ij}$$

In addition to the QOL domain assessments, a study may have observable marker processes related to the health status of the subject that can be informative about health status and survival. Technically, these supplementary marker processes may be treated as QOL domain assessments and incorporated in the composite QOL index as additional regression variables. Increases in ρ^2 that are provided by these supplementary markers represent a gain in the ability of the composite QOL index to track the latent health status of the subject.

The interpretation of the composite QOL index brings into play all of the issues of multiple regression, such as multicollinearity and regression model choice. With respect to multicollinearity, for example, the explanatory significance of one QOL domain measure may depend on which other domain measures are in the composite QOL index; for instance, regression coefficient γ_k reflects the marginal contribution of QOL domain process $Q_{(k)}(t)$ to the composite QOL index. With respect to model choice, it may happen that particular transformations or functional forms of the QOL domain assessments are better than others in defining the relation with health status and survival.

5. Cumulative QOL and Health Status

We now return to consider a single QOL process $\{Q(t)\}$. The sample path traced by this process over a subject's remaining life describes the (residual) lifetime QOL experience. In QOL research, the following integral represents lifetime QOL or, with suitable scaling, quality-adjusted lifetime. We shall refer to this integral as *cumulative quality of life* or CQOL for short.

$$\text{CQOL} = \int_0^S Q(t)dt \quad \text{for lifetime } S. \tag{1}$$

The larger is CQOL, the better is the subject's lifetime QOL. Note, however, that the definition of CQOL in (1) makes sense only if the sample paths of $\{Q(t)\}$ remain positive. A substantial literature has developed around the CQOL concept and the various statistical problems it poses. See, for example, Glasziou, Cole, Gelber, Hilden and Simes (1998), and Zhao and Tsiatis (1997, 1999, 2000).

Prompted by an idea proposed by Cox (1999) and motivated by the concept of CQOL, we propose to interpret the area between the health status sample path and the failure threshold at zero (the horizontal axis) as (residual) lifetime *cumulative health status*, or CHS for short. That is,

$$\text{CHS} = \int_0^S H(t)dt \quad \text{for lifetime } S.$$

Figure 2 illustrates the CHS concept. In this situation, the fact that S is a first passage time ensures that $H(t)$ remains positive in the interval $(0, S)$. By definition, the larger is lifetime CHS, the better is the survival component of lifetime health experience of the subject. In other words, better without reference to the palliative component.

Figure 2. Time path of health states from initial level h_0 until failure at time S. Area under the curve constitutes lifetime CHS.

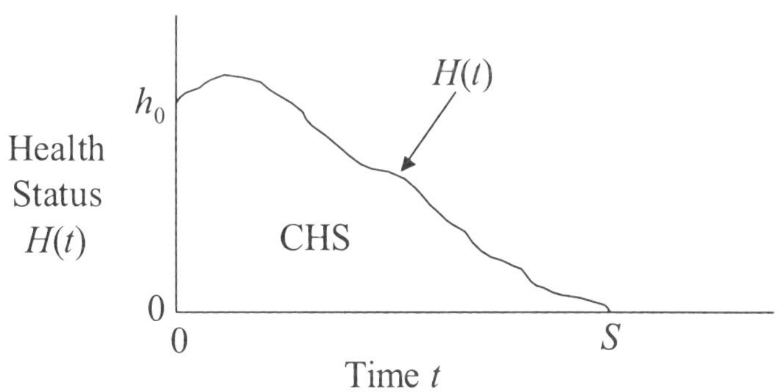

The efficacy of medical treatment, health care and palliative care programs can be judged by examining the expected values of CQOL and CHS for different populations of subjects. These expected values depend on the distributional form of the joint process $\{H(t), Q(t)\}$. To illustrate these expected values for a particular process, we have derived them for a Wiener process. For a Wiener process, the expected values of lifetime CQOL and lifetime CHS are given by

$$E\{\text{CQOL}\} = q_0 E(S) + \frac{\mu_Q}{2} E(S^2) + \beta|\mu_H|\text{var}(S) \quad \text{for } \mu_H < 0, \tag{2}$$

$$E\{\text{CHS}\} = \frac{|\mu_H|}{2} E(S^2) \quad \text{for } \mu_H < 0. \tag{3}$$

Here β is the slope coefficient in a regression of QOL increments (Δq) on health status increments (Δh) and is related to the process parameters as follows: $\beta = \sigma_{HQ}/\sigma_{HH}$. Thus, β is capturing the influence on $E\{\text{CQOL}\}$ of the correlation between the health status and QOL processes. For a Wiener process, the first passage time to the failure threshold follows an inverse Gaussian distribution. From properties of this distribution, we also have

$$E(S) = \frac{h_0}{|\mu_H|}, \quad \text{var}(S) = \frac{h_0 \sigma_{HH}}{|\mu_H|^3}, \quad E(S^2) = \text{var}(S) + E(S)^2. \tag{4}$$

We provide no proof of these results here. We note that both $E(\text{CQOL})$ and $E\{\text{CHS}\}$ are undefined (infinite) if $\mu_H \geq 0$.

The preceding formulas for $E(\text{CQOL})$ and $E\{\text{CHS}\}$ show how the process parameters and initial levels of health status and QOL affect lifetime QOL and health experience. To illustrate, we re-express $E(CHS)$ explicitly in terms of the parameters as follows.

$$E\{\text{CHS}\} = \frac{h_0^2}{2|\mu_H|}\left(1 + \frac{\sigma_{HH}}{h_0|\mu_H|}\right) \quad \text{for } \mu_H < 0. \tag{5}$$

Note how expression (5) simplifies if σ_{HH} is zero. If the $\{H(t)\}$ process has no variability, the health status sample path is linear and downward slopping (for $\mu_H < 0$) and $E\{\text{CHS}\}$ is the triangular area defined by h_0 and the expected survival time h_0/μ_H. The form of (5) also shows that the influence of the process variability σ_{HH} is moderated by the product $h_0|\mu_H|$. The larger is h_0 or $|\mu_H|$, the smaller is the effect of process variability on $E\{\text{CHS}\}$.

A similar examination of $E(\text{CQOL})$ also provides insights. For example, if the QOL and health status processes were uncorrelated, implying that $Q(t)$ had no survival component, then $\sigma_{HQ} = 0$, $\beta = 0$ and the last term in (2) would be zero. This last term captures the pure contribution of the survival component to CQOL. Note, however, that even if QOL had only a palliative component, survival time per se would still contribute to $E(\text{CQOL})$ through the fact that the benefits of palliation would accumulate over the lifetime S of the subject. This latter contribution is evident from the presence of the terms $E(S)$ and $E(S^2)$ in the leading two terms on the righthand side of (2).

6. Case Example

We present a small case example based on the realistic but artificial data set presented in Table 1. We use an artificial data set because QOL studies available to us have not concentrated on the link between QOL and survival.

The data set in Table 1 shows outcomes for $n = 30$ subjects divided randomly into treatment and control groups of equal size. The first column gives the *case* number of the subject. The second column gives an indicator outcome (*fail*) that is 0 if the subject's time is censored and 1 if it is the actual survival or failure time. The third column gives the censoring or survival *time* (in months). The fourth and fifth columns give outcomes for a global QOL assessment that is made at the outset of the study and at the point in time nearest to the censoring or survival time of the subject. For simplicity, the assessment is a rating on a 10-point scale from best (10) to worse (1). The fourth column shows the change in the QOL assessment from the initial assessment to the final assessment (*qchg*). It can be seen that most changes are negative, reflecting deteriorating quality of life. The fifth column gives the initial QOL assessment (*q0*). This value will be used as a covariate, together with the treatment indicator *treat*.

Table 1. Case example data

Control (*treat* = 0)					Treatment (*treat* = 1)				
case	*fail*	*time*	*qchg*	*q0*	*case*	*fail*	*time*	*qchg*	*q0*
1	1	4	−3	4	16	1	104	−4	5
2	1	24	−4	7	17	1	70	−5	6
3	0	13	0	10	18	1	83	−7	10
4	1	39	−7	9	19	0	39	2	7
5	1	52	−6	8	20	1	59	−3	7
6	1	39	−2	8	21	0	118	−3	9
7	0	23	−7	10	22	1	67	−5	9
8	0	45	−5	8	23	0	19	1	9
9	1	25	−7	9	24	0	88	−1	8
10	0	37	2	7	25	0	67	−4	10
11	1	43	−9	10	26	0	98	−1	9
12	0	39	−1	10	27	0	34	−6	7
13	0	37	−7	10	28	1	108	−4	9
14	1	36	−5	6	29	0	41	−2	10
15	0	5	0	7	30	1	33	−1	6

The data are assumed to arise from a bivariate Wiener process. Although the QOL assessment scale is a highly discrete finite interval, the analysis proceeds without transformations or refinements to demonstrate the basic methodology in a simple manner. The data have been analyzed using the initial QOL assessment *q0* as a covariate for the initial health status h_0 and the treatment variable *treat* as a covariate for the two mean parameters μ_H and μ_Q. The maximum likelihood estimates for the regression parameters have been obtained using the *ml* routine in Stata and are reported in Table 2. Observe that logarithmic link functions have been used for the h_0 and σ_{QQ} parameters and the logit link function has been used for the correlation coefficient ρ. The label *cons* represents the intercept estimate for each regression function. The following points are noteworthy:

1. The treatment effect is significant (at the 0.05 level) for both mean parameters, indicating that treatment impacts both the survival component of QOL and QOL itself. Treatment raises both mean parameters, implying greater lifetime CHS and improved overall QOL assessments.

2. Treatment was not expected to affect h_0 for this data set and tests (not presented here) confirm that none of h_0, σ_{QQ} or ρ have significant treatment effects at the 0.05 level.

3. The point estimates of ρ^2 for both control and treatment groups is 72%; a result that indicates that the survival component is the major component of the QOL assessment, accounting for about three fourths of its variability. The remaining one fourth is accounted for by the combined palliative and noise components.

4. The estimated mean survival time under treatment and control can be estimated from the parameter estimates in Table 2 and the equation for $E(S)$ in (4). We consider a hypothetical subject with an inital QOL assessment of 10 (i.e., $q0 = 10$). The estimated means are 151 and 59 months, respectively. Thus, treatment is estimated to almost triple life expectancy for this hypothetical subject. We note that both life expectancy estimates are values that lie somewhat beyond the range of the observed survival data. Thus, we are relying here on the validity of the underlying assumption that the joint process is a Wiener process.

5. To illustrate $E\{\text{CHS}\}$, we again consider a hypothetical subject with an inital QOL assessment of 10 (i.e., $q0 = 10$). The estimated lifetime $E\{\text{CHS}\}$ for this subject, calculated from (3) using the maximum likelihood estimates of the parameters, are 2191 and 733 health status unit-months for treatment and control, respectively. Thus, treatment almost triples expected lifetime CHS in this example.

   To illustrate $E\{\text{CQOL}\}$ for the same hypothetical subject, we have substituted the maximum likelihood estimates in (2) and obtained 1300 and 395 QOL unit-months for treatment and control, respectively. Again, we see that treatment here has a major impact on CQOL for this type of subject; more than tripling expected lifetime CQOL. The units of the $E\{\text{CHS}\}$ and $E\{\text{CQOL}\}$ measures are incommensurate but a comparison of their ratios is meaningful. The fact that both ratios are close to 3 indicates that they have been affected equally by treatment. A closer examination of the measures shows that the improvements in $E\{\text{CHS}\}$ and $E\{\text{CQOL}\}$ with treatment are largely driven by the near tripling of life expectancy.

Table 2. Maximum likelihood parameter estimates (maximum log-likelihood value equals −137.053)

Parameter	Covariate	Estimate	Std. Err.	z	$P > \|z\|$
$\ln(h_0)$					
	q0	0.19550	0.02773	7.051	< 0.001
	Constant	1.14499	0.24339	4.704	< 0.000
μ_H					
	treat	0.22951	0.07093	3.236	0.001
	Constant	−0.37644	0.08169	−4.608	< 0.001
μ_Q					
	treat	0.09049	0.02654	3.409	0.001
	Constant	−0.13232	0.02206	-6.000	< 0.001
$\ln(\sigma_{QQ})$					
	Constant	−1.49502	0.24166	-6.187	< 0.001
$\text{logit}(\rho)$					
	Constant	2.50216	0.45290	14.357	< 0.001

7. Concluding Remarks

The proposed methodology calibrates QOL assessment instruments and allows a determination of the relative magnitudes of the survival and palliative-noise components in longitudinal QOL assessments. The methodology also allows the concept of QOL to fit comfortably within the framework for traditional survival data analysis. The model has the advantage of being able to accommodate QOL domain measures as well as health status markers in the form of a composite QOL index that has maximum correlation with health status and survival. The model can incorporate covariates using a variety of functions to link them to the process parameters.

Explicit results are available using the bivariate Wiener model proposed by Whitmore *et al.* (1998) and Lee *et al.* (2000). The expressions for $E\{\text{CQOL}\}$ and $E\{\text{CHS}\}$ show how the different parameters of the joint QOL and health status process impact lifetime cumulative quality of life and health status.

The current paper does not present the complete methodology for handling applications with longitudinal data for more than two time points. Lee and Whitmore (2000b) describe an approach to parameter estimation in this situation but full-scale implementation in large studies still presents some technical challenges. Other issues that remain to be studied include predictive inference and model checking procedures. Also, further research is required to provide guidance on model checking and transformations of the QOL assessments to satisfy distributional assumptions. For checking of assumptions underlying the bivariate Wiener model, the observations in Lee and Whitmore (2000a) are relevant.

ACKNOWLEDGEMENTS

We acknowledge with thanks the financial support provided for this research by the National Institutes of Health grant HL40619-09 (Lee) and by a grant from the Natural Sciences and Engineering Research Council of Canada (Whitmore).

REFERENCES

Cox, D. R. (1999). Some remarks on failure-times, surrogate markers, degradation, wear and the quality of life. *Lifetime Data Analysis* **5**, 307–314.

Glasziou, P.P., Colc, B.F., Gelber, R.D., Hilden, J., Simes, R.J. (1998). Quality adjusted survival analysis with repeated quality of life measurements. *Statistics in Medicine* **17**, 1215–1229.

Lee, M.-L.T., V. DeGruttola and D. Schoenfeld (2000). A model for markers and latent health status. *J. Royal. Statist. Soc., Series B* **62**, 747–762.

Lee, M.-L.T. and G. A. Whitmore (2000a). Assumptions of a Latent Survival Model. In: *Proceeding of the Conference on Goodness of Fit*, 1999, Paris, France, forthcoming.

Lee, M.-L.T. and G. A. Whitmore (2000b). Distribution-free inference methods for latent disease progression and survival. Technical paper, Channing Laboratory, Harvard Medical School.

Whitmore, G. A., Crowder, M.J. and Lawless, J.F. (1998). Failure inference from a marker process based on a bivariate Wiener model. *Lifetime Data Analysis* **4**, 229–251.

Zhao, H. and A. A. Tsiatis (1997). A consistent estimator for the distribution of quality-adjusted survival time. *Biometrika* **84**, 339–348.

Zhao, H. and A. A. Tsiatis (1999). Efficient estimation of the distribution of quality-adjusted survival time. *Biometrics* **55**, 231–236.

Zhao, H. and A. A. Tsiatis (2000). Estimating mean quality-adjusted lifetime with censored data. *Sankyha, Series B* **62**, 175–188.

APPLYING SURVIVAL DATA METHODOLOGY TO ANALYZE LONGITUDINAL QUALITY OF LIFE DATA

LUCILE AWAD,[1] EMMANUEL ZUBER[1] AND MOUNIR MESBAH[2]

[1]*Aventis and* [2]*Université de Bretagne-Sud*

In metastatic cancer studies, the deterioration of the patient's health status is often observed during the trial either because of the toxicity of treatment or the progression of disease. This deterioration is very likely to be reflected in the patient's quality of life. Therefore, when analyzing the global health status/quality-of-life (QL) score of the EORTC QLQ-C30 instrument, an event, QL deterioration can be defined in terms of health states. Deterioration could be characterized by an absorbing state (similar to death when analyzing survival time). We define only two kinds of events, so repeated measures of QL are easily converted into time-to-event data, and the Kaplan-Meier method and log-rank tests can be used for analysis. We apply this methodology to data from a clinical trial of treatments for metastatic colorectal cancer.

1. Introduction

The aim of clinical trials conducted in oncology is to estimate the efficacy and the safety of new chemotherapies. An important endpoint is the patient's perception of his/her global quality of life. This endpoint integrates the impact of both efficacy and safety of the drug from the patient's perspective (Cox *et al.*, 1992).

Despite the growing importance of quality of life outcomes in medical research in general and in cancer clinical trials in particular, methods of analysis of these data remain an issue. In quality-of-life analysis, missing data cannot be considered as missing at random, as they are most likely related to the worsening of the patient's condition or to death. No consensus exists on the way of dealing with missing data. Therefore it is important to use a palette of statistical methodologies.

Clinical end-points such as time to progression or time to treatment failure are definitive events generally occurring during the study. These data can be analyzed using survival analysis methods. Similarly, an event corresponding to a "quality-of-life deterioration" can be defined. The goal of this paper is to present this methodology and its application to data from a clinical trial of treatments for metastatic colorectal cancer (Douillard *et al.*, 2000). We compare and contrast our results with results based on more classical analyses of quality-of-life data.

2. Methods

2.1 Quality of Life Instruments and Data

The European Organization for Research and Treatment of Cancer (EORTC) QLQ-C30 instrument (Aaronson *et al.*, 1993) has been widely used to evaluate the quality of life of cancer patients. It is a 30-item questionnaire completed by patients. Following EORTC

M. Mesbah et al. (eds.), Statistical Methods for Quality of Life Studies, 231–243.

guidelines, linear transformations are used to obtain 15 scales for analysis. These scales include five functional scales, nine symptom scales and one global scale, the global health status/quality-of-life scale (QL). For the five functional scales and the QL scale, a high score indicates a high level of functioning. On the contrary, a high score on a symptom scale is related to a high level of symptoms. The EORTC (Fayers *et al.*, 1995) and other authors (McLachlan *et al.*, 1998 and Beitz, Gnecco and Justice, 1988) recommend using the QL scale as an overall summary of the patient's quality of life. The QL scale is preferable to a composite summary of the other scales (Osoba, 1994). It indeed corresponds to a self-assessed summary measure of the patient's quality of life, based on two separate ratings of his/her overall health and quality of life during the past week. The QL score takes 13 possible values ranging from 0 to 100, by 8.3.

Among the analyses performed on the 15 scales in the colorectal cancer clinical trial, a specific analysis was performed on the QL scale to assess both the efficacy and safety of the drug. Repeated measures of QL were recorded at various time points during the study: before randomization, during treatment (usually before each cycle of treatment), and during follow-up.

2.2 Time to Event Analyses

To allow for a time-to-event analysis, repeated measures of QL can be transformed into survival data by defining an absorbing state that represents deterioration of quality of life. We define QL deterioration as a decrease in QL score from baseline without any return to a better state during the study. Because there are no established criteria for choosing a specific level of deterioration, we used four levels for the analysis: 5%, 10%, 20%, and 30%. Table 1 shows how these levels of deterioration correspond to changes on the two individual items comprising the QL score. Changes are shown for low medium and high values of QL at baseline. For the 5% level of deterioration, any maintained decrease will be considered as an event. For the other levels of deterioration, the better the QL state at baseline, the greater the decrease that is required for the change to be considered an event. We did not consider levels of deterioration greater than 30% because of the small number of events occurring.

We define two endpoints: "QL-deterioration-free-survival" and the "time to deterioration of QL." For the first endpoint, the event of interest is the occurrence of either a QL deterioration or the death of the patient, whichever occurs first. For the second end-point, the event is the QL deterioration, but death is considered as an event only if it occurs within a predefined period following the last QL assessment. This is analogous to using death as a surrogate for QL deterioration. By convention, death is considered as an event when it occurs within a period of time defined by 1.5 times the period between two assessments as planned in the study protocol. Otherwise, the patient is considered lost to follow up for QL and is censored at the date of last assessment.

The first endpoint is a composite endpoint of QL deterioration and death. The second endpoint focuses on the QL deterioration but takes into account the information of death assuming that if death occurs within a relatively short period of time after a QL assessment, the QL of the patient might have deteriorated within this period of time. Using these two definitions, the longitudinal QL data are transformed into time-to-event data and can be analyzed using methodology appropriate for survival analysis. Kaplan-Meier probabilities can be estimated and the log-rank test can be used to compare

Table 1. Levels of QL deterioration from baseline in absolute QL units depending on the baseline score. One level on one item = 8.3 units on the QL scale).

<table>
<tr><th rowspan="2">Level of QL deterioration</th><th colspan="3">Baseline QL score</th></tr>
<tr><th>33.3 (low)</th><th>66.7 (medium)</th><th>100 (high)</th></tr>
<tr><td></td><td colspan="3">Absolute change in QL
Description of change</td></tr>
<tr><td>5%</td><td>1.7 QL units</td><td>3.3 QL units</td><td>5 QL units</td></tr>
<tr><td></td><td colspan="3">= Any change of at least 1 level on either item</td></tr>
<tr><td>10%</td><td>3.3 QL units</td><td>6.6 QL units</td><td>10 QL units</td></tr>
<tr><td></td><td colspan="2">= Any change of at least 1 level on either item</td><td>= Any change of at least 2 levels on one item, or of 1 level on both items</td></tr>
<tr><td>20%</td><td>6.6 QL units</td><td>13.3 QL units</td><td>20 QL units</td></tr>
<tr><td></td><td>= Any change of at least 1 level on either item</td><td>= Any change of at least 2 levels on one item, or of 1 level on both items</td><td>= Any change of at least 3 levels on one item, or of 1 level on one item and 2 levels on the other item</td></tr>
<tr><td>30%</td><td>10 QL units</td><td>20 QL units</td><td>30 QL units</td></tr>
<tr><td></td><td>= Any change of at least 2 levels on one item, or of 1 level on both items.</td><td>= Any change of at least 3 levels on one item, or of 1 level on one item and 2 levels on the other item</td><td>= Any change of at least 4 levels on one item, or of 1 level on one item and 3 levels on the other, or 2 levels on both items.</td></tr>
</table>

treatment groups. To take into account that missing values were very likely to be related to the bad condition of the patient, when a deterioration was observed after a missing value, it was assumed that the deterioration had occurred at the time of the missing value.

The Kaplan Meier analysis includes only patients with at least a baseline score. This may induce a selection bias. Therefore, we compared QL over time in patients with and without a baseline QL score. Table 2 shows the definitions used in the analysis.

All the analyses were performed on evaluable questionnaires only. To be considered evaluable on treatment, a questionnaire had to be filled more than 5 days after the latest infusion, and before any further infusion. In the protocol, questionnaires were intended to be completed before the infusions to avoid the effects of acute toxicities following treatment administration (these toxicities were analyzed separately). In addition, questionnaires without a date of assessment or that were completed after the cut-off date were not evaluable. All questionnaires completed before the first infusion were considered as evaluable baseline questionnaires.

In addition to the Kaplan-Meier analyses, we performed more classical quality-of-life analyses, including analysis of compliance and analysis of variance on the QL scores. We used repeated measures analysis of variance to study the evolution of the QL score over time. We used a mixed effects model, assuming a normal distribution for the QL scores. Treatment and the treatment-by-time interaction were the fixed effects, time was a

Table 2. Definitions for Kaplan-Meier analyses

Component	Definition
Baseline	Date of randomisation
Population	Intent to treat population, in patients with a QL scale measure at baseline
Event	Definitive deterioration QL, by 5%, 10%, 20%, or 30% Death* if no deterioration of QL
Date of event	Date of QL deterioration Date of death
Censoring Reason	No event prior to the cut-off date Lost to follow-up for QL†
Censoring date	Date of last QL evaluation Cut-off date if no event occurs prior to the cut-off date

*Death is an event whenever it occurs before a definitive deterioration or if it occurs ≤ 1.5 × the time between two protocol assessments from the last QL assessment.
†Declared lost to follow up by the investigator at study discontinuation or no QL evaluation within the last 10 weeks on treatment

repeated factor, and patient-within-treatment-group was a random factor. The most suitable covariance structure was chosen according to Akaike's information criterion (AIC) and Schwartz' Bayesian criterion (SBC), between unstructured, compound symmetric and autoregressive of order 1. The hypothesis of no treatment effect was tested at a 5% two-sided significance level.

A certain paucity of data was expected beyond a certain time point, making interpretation of the observed quality-of-life patterns difficult. Therefore, we limited the repeated measures analysis to time points at which at least 10% of patients in each treatment group provided evaluable questionnaires. In some cases, multiple evaluable questionnaires for a patient occurred within a single time interval. In these cases, we used the mean of the evaluable QL scores within the time interval.

To study whether data missingness was informative of the patient's quality of life, we analyzed the relationship between missing data and bad clinical condition or reason for study dropout. The cumulative number of missing QL scores by treatment group was tabulated against the concomitant occurrence, in the same time interval, of one of the following: (1) death, (2) occurrence of progressive disease, (3) occurrence of a grade 3 or worse adverse event, (4) progressive disease and a grade 3 or worse adverse event occurring in the same time interval, or (5) the patient withdraws consent to participate.

2.3 Clinical Studies

The QLQ-C30 instrument has been used to measure quality of life in three randomized phase III studies conducted in metastatic colorectal cancer. The objective of the first study (V301) was to show that a new drug (irinotecan) administered after failure of treatment with fluorouracil prolonged the survival of the patients in second line metastatic colorectal cancer (Cunningham *et al.*, 1998). This study compared irinotecan plus best supportive care (BSC) to BSC alone. In the second study (V302), irinotecan was compared to fluorouracil as second-line treatment for metastatic colorectal cancer (Rougier *et al.*, 1998). In the third study (V303), irinotecan plus fluorouracil (CPT-11 + 5-FU was compared to fluorouracil alone (5-FU) as first-line treatment for metastatic colorectal cancer (Douillard *et al.*, 2000). The primary end-points were overall survival for V301 and V302, and response and time to progression for V303.

The schedule of assessment was different in the three studies as the patients were followed for their quality of life until death or for a maximum of one year for V301 and V302, whereas in V303, the questionnaire was administered only during treatment. It is important to emphasize that survival was prolonged by the administration of irinotecan in each of the three studies. Therefore, it was important to show that this survival gain was not obtained at the price of a deterioration of the patient's quality of life. Additionally, due to the survival difference between the treatment groups, it was clear that the analysis of variance comparison will be biased in favor of the group with the worst survival.

In this paper, we present in detail only the methodology used in the analysis of V303. Results for V301 and V302 are briefly discussed in Section 4. Two possible fluorouracil regimens were chosen by the clinical center according local clinical practice or preference. One regimen consisted of administration of drug every two weeks. The other regimen consisted of 6 infusions every 7 weeks.

In V303, the quality-of-life questionnaire was to be completed within 8 days after randomization, before the first treatment, and before treatment for each treatment cycle (every 6 to 7 weeks) while patients were on treatment. The Kaplan-Meier analysis applied to the data from this study uses the definition where death is an event only if it occurs sufficiently close in time to the last QL assessment. Indeed, death was only considered in patients without a prior deterioration, and if it occurred within 10 weeks of the last QL score available for the patient. That is, death was considered only when it could replace a QL evaluation given the period between two assessments defined in the protocol (6 to 7 weeks, to which a security margin of 3 weeks was added).

3. Results

One hundred ninety-eight patients were randomized to CPT-11 + 5-FU, and 187 were randomized to 5-FU alone. The results of the clinical end-points (response rate, time to progression and survival) were in favor of CPT-11 + 5-FU. In particular, survival was prolonged. These results are reported elsewhere in detail (Douillard *et al.*, 2000).

A high percentage of the 643 questionnaires received in the CPT 11 + 5-FU group and of the 518 received in the 5-FU alone group was evaluable (94% and 92%, respectively). The averaging of multiple questionnaires in the same time interval caused a slight reduction of the degrees of freedom for the analysis. The equivalent of 570 distinct questionnaires were eventually considered in the CPT-11 + 5-FU group, and 448 in the 5-FU alone group. Of the total number received, this represents 89% and 87% in the two treatment groups, respectively. These percentages would have been 92% and 90%, respectively, if we had used protocol cycles for the questionnaire averaging instead of time intervals. Therefore, only a limited number of degrees of freedom were lost because of the definition of the time intervals (22 intervals for the CPT-11 + 5-FU group, and 20 intervals in the 5-FU alone group).

3.1 Time to Event Analyses

The Kaplan-Meier estimate of the survival distribution of the time to QL deterioration in the CPT-11 + 5-FU group was consistently above that of the 5-FU alone group, regardless of the level of deterioration considered (Figure 1).

Figure 1. Time to QL deterioration for CPT-11 + 5-FU (*N* = 154) versus 5-FU alone (*N* = 138)

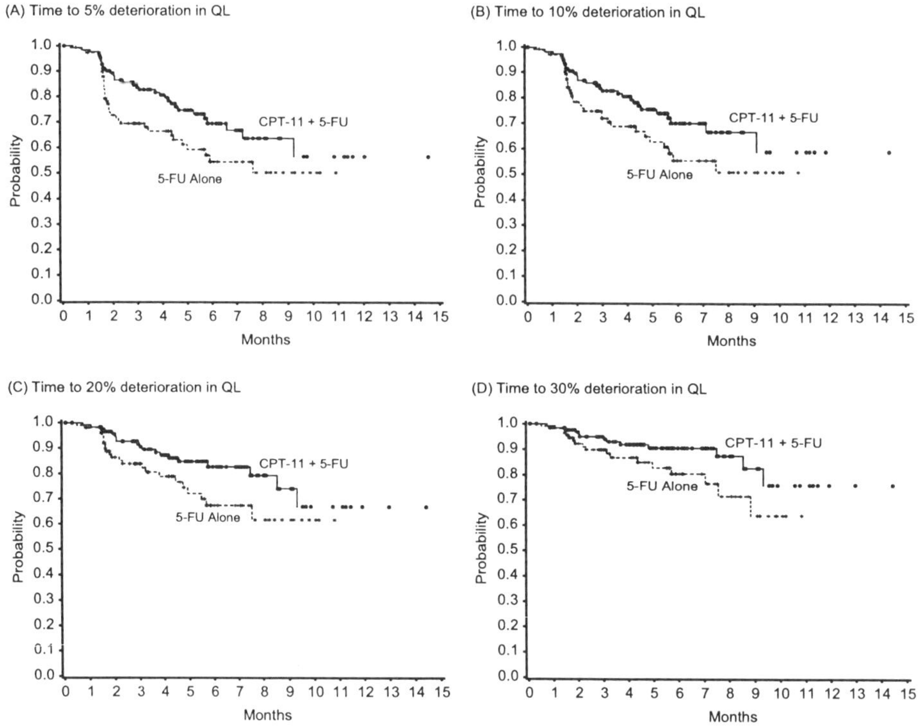

The log-rank test was statistically significant for the 5% and 20% deterioration levels ($p = 0.03$ and $p = 0.04$, respectively), and the trend was similar for the 10% and 30% deterioration levels ($p = 0.06$ in both cases), which indicates increased time to deterioration of QL for CPT-11 + 5-FU. Censoring was mainly due to the absence of event at the cut-off date. The proportion of patients lost to follow up for QL (as defined in Section 2) was always below 33% in the CPT-11 + 5-FU group and always below 22% in the 5-FU alone group.

The aim of this analysis was to focus on the QL score and not to mix the information with survival. Therefore we analyzed the proportions of deaths in the QL events of the Kaplan-Meier analysis. Table 3 shows the proportion of deaths in the number of events at all levels of deterioration (below 10% in both treatment groups at deterioration levels of 5% and 10%, below 17% at the 20% deterioration level, and below 24% at the 30%

deterioration level), indicating that quality of life and not survival was the primary cause of the treatment effect observed.

Table 3. Events in the analyses of the time to QL deterioration from baseline

Level of QL deterioration	Treatment group	Number of events	Deaths (%)	QL Deteriorations (%)
5%	CPT-11 + 5-FU	33	3 (9)	30 (91)
	5-FU alone	40	3 (8)	37 (93)
10%	CPT-11 + 5-FU	30	3 (10)	27 (90)
	5-FU alone	35	3 (9)	32 (91)
20%	CPT-11 + 5-FU	19	3 (16)	16 (84)
	5-FU alone	24	4 (17)	20 (83)
30%	CPT-11 + 5-FU	13	3 (23)	10 (77)
	5-FU alone	18	4 (22)	14 (78)

3.2 Analysis of Compliance

The study protocol specified that a QLQ-C30 questionnaire had to be completed by each patient before each treatment cycle. We calculated compliance with this protocol as the ratio of the number of patients with at least one evaluable questionnaire per cycle to the number of patients in the treatment cycle, as defined in the protocol. The overall compliance was 62% in the CPT-11 + 5-FU group and 59% in the 5-FU alone group. Table 4 shows the compliance over time. As expected, attrition was due to the decrease in the number of patients on treatment, and the decrease in compliance increased with the cycle number. Compliance was above 50% in both treatment groups for the first three cycles of treatment.

At baseline, compliance was of 83% in the CPT-11 + 5-FU group versus 77% in the 5-FU alone group. Compliance was stable for the first three treatment cycles and then lower but still nearly stable for the next four cycles. In the 5-FU alone group, compliance was 56% and 53% at cycles 2 and 3 (versus 65% and 61% for the CPT-11 + 5-FU group). We conclude that compliance was comparable in both treatment groups for the four next cycles.

A small and identical number of patients in each treatment group had QL data while on treatment without a score at baseline (18 patients, representing less than 10% of the initial population in each group). The trends with and without a baseline score were very similar in both groups, although the curve for patients without a baseline score in the CPT-11 + 5-FU group was below the corresponding curve for the 5-FU alone group. The small number of available scores from the patients without a baseline score, which did not exceed 7% of the initial population in both groups in each time interval, prevented any further interpretation.

Table 4. Compliance in the completion of QLQ-C30 forms

	CPT-11 + 5-FU			5-FU alone		
Cycle	Number in the cycle	Number evaluable	Compliance (%)	Number in the cycle	Number evaluable	Compliance (%)
Baseline	198	165	83	187	143	77
Cycle 1	198	120	61	187	112	60
Cycle 2	166	108	65	145	81	56
Cycle 3	140	85	61	110	58	53
Cycle 4	110	51	46	76	35	46
Cycle 5	64	30	47	41	20	49
Cycle 6	40	16	40	26	12	46
Cycle 7	19	8	42	14	6	43
Cycle 8	10	7	70	3	1	33
Cycle 9	6	1	17	0	0	0
Cycle 10	3	1	33	0	0	0
Cycle 11	1	0	0	0	0	0
Overall	955	592	62	789	468	59

3.3 Time Interval Definition

Because the durations of a protocol cycle, and therefore the frequency of quality-of-life evaluation, were different for the two 5-FU regimens used (every 7 weeks versus every 6 weeks), the analyses (other than the analyses of compliance and of the time to deterioration of the QL score) were performed according to time interval. The baseline interval was the time before the first infusion of the first cycle. While on treatment, the time intervals corresponded to 7-week periods (49 days), except for the first on-treatment interval. For the first on-treatment time interval, a 3.5-week lag (25 days) was added to the 7-week period, to make it a 10.5-week period (49 + 25 = 74 days). This allowed the questionnaires in the same time interval to be more synchronous for the two 5-FU schedules. Time interval 1 was from the first infusion (day 1 of week 1, excluded) to day 5 of week 11 (included). Time interval 2 was from day 5 of week 11 (excluded) to day 5 of week 18 (included). In general, the n-th time interval was from day 5 of week $[4 + 7(n - 1)]$ (excluded) to day 5 of week $(4 + 7n)$ (included).

3.4 Analysis of Variance

Although all the data are shown on Figure 2, the model for the primary analysis of variance was applied to the first four on-treatment time intervals only. The QL patterns observed on fewer questionnaires would indeed not be representative of the initial population. We used a compound symmetric covariance structure for the repeated measures mixed model. It led to the lowest absolute values for both AIC and SBC criteria as compared to unstructured or autoregressive (order 1) matrices. In addition, convergence was reached in 3 iterations instead of 6 with the unstructured matrix, which indicated less over-parameterization with the simpler compound symmetric model. Despite the observed better trend in the CPT-11 + 5-FU group, the test of a treatment effect from the repeated measures analysis of variance was not significant ($p = 0.5$).

Figure 2. Evolution over time of QL

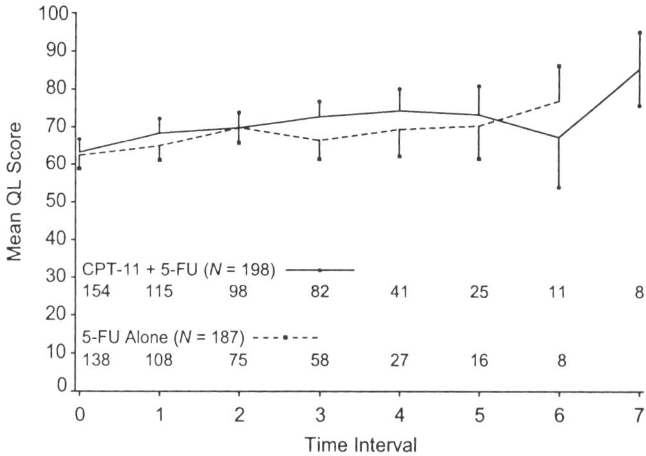

3.5 Study of Data Missingness

The number of evaluable QL scores was comparable in both treatment groups, although always slightly higher in the CPT-11 + 5-FU group, both in absolute number and in percentage of the initial population. As expected from the clinical analysis, the primary reason for data missingness in both groups was the progression of the disease, which was more frequent in the 5-FU group. Conversely, a little more missing data could be related to grade 3 or worse adverse events with CPT-11 + 5-FU. The number of missing observations due to the withdrawal of the patient's consent also seemed higher in the CPT-11 + 5-FU group. These findings were consistent with the reasons for treatment discontinuation.

It may be assumed that the patients with missing data for progressive disease or adverse events had a worse QL score. Conversely, the same assumption could not be made so easily for missing data due to consent withdrawal. Some patients indeed withdrew their consent because they were feeling well and did not see further benefit from chemotherapy. The relationship between data missingness and the possibly low values of the missing QL scores for progressive disease or adverse events suggested that the missingness mechanism was not at random. In addition, the number of missing observations for these reasons seemed to be unbalanced between the treatment groups.

4. Discussion

Obviously when there is a survival difference between the treatment groups, the analysis of variance cannot be considered adequate for comparing QL. It is indeed biased in favor of the group with the poorer survival. This can be generalized to data missing not at random, as was the case in this study. Another criticism is that the analysis of variance does not take deaths into account. On the contrary, time-to-event analyses explicitly account for deaths. Also, the time-to-event analyses avoid the need for time intervals, which can be difficult to define in some cases. The absence of a treatment effect in the analysis of variance we presented in this paper, contrasts with the results of the time to

QL deterioration analysis. This should be related to the fact that in the mixed model analysis, missing data are ignored, even when they are related to a bad QL status.

The results of the deterioration-free-survival analyses performed on the V301 and V302 studies can be summarized as follows. In V301 all log-rank tests comparing the irinotecan group to the no irinotecan group were significant with $p < 0.001$. In V302, the irinotecan group showed curves always above that of the no irinotecan group, but all the comparison were not significant. For these three studies, the results of the QL analyses seem quite consistent with their respective clinical results.

Mixed models for longitudinal repeated measures are currently very popular. Nevertheless, the occurrence of death, and its relationship with missing data need to be taken into account, and this makes the analysis more complicated than a classical longitudinal analysis. Longitudinal data with non-random missingness, even without occurrence of death is an issue. Various more-sophisticated methods and models are presented by other authors (Billot and Mesbah, 1999; Heutte and Huber-Carol, 2002; Dupuy and Mesbah, 2002; and Cole and Kilbridge, 2002).

The endpoint "time to QL deterioration" takes the missing data into account in a specific manner. It appears more sensitive to treatment effects in presence of missing data. As it has been defined, this endpoint has the advantage that missing data occurring before or after deterioration does not impact it. Indeed, if deterioration was observed after a missing value, it was assumed that the first deterioration had already occurred at the time the missing value was expected. This could be related to a last observation carried forward (LOCF) imputation of the missing data coupled with a procedure carrying backward the first observation after deterioration. Thus, it corresponds to a sophisticated kind of imputation, which considers that the endpoint is at least deteriorated by the same amount as the observed deterioration. Of course, this holds as long as it can be assumed that a missing observation is very likely to be related to deterioration.

In addition, missing data due to death are specifically taken into account in this endpoint. For this analysis, it is important to define reasonably large intervals, within which death is taken as an event to avoid censoring a death following closely a QL assessment but without prolonging too much the time to deterioration if no assessment has been performed during a long period.

4.1 Definitions of the Time to Event Endpoint

It was more logical to use "time to QL deterioration" for the analysis of V303 because the patients were followed on treatment only. Because patients were followed for their quality of life until death, the endpoint "QL-deterioration-free-survival" was used for V301 and V302. It seems more appropriate to use this endpoint when the objective is to show that a treatment prolongs survival without deterioration of the quality of life. "Time to QL deterioration," on the other hand, focuses on quality of life *per se*.

Another possibility would be to use the competing risk methodology, with death being considered as a competing risk for QL deterioration. However, using this method would imply making the assumption of a same survival in the two treatment groups. When the objective of the study is to show a difference in survival, this methodology is not applicable. However, if the objective of the trial is to show that there is no difference in survival, but that the quality of life is better in one of the groups, this could be an appropriate method.

The definition of QL deterioration is a weak definition in the sense that if only one measure of QL shows deterioration at the end of the study, it is considered a deterioration even though it is not confirmed by a further assessment. This should be put in the context of metastatic cancer. Usually if the patient has a worsening status at the end of the study without any other measure of QL, it can be assumed that the deterioration is continuous.

4.2 Relationship to Corresponding Clinical Endpoints: Overall Survival and Time to Progression

The two endpoints based on quality of life are very similar to the two time-to-event analyses usually performed on the time until progressive disease. The time to deterioration of QL is analogous to the time to progression, and "QL-deterioration-free-survival" is analogous to progression-free survival. When the parameter of interest is progression-free survival (time to progression or death, whichever occurs first), it is important to have regular tumor assessments unless the end-point would be artificially prolonged until death. This remark also holds for "QL-deterioration-free-survival."

4.3 Conclusion

Among the possible analyses of quality of life, the time to event analyses have good properties. The choice of the relevant analysis depend form the objective of the trial. If the objective is to show a survival advantage without quality of life deterioration, the endpoint "QL-deterioration-free-survival" can be used. If the objective is to show an improvement of both survival and quality of life, then the "time to QL deterioration" parameter might be preferable. When applied to the QL score of the QLQ-C30 questionnaire, this type of analysis has been shown to be sensitive. The analyses were highly significant in the V301 study when comparing the irinotecan treatment to best supportive care. They were also significant or not far from significant when applied to the V303 study.

A third possibility would be the time to deterioration with death being a competing event. This endpoint would be appropriate if the objective were to show a similar survival with an improved quality of life. In that case, another possibility could be to analyze the effect of treatment on quality of life, *knowing the effect of treatment* on survival. Some authors suggest performing a classical longitudinal analysis adjusted for the survival duration. This simple kind of analysis answers a surrogate question: what is the effect of treatment on quality of life, if the treatment groups were equivalent in terms of survival. This type of analysis would not be appropriate if there were differences in survival between the groups. For instance if one treatment is better than another in terms of survival, then when we adjust for the survival duration, we will disadvantage that better treatment group, because quality of life and the survival duration are highly positively related. A better solution might be to *jointly* analyze quality of life and survival, taking into account the pre-requested results about treatment effect on survival duration.

A more sophisticated solution should be to model and to estimate the joint distribution of the longitudinal quality of life outcome and the survival process. A growing recent literature, described by Dupuy (2002), deal with that issue. Multi-state Markov or semi-Markov models (Heutte and Huber-Carol, 2002) may be also used, if we can easily translate quality-of-life scores into states.

All these appealing methods need specific software and careful computer programming. Furthermore, interpretation of results is not straightforward. Our solution has the main advantage to be easy to implement and to interpret. Clinicians are familiar with Kaplan-Meier curves. All general statistical software nowadays includes survival methods with Kaplan-Meier estimates and the log-rank test.

As there does not seem to be a logical choice for a unique level for the deterioration, we recommend using a range of different levels. The consistency of the results is important for the strength of the conclusion. In fact, it would be justified to use a higher significance level than 0.05 for each of the tests. Further research is aimed at building a global significance test, integrating the results of a set of deterioration levels.

REFERENCES

Aaronson, N.K., Ahmedzai, S., Bergman, B., Bullinger, M., Cull, A., Duez, N.J., Filiberti, A., Flechtner, H., Fleishman, S.B., De Hues, J.C.J.M., Kaasa, S., Klee, M., Osoba, D., Razavi, D., Rofe, P.B, Schraub, S., Sneeuw, K., Sullivan, M. and Takeda, F. for the European Organization for Research and Treatment of Cancer Study Group on Quality of Life (1993). The European Organization for Research and Treatment of Cancer QLQ-C30: a quality-of-life instrument for use in international clinical trials in oncology. *Journal of the National Cancer Institute* **85**, 365–376.

Beitz, J., Gnecco, C. and Justice, R. (1998). Quality-of-life end points in cancer clinical trials: the US Food and Drug Administration Perspective. *Journal of the National Cancer Institute Monographs* **20**, 7–9.

Billot, L. and Mesbah, M. (1999). *"Analyse d'un essai de Qualité de Vie longitudinal en cancérologie avec prise en compte des abondans"* in Actes des Journées Vannes-Bordeaux. (Proceedings).

Cole, B.F. and Kilbridge, K.L. (2002). Quality-adjusted survival analysis in cancer clinical trials. In: Mesbah, M., Cole, B.F. and Lee, M.L.T. (eds.), *Statistical Methods for Quality of Life Studies: Design, Measurements and Analysis*, Boston: Kluwer.

Cox, D.R., Fitzpatrick, R., Fletcher, A.E., Gore, S.M., Spiegelhalter, D.J. and Jones, D.R. (1992). Quality-of-life assessment: can we keep it simple? *Journal of the Royal Statistical Society, Series A* **155**, 353–393.

Cunningham, D., Pyrhönen, S., James, R.D., Punt, C.J.A., Hickizsh, T.P., Heikkila, R., Johannesen, T.B., Starkhammar, H., Topham, C.A., Awad, L., Jacques, C. and Herait, P. (1998) Randomised trial of iritonecan plus supportive care versus supportive care alone after fluorouracil failure in patients with metastatic colorectal cancer. *Lancet* **352**, 1413–1418.

Douillard, J.Y., Cunningham, A.D., Navarro, M., James, R.D., Karasek, P., Jandik, P., Iveson, T., Carmichael, J., Alakl, M., Gruia, G., Awad, L. and Rougier, P. (2000) Irinotecan combined with fluorouracil compared with fluorouracil alone as first-line treatment for metastatic colorectal cancer: a multicenter randomized trial. *Lancet* **355**, 1041–1047.

Dupuy, J.F. (2002) Joint modeling of survival and nonignorable missing longitudinal quality of life data. In: Mesbah, M., Cole, B.F. and Lee, M.L.T. (eds.), *Statistical Methods for Quality of Life Studies: Design, Measurements and Analysis*, Boston: Kluwer.

Dupuy, J.F. and Mesbah, M. (2002). Joint modeling of event time and nonignorable missing longitudinal data. *Lifetime Data Analysis* (to appear).

Fayers, P., Aaronson, N., Bjordal K., Curran, D. and Groenvold, M. for the EORTC Quality of Life Study Group (1999). *EORTC QLQ-C30 Scoring Manual, 2nd Edition*. Brussels: European Organization for Research and Treatment of Cancer.

Heutte, N. and Huber-Carol, C. (2002). Semi-Markov models for quality of life data with censoring. In: Mesbah, M., Cole, B.F. and Lee, M.L.T. (eds.), *Statistical Methods for Quality of Life Studies: Design, Measurements and Analysis*, Boston: Kluwer.

McLachlan, S.A., Devins, G.M. and Goodwin P.J. (1998). Validation of the European Organization for Research and Treatment of Cancer quality-of-life questionnaire (QLQ-C30) as a measure of psychological function in breast cancer patients. *European Journal of Cancer* **34**, 510–517.

Osoba, D. (1994). Lessons learned from measuring health-related quality of life in oncology. *Journal of Clinical Oncology* **12**, 608–616.

Rougier, P., van Cutsem, E., Bajetta, E., Niederle, N., Possinger, K., Labianca, R., Navarro, M., Morant, R., Bleiberg, H., Wils, J., Awad, L., Herait, P. and Jacques, C. (1998). Randomized trial of iritonecan versus fluoracil by continuous infusion after fluoracil failure in patients with metastatic colorectal cancer. *Lancet* **352**, 1407–1412.

LATENT CLASS MODELS TO DESCRIBE CHANGES OVER TIME: A CASE STUDY

HANS C. VAN HOUWELINGEN

Leiden University Medical Center

By means of a case study we describe the statistical analysis of repeated measures as they may be found in a typical quality-of-life trial that studies the effect of some intervention on quality-of-life. We will show that latent class models are a very useful to tool to discover patterns in the follow-up data. Once the patterns have been found, data-driven summary statistics can be defined that are more useful than simple pre-defined measures of response.

1. Introduction

In cancer as in other chronic diseases therapeutic interventions are not so much aimed at prolonging the life of the patient but more at improving his/her quality of life. Clinical studies designed to assess the impact of the intervention on the quality-of-life results in large data-sets with many repeated measurements per patient. Statistical analysis of such data is far from easy: the data can be quite noisy and it is not clear what kind of patterns can be expected in the data. The simple solution is to summarize the effect of the intervention in one single measure of response that is defined before the data were actually collected. Such a simplification is not quite fair in the light of all efforts made by patients and researchers to collect the data. In this paper we advocate to analyze the data more thoroughly. To exemplify our approach we present a detailed case study of a large clinical trial aimed at palliating painful bone-metastases by radiotherapy. Where possible, we demonstrate our approach graphically. In section 2 we describe the trial and the data in more detail. In section 3 we discuss the handling of missing data. Disentangling signal and noise by fitting so-called mixed models is discussed in section 4. In section 5 latent class models are introduced as a tool to discover patterns in the data. Finally, conclusions, refinements and future developments are briefly discussed in section 6.

2. Description of the Trial and Data

The Dutch Bone Metastasis Study is a large study (about 1000 patients) aimed at comparing two different radio therapy regimens for patients with painful bone metastasis. See Steenland *et al.* (1999) for a full description of the trial. Patients with incurable cancer often develop bone metastasis in a late stage of their disease. These bone metastases are very painful. To relieve the pain, the patient is treated by irradiation of the metastasis. The standard treatment has six daily doses of 4 Gy and the new treatment has only one daily dose of 8 Gy. The latter is less burdensome for both patient and hospital. The hope (to be confirmed by this trial) is that the daily 1×8 Gy regimen is as effective as the 6×4 Gy regimen. Apart from the radio therapy patients can take pain relief

M. Mesbah et al. (eds.), Statistical Methods for Quality of Life Studies, 245–259.

medication. If absolutely necessary due to unbearable pain, the patient can have a second radio therapy treatment. The survival prospects of these patients are very poor and, therefore, the main reason of dropout is death from the primary tumor. The pain is weekly measured on a self-administered 11 point-scale (0-10) during the first 13 weeks (numbered 0-12) and monthly thereafter. Here we restrict attention to the first 13 measurements. The inclusion criterion is that the pain score pre-entry (before week 0) is at least two. The type of the primary tumor is an important explanatory variable in this study. The total number of patients entered is given in Table 1. During the first 13 weeks the numbers drop to 326 patients in the 6×4 Gy group and 330 patients in the 1×8 Gy group. Most missing data are because of drop out, but there are some occasional missing data in between as well.

Table 1. Numbers of patients entered into the study

	Radiation Dose		
Tumor Type	6×4 Gy	1×8 Gy	Total
Lung	138	134	272
Breast	212	228	440
Prostate	132	124	256
Other	72	74	146
Total	554	560	1,114

The overall drop in pain is nicely shown in the box-plots of Figure 1. It clearly shows the discrete character of the data. For the sake of our exposition, we will treat them as being multivariate normal. Our approach can be extended to ordinal data, but that is beyond the scope of this paper. We computed, but do not show, the crude means (without correction for dropout) per subgroup over time. They show a similar drop. At first sight, there is no difference between the treatment groups, but a clear difference between the primary tumor groups. Breast cancer patients show the lowest pain scores, prostate cancer patients have an intermediate position, and patients with lung and other cancers show the highest average pain scores.

It is interesting to see how the average course over time depends on the starting value as shown in Figure 2. The study protocol of the trial speaks of evaluation of the data on the basis of (1) time till response (decrease of 2 points), (2) time till relapse (back at starting level) for responders, and (3) duration of remission for responders. These definitions show a need for models for the natural course of pain after start of the treatment. They do not speak about average pain, total pain or pain at specific time-point. They are based on the point of view of the therapist and focus on "does it help." Statistical modeling should help in advancing the clinical understanding of what is going on.

In the analysis of "time to response," drop out leads to censored outcomes that are easily handled by the standard techniques for survival data. Intermittently missing observations are harder to handle. When studying time to relapse and duration of remission, dropout is a nuisance as well, because patients that drop out before response might have had a response later on. So, the first problem to be solved is the handling of missing data.

Figure 1. Box plots of pain scores

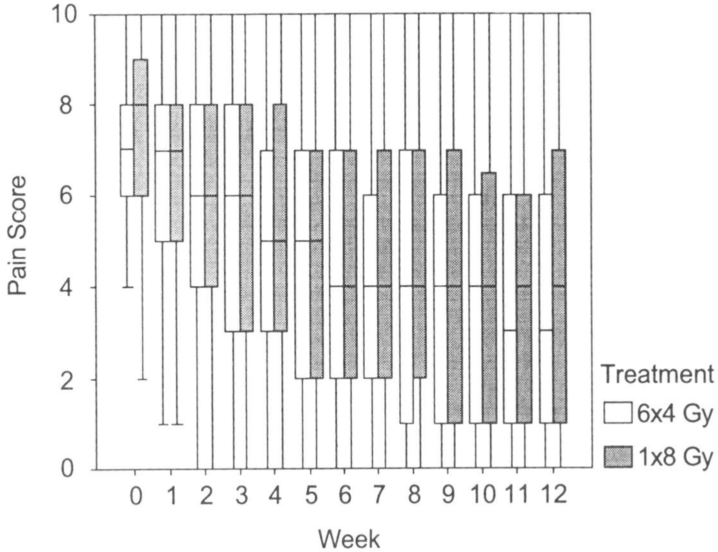

Figure 2. Mean pain score over time by baseline pain score

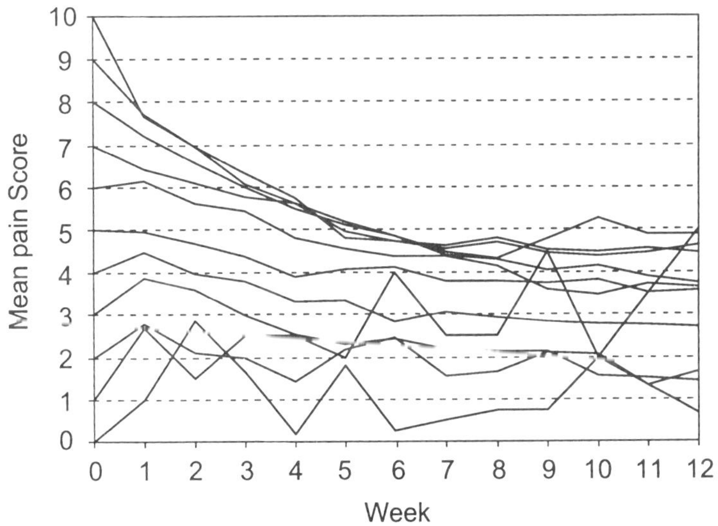

3. Missing data

Basically, there are two ways to handle missing data. The first one is to impute missing data by some educated guess. That is possible for the intermittent missing data, but very hard for the drop outs. The other way is to assume that the data are missing at random (MAR) as defined by Little and Rubin (1987) and to analyze all available data by maximum likelihood. Missing at random assumes that the probability that observations are missing does not depend on those potential observations but on the actually observed data. Particularly, it assumes that drop out depends on the past observations and not on the present or the future observations. Since in this data set drop out is mainly due to the primary tumor and not to the bone metastasis, we think it safe to work under this assumption. It should also be noted that using maximum likelihood methodology implies that we rely on the multivariate normal model. Since we have plenty of data, we can afford to fit multivariate normal models to our data (in all relevant subgroups) without specification of any model for the means or the covariances as a function of follow-up time (week). The parameters estimated in this procedure are the population parameters if no drop out occurs. Data of patients that drop out are implicitly imputed by the predictions from the past observations. Therefore, means estimated this way may differ from the crude means of all available data if missing does depend on the past. In this data set there is hardly any difference. The multivariate normal model can be fitted by standard software as SAS, but we preferred to write our own program in Gauss based on the EM algorithm. We do not give computational details, but refer the reader to useful material as Laird, Lange and Stram (1987), McLachlan and Krishnan (1997) or Meng and Van Dijk (1997) for further details. The results for the total data set are shown in Figures 3, 4 and 5.

As said before, the overall mean in Figure 3 is very close to the crude mean. Figure 4 shows that the standard deviations increase over time as could be expected from a group of patients that is selected to be homogeneous at entry. Furthermore, Figure 5 shows a nice ridge on the covariance matrix indicating pure noise that hopefully can be separated from the signal. We will come back to that in the next section.

The interesting part in this section is that we, in some sense, know everything about the distribution of the pain measurements and can ask any question we want of the multivariate normal distribution. These questions can easily be answered by simulating

Figure 3. Mean pain score over time and 95%-confidence bands

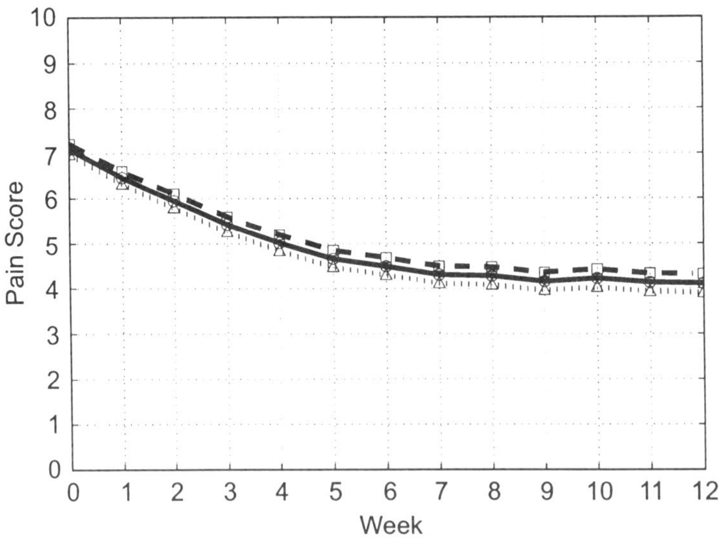

Figure 4. Standard deviation of the pain score over time

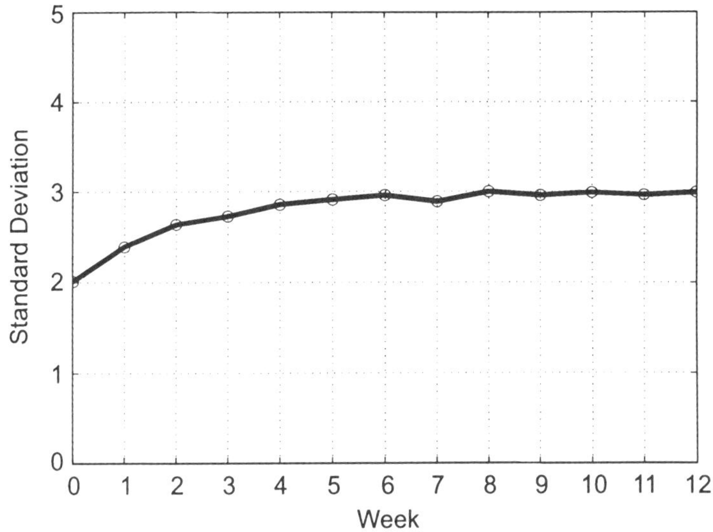

Figure 5. Covariances of the pain scores

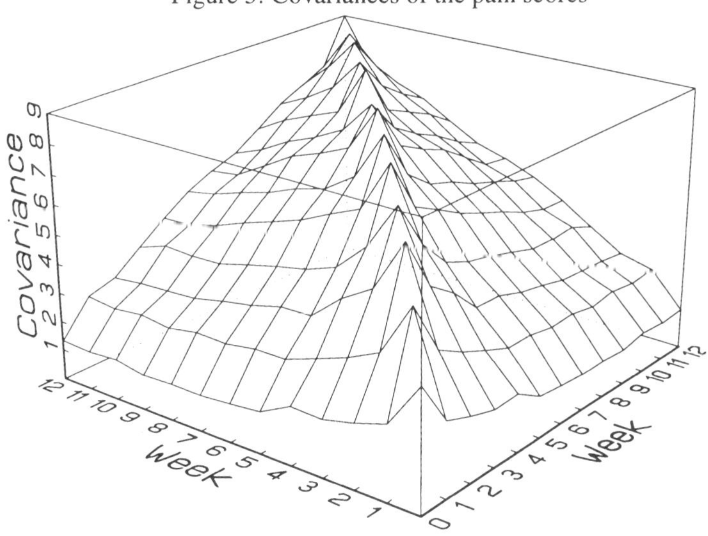

Figure 6. Survival curves for the time to response and the time to relapse. Solid lines are for 1×8 Gy, and dashed lines are for 6×4 Gy

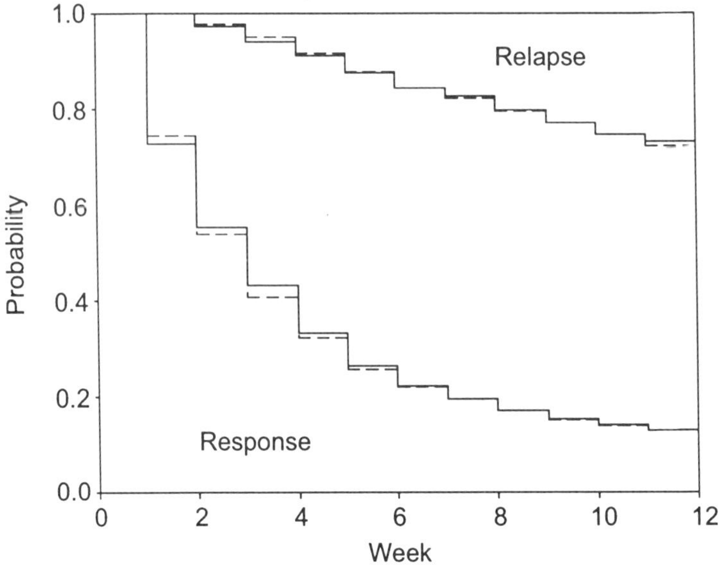

Figure 7. Mean pain score according to tumor type

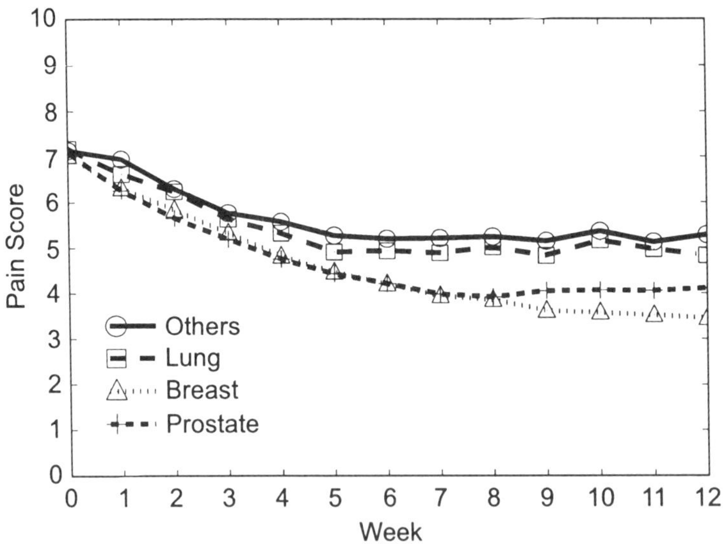

from the distribution. So we can, for example, compute the time-to-response distribution in the two treatment groups, after fitting multivariate normals to each group separately. Similarly, we can compute the time-to-relapse distribution for all patients that show a response within the first 13 weeks. The resulting survival curves are shown in Figure 6.

The lower curves in Figure 6 show the time to response, and the upper curves the time to relapse. There is hardly any difference between the two treatment groups. Actually, there is some difference between the tumor type groups that could best be visualized from their estimated means as shown in Figure 7. Summarizing, if one believes that the data are missing at random and that they have a multivariate normal distribution, the latter model can be fitted easily on data sets of this size by means of the EM-algorithm and all questions about probabilistic behavior of the outcome over time can be answered by computation or simulation. However, that does not give much insight. To get more insight we should try to separate signal from noise.

4. Separating signal from noise

The next step is the separation of signal and noise. Let us first consider the case of no missing values. All observation vectors are of the same length, l, say. For the data of patient i, we can write

$$Y_i = \mu_i + \theta_i + e_i.$$

Here, the vector Y_i denotes the observed measurements of the i-th patient, μ_i is the mean value (possibly depending on covariates like treatment and tumor type), and the vector θ_i denotes the patient-specific signal. The latter is supposed to lie in a low-dimensional space of dimension r, that is we can write $\theta_i = Fu_i$, with patient-specific u_i having the $N(0,\tau^2 I_r)$ distribution. Here, F is an unknown $1 \times r$ matrix defining the space in which the θ_i can be found. Finally, the vector e_i denotes the noise that is independent of θ_i and has the $N(0,\sigma^2 I)$ distribution. If there are missing observations, the model can be obtained by skipping the rows of Y_i, μ_i, θ_i, F and e_i that correspond with the missing positions.

The problem of estimating the unknowns F, τ^2 and σ^2 is the problem of classical factor analysis. The result of applying factor analysis to the estimated covariance matrix in the model without subgroups ($\mu_i \equiv \mu$) gave $r = 4$ as a reasonable dimension for the factor space. Figure 8 gives the plots of the columns of F (known as factor loadings) against time. These curves are usually called the principal curves (See Berkey, Laird, Valadian and Gardner, 1991). The first curve is corrected slightly to be monotonic. All principal curves can be smoothed manually or by some smoothing algorithm, but we stick to the crude principal curves shown in Figure 8.

Instead of redoing the factor analysis with covariates affecting the mean vector μ, we use the principal curves of the model for the total group as the starting point for a random effects model. That is, we consider the matrix F as given and we write

$$Y_i = X_i\beta + F_i u_i + e_i.$$

Here, e_i denotes the noise with variance σ^2, F_i denotes the principal curves at the observation points, u_i for the patient-specific random effects that are taken to be independent $N(0,\Sigma_u)$, and X_i denotes the patient-specific design matrix. We use the principal curves in F and the constant to model the time-effects. This is not a matter of principle, but merely a matter of convenience. It means that in the model for the pooled

Figure 8. Principal curves derived from the factor analysis of the covariance matrix

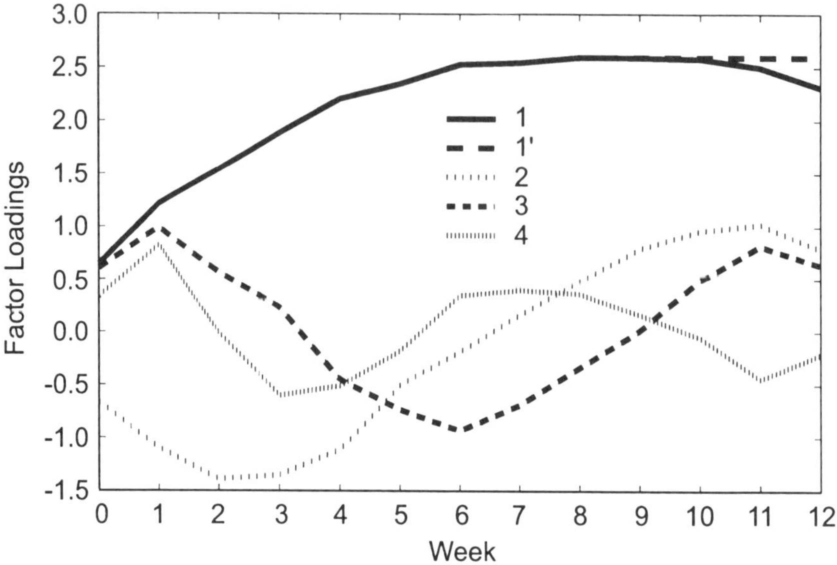

group, X_i, is just F_i extended with a column of ones: $X_i = [F_i \mid 1]$. Furthermore, covariates such as treatment and tumor type and their interactions with the basis time functions can be included by lengthening β and extending the number of columns of X_i in the usual way. The model we have now is just the random effects model of Laird and Ware (1982). Again, it can be easily fitted by the EM algorithm.

The mean curves estimated this way hardly differ from the mean curves in the saturated (full) model of Section 3. The interesting thing is that we can split up the covariance matrix in a part stemming from the signal ($F\Sigma_u F'$) and a part ($\sigma^2 I$) due to the noise. A plot like Figure 5 of the total covariance matrix $F\Sigma_u F' + \sigma^2 I$ would show a ridge similar to the one in Figure 5. This splitting up of the covariance matrix enables us to answer all questions about the distribution of the signal. The most interesting question is what the distributions of time to response and time to relapse are if we define them in terms of the signal instead of the crude observations. Notice, that we are not able to remove the noise from the individual data, but that we do know the probabilistic behavior of the signal, provided we believe our model. The resulting distribution of signal-based time-to-response and time-to-relapse are shown in Figure 9 for the two treatment groups. Comparing it with Figure 6, we see that there is less response since response due to random fluctuation is removed and that there is hardly any relapse left. So, most observed relapses are purely due to random fluctuation. Apparently, the concept relapse should be handled with very much care. We can also draw random curves from the multivariate normal signal model in the hope to see some system in the curves. Unfortunately, that gives rather a messy picture (not shown) and little information. In some sense, the multivariate normal distribution is much too continuous. If we expect clear patterns we should build that into the model. The next section discusses how to do that.

Figure 9. Survival curves for the time to response and the time to relapse based on the signal only. Solid lines are for 1×8 Gy, and dashed lines are for 6×4 Gy

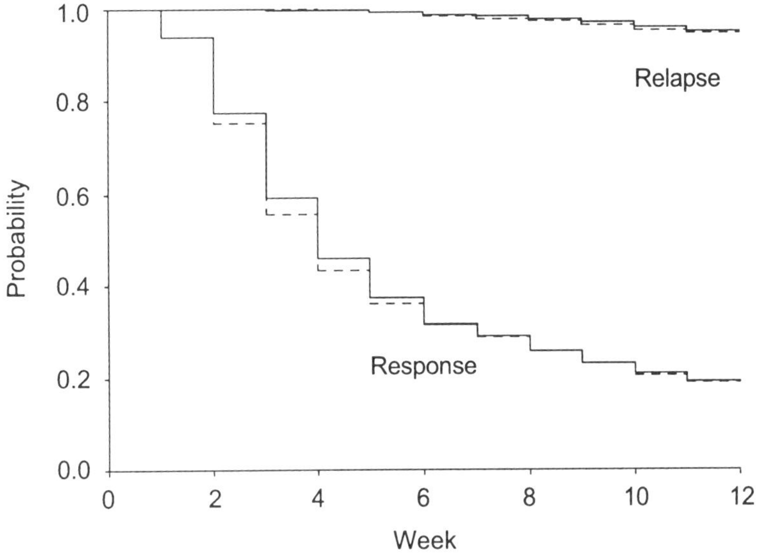

5. Latent Class Models

Instead of considering a continuous random effects model we look for a few distinctive patterns as in Skene and White (1992). To reduce the dimension of the problem we seek the patterns in the same space as the random effects model, that is the space generated by the l × (r+1)-matrix C consisting of the constant and the principal curves F of Figure 8, $C = [F|1]$. That leads to a mixture model with k latent classes for the complete observations of patient i

$$Y_i \sim \sum_{j=1}^{k} \pi_j N(C\xi_j, \sigma^2 I).$$

The typical curves for each class are given by the $C\xi_j$. The observations vary around it with independent noise with variance σ^2. The unknown parameters in this model are k (the number of classes), the class probabilities π_j, the r-vectors $\xi_1,\ldots, \xi_k$ that determine the location of the classes and the residual variance σ^2. The classes are thought to be independent of the covariates, but the class probabilities might depend on the covariates. We will come back to that aspect later. For the time being we ignore the covariates and consider the pooled group. This model is very close to old-fashioned cluster analysis. Describing it as a latent class model has the nice feature that it allows for missing data as long as they are missing at random. Again, missing data are taken care of in the model by skipping the rows that corresponds to unobserved components of Y.

The search for typical curves and mixing probabilities is rather straightforward by EM-algorithm. Actually, it is one of the first applications of the EM-algorithm. The

Figure 10. Typical curves for a two-classes model ($k = 2$) for the original data

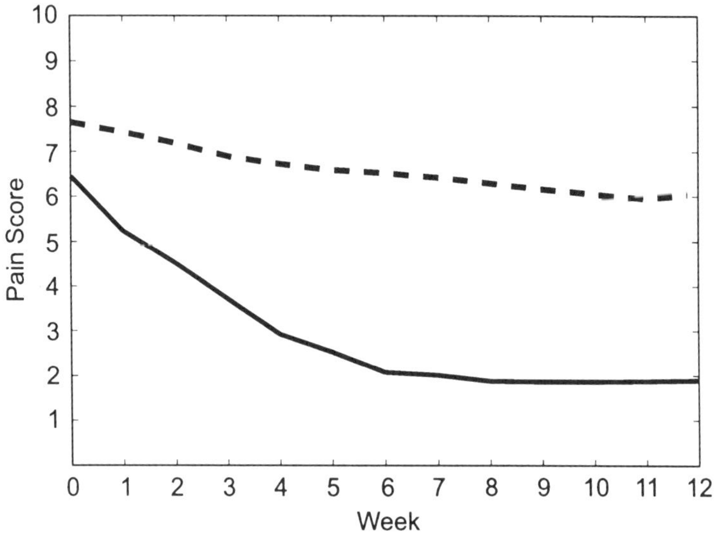

typical curves for $k = 2$ are shown in Figure 10. It shows two different patterns. One starting at a high level and not changing very much and another one starting at a lower level and apparently responding to treatment. Although this solution looks interesting, it does not fit very well. (Fit can be measured by the residual variance or by the likelihood of the model. Usually this two measures lead to the same conclusions about the number of classes that is needed.). For our data, we need a very high value of $k > 20$ to obtain a reasonable fit. The intuitive reason is that we model starting value and changes over time simultaneously. It is better to split the two problems and to consider the changes in the Y's instead of the original observations. A straightforward approach is to subtract the starting value of the subsequent observations. That is feasible if one realizes that subtraction of the first observation changes the covariance structure of the error. However, we run into trouble with this approach if the first observation is missing. To avoid that problem we write the latent class model for the changes as

$$Y_i \sim \sum_{j=1}^{k} \pi_j N(\alpha_i 1 + F^* \eta_j, \sigma^2 I).$$

Here α_i stands for the true unknown starting value for patient i. It is treated as a pure nuisance parameter that can vary from patient to patient. The adjusted design matrix F^* does not contain the constant anymore and is obtained by subtracting the starting value from all principal curves in F. Consequently, the first row of F^* contains only zero. As before, missing values (even of the starting value) can be handled easily by skipping rows. This model is also easy to fit by the EM-algorithm. The results for $k = 2$ and $k = 4$ are shown in Figure 11 and Figure 12. The solution of Figure 11 gives a simple solution

Figure 11. Typical curves for a two-classes model ($k = 2$) for the changes from baseline. The mixing proportions are 0.60 and 0.40.The residual variance is 2.43.

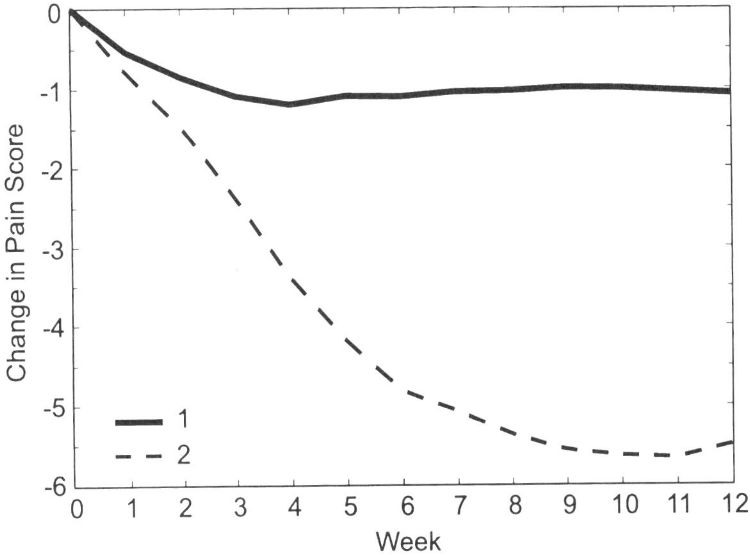

Figure 12. Typical curves for a four-classes model ($k = 4$) for the changes from baseline. The mixing proportions are 0.42, 0.27, 0.20 and 0.11. The residual variance is 2.06

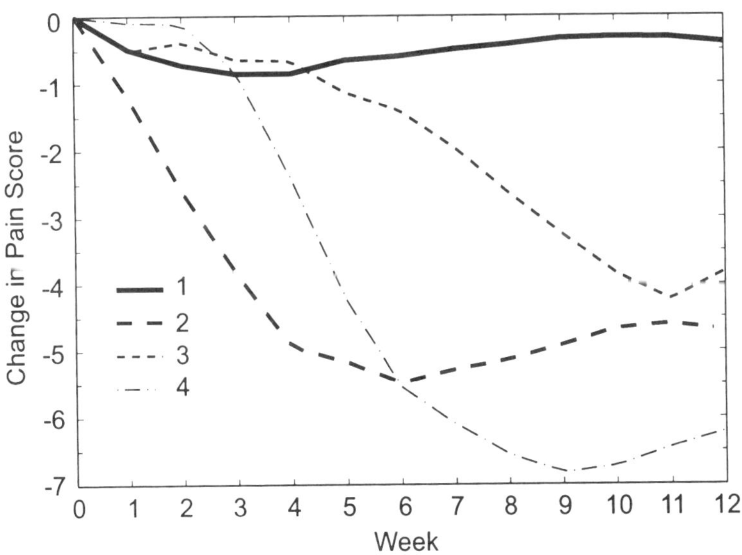

in two classes, one with a slow and limited improvement and one with a rapid improvement. Observe that neither curve shows any relapse. However, this model is also a bit too simple in terms of the fit of the model. A very good fit in terms of likelihood is obtained with $k = 8$, but the model of Figure 12 with $k = 4$ gives a reasonable fit and is very easy to interpret.

In Figure 12, the latent classes can be interpreted as 1 = no response, 2 = immediate response, 3 = late response and 4 = intermediate response. The more natural order is immediate response, intermediate response, late response and no response. For each patient in the data set with at least two observations we can compute the posterior probabilities of belonging to each of these classes. With these posterior probabilities we can first perform a crude check of whether the latent classes are really there (i.e., that is the clusters do not overlap). In the ideal case, the posteriors should all be zero or one. This is checked in Figure 13. The result seems to be very promising.

Figure 13. Histograms of the posterior distributions

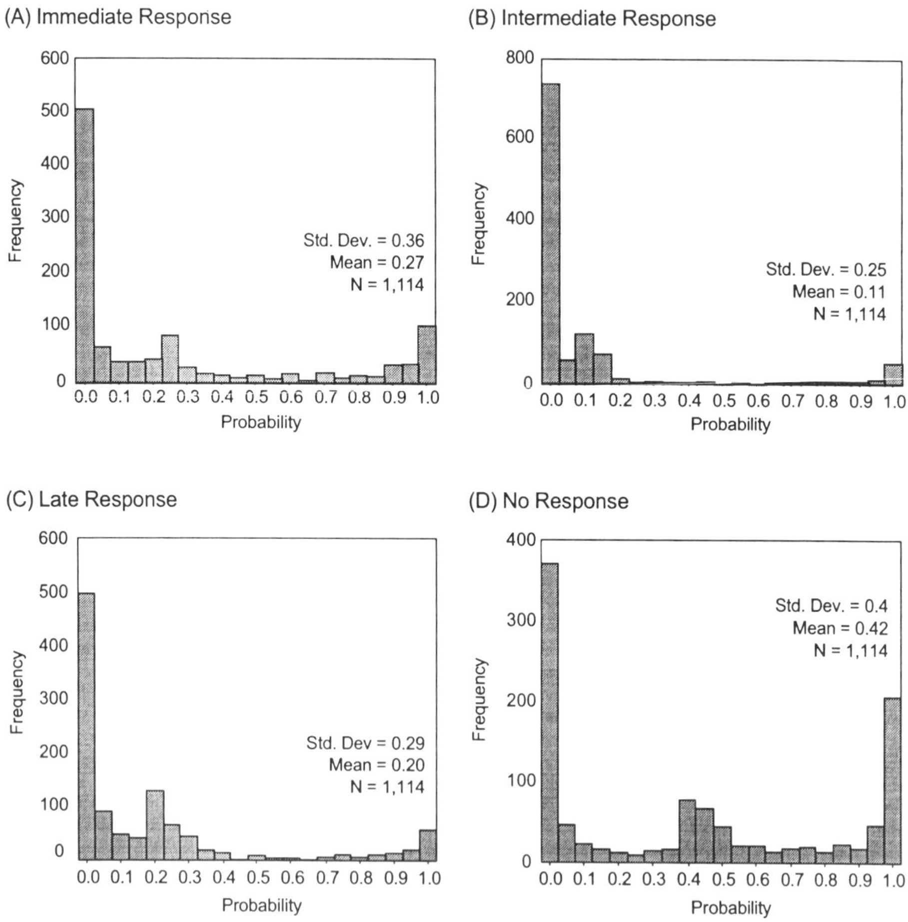

Figure 14. Mean posterior probability by subgroup

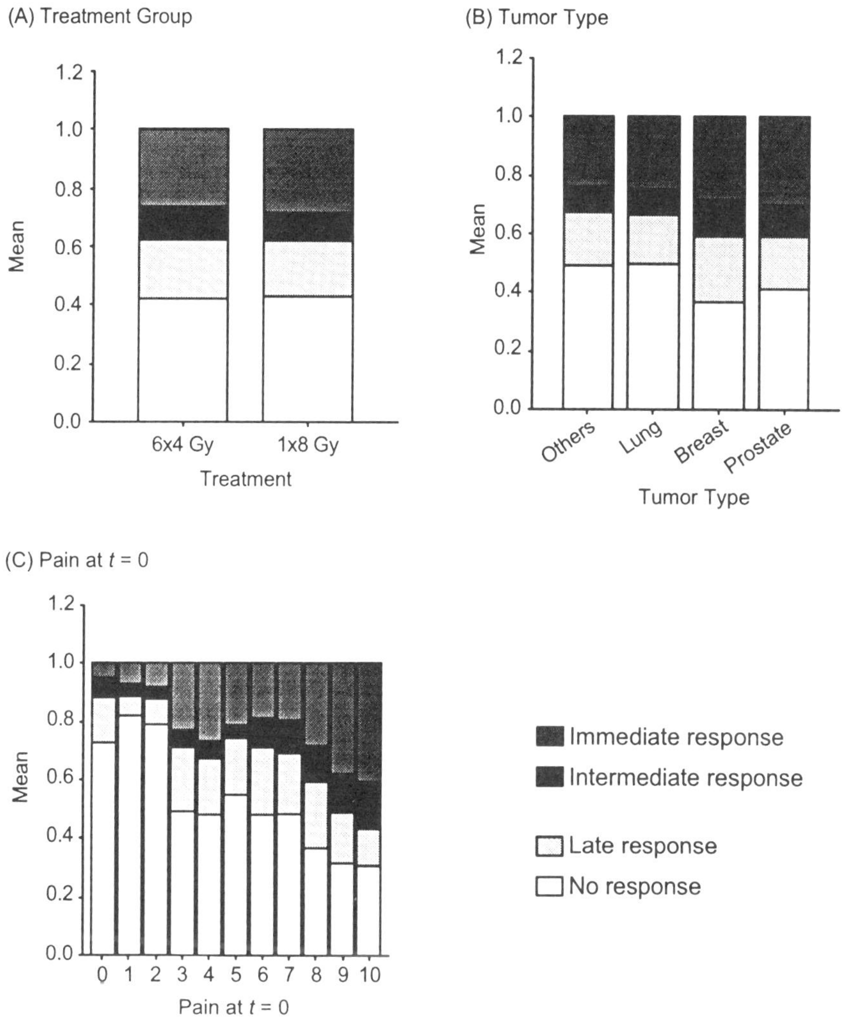

A second question is in how far the mixing probabilities depend on covariates. A sophisticated way of answering that question is by including covariates in the mixing probabilities via a polytomous logistic regression model. It is possible to fit such models, but in this paper we restrict attention to more exploratory ways of analyzing the covariate effect. A very simple way is to force every patient into one of the k classes (as usually is done in cluster analysis) and then compare the clusters with respect to the distribution of the covariates. A less simple approach is to use the posterior probabilities of the pooled model as computed above and to study the relation between the posterior probabilities and the covariates. This can be done graphically or analytically. The graphical results of Figures 14 show the mean posterior probabilities in the subgroups. Apparently, the response does not depend on treatment (Figure 14A), but does depend on the tumor type (Figure 14B) and the starting value (Figure 14C).

An analytical alternative is to perform an AN(C)OVA on each of the posterior probabilities. The results for the probability of no response are shown in Table 2 and support the inference made from the graphs. These findings indicate that this approach is able indeed to find patterns in the data and to relate them to the covariates. It is a hopeful start for further development of this analysis strategy.

Table 2. ANOVA on the posterior probabilities of no response

Source	Sum of squares	DF	Mean square	F	p-value
Corrected model	13.527	8	1.691	11.567	< 0.001
Intercept	45.909	1	45.909	314.050	< 0.001
Start	9.041	1	9.041	61.846	< 0.001
Tumor type	4.047	3	1.349	9.229	< 0.001
Treatment	0.221	1	0.221	1.514	0.2
Tumor type by treatment interaction	0.737	3	0.246	1.680	0.2
Error	155.541	1,064	0.146		

6. Discussion

Thompson Beacon and England (1998) analyzed a very similar data set using generalized estimating equations in combination with cubic splines. Their approach focused on estimating the mean curve over time, taking the correlation between observations as a nuisance parameter. In our analysis, the focus is on grasping the shape of the response curves over time. This is very close to modelling the correlation between the observations. As always, estimating correlations and latent structure is much harder than estimating the mean.

Our approach found a particular pattern in the data and distinguished between four response categories: immediate response, intermediate response, late response and no response. This is similar to studying the time-to-response as suggested in the study protocol. The main difference is that we used all data from a patient to classify the patient into a response category rather than a simple response definition such as a two-point drop in score.

The shapes we obtained are purely data driven. We would like to incorporate more medical information about the shape of the curves into the model or use very simple shapes like the hockey-stick or the bath-tub curve. This would lead in a natural way to finite mixtures of highly non-linear models. Such models are quite hard to fit. Finding good algorithms to fit such models is the subject of ongoing research subsidized by the Dutch Cancer Society.

REFERENCES

Beacon, H.J., Thompson, S.G and England, P.D. (1998). The analysis of complex patterns of longitudinal binary response: an example of transient dysphagia following radiotherapy. *Statistics in Medicine* **17**, 2551–2561.

Berkey, C.S., Laird, N.M., Valadian, I. and Gardner J. (1991). Modelling adolescent blood pressure patterns and their prediction of adult pressures. *Biometrics* **47**, 1005–1018.

Laird, N.M., Lange, N. and Stram, D. (1987). Maximum Likelihood computations with repeated measures: application of the EM algorithm. *Journal of the American Statistical Association* **82**, 97–105.

Laird, N.M. and Ware, J.H. (1982). Random-effects models for longitudinal data. *Biometrics* **38**, 963–974.

Little, R.J.A. and Rubin, D.B. (1987). *Statistical Analysis with Missing Data*, New York: Wiley.

McLachlan, G.F. and Krishnan, H. (1997). *The EM Algorithm and Extensions*, New York:Wiley.

Meng, X.-L. and Van Dyk, D. (1997). The EM algorithm–an old folk-song sung to a fast new tune. *Journal of the Royal Statistical Society Series B* **58**, 511–567.

Skene, A.M. and White, S.A. (1992). A latent class model for repeated measurement experiments. *Statistics in Medicine* **11**, 2111–2122.

Steenland, E., Leer, J., van Houwelingen, H., Post, W.J., van den Hout, W.B., Kievit, J., de Haes, H., Martijn, H., Oei, B., Vonk, E., van der Steen-Banasik, E., Wiggenraad, R.G.J., Hoogenhout, J., Warlam-Rodenhuis, C., van Tienhoven, G., Wanders, R., Pomp, J., van Reijn, M., Mierlo, T. and Rutten, E. (1999). The effect of a single fraction compared to multiple fractions on painful bone metastases: a global analysis of the Dutch Bone Metastasis Study. *Radiotherapy and Oncology* **52**, 101–109.

Chapter 5

Quality-Adjusted Survival Analysis and Related Methods

PREVALENCE ANALYSIS OF RECURRENT AND TRANSIENT HEALTH STATES IN QUALITY OF LIFE STUDIES

ANDREW KRAMAR[1] AND REMI LANCAR[2]

[1] *Val d'Aurelle Regional Cancer Centre* [2] *INSERM SC4*

We present methods for analyzing quality of life data through the use of weighted prevalence functions when data allow a classification of scores into discrete states of health. Individual longitudinal data is transformed from an event history model into a non-parametric setting to provide a simpler interpretation in terms of probabilities. We discuss similarities and differences with quality adjusted survival methodology and illustrate the methods with an example.

1. Introduction

Many quality of life (QoL) scales use categorical measurements to summarize the "health" state of an individual at baseline and at either pre-specified or random time points depending on the study requirements. Information is collected on many variables, which are usually subdivided into specific sub-categories relating to functions (physical, role, emotional, cognitive, social), symptoms (fatigue, pain, etc.) or organs (heart, brain, bladder, etc.) depending on the clinical question of the study. One such scale has been developed by the European Organisation for Research and Treatment of Cancer (EORTC) with its quality-of-life questionnaire QLQ-C30, which is now being widely used in clinical trials in oncology (Aaronson *et al.*, 1996). Late effects of therapy are major endpoints in oncology studies that evaluate radiation or chemotherapy treatments. It is known from radiobiology that increased dose rates influence late effects to a greater extent than early effects. So in trials that compare different doses, it is imperative to use late effects scoring systems and to follow patients regularly in order to capture these effects. Techniques for measuring late effects associated with radiotherapy have recently been proposed by a concerted effort of the EORTC and the Radiation Therapy Oncology Group (RTOG). With this system, late effects are coded with subjective, objective, management and analytical (SOMA) components for the evaluation of late effects on normal tissue (LENT) (Pavy *et al.*, 1995). Scoring systems have also been developed for specific cancer sites. Examples are the French-Italian Glossary for gynecological cancers (Chassagne *et al.*, 1993) and head and neck cancers (DAHANCA). No matter which scale is used, each question usually relates to a specific category, and each category can have a varying number of questions, usually scored from 1 to n, with n ranging from 2 to 7 depending on the scales used.

The EORTC QLQ C-30 (version 1.0) is a 30-item questionnaire with 7 questions requiring a yes/no answer, 21 questions with 4 possible answers (not at all = 1, a

M. Mesbah et al. (eds.), Statistical Methods for Quality of Life Studies, 263–274.

little = 2, quite a bit = 3, and very much = 4), and 2 questions with 7 possible answers (ranging from very poor = 1 to excellent = 7). A more recent version now has the first 28 items on a 1 to 4 scale. The overall standardized summary measure (QL) based on the last two items represents global health status/QoL. It is computed as $QL = 100 \times ([Q_{29} + Q_{30}]/2 - 1)/6$, where Q_{29} and Q_{30} denote the respective responses to questions 29 and 30 on the questionnaire. The computation transforms the data to a scale ranging from 0 to 100 in steps of 8.33. If only one of the two questions is answered, QL is computed as $QL = 100 \times (Q_x - 1)/6$, where x is 29 or 30 depending on which question was answered. The QL score is usually analyzed using methods for means. Often a comparison is made between treatment groups.

The SOMA/LENT scales were developed to exhaustively represent a total of 38 topographic sites. Particular sites can be chosen depending on the patient's primary cancer and the treatment target area. The scales have been separated into parts relating to the patient's evaluation (S), and the clinician's evaluation (O) of the symptoms and signs. However, their use is not yet well integrated in the medical community and there are no present recommendations as to how summary statistics should be obtained. The first suggested approach was to take an average of all items, but this was later criticized since it was possible to obtain mean scores with completely different patient profiles, which could miss important grade 4 components of the scales (Denekamp, 1996). Work still needs to be done to define the mechanism by which the various scores can be summarized. There is still much variability in the use of these scales since they are not oriented as questions, but rather as signs and symptoms recorded in boxes, depending on severity.

In any case, one of the major obstacles in using one scale or another depends to a great extent on how these scores are summarized in interpreting the results. Most clinicians know how to interpret percentages and mean values for a tangible quantitative variable in a group of patients, such as blood pressure, a biological measurement or performance status (King, 1996). Mean QoL scores are a bit more difficult to interpret even though high scores are usually constructed to reflect a better well being. However, it may be just as important to focus on maximum scores or on another combination of scores to categorize patients into mutually exclusive health states. Then the prevalence of a particular health state at a specific point in time has a much simpler interpretation since it represents the proportion of patients in a particular health state among those patients still alive and followed.

We present an approach for the analysis of health-related QoL data through the use of weighted prevalence functions for longitudinal data. We illustrate the methods in an example and discuss similarities and differences with quality adjusted survival methodology.

2. Methods

No matter which QoL scales are used, we assume that measurements occur at regularly planned or unplanned intervals before, during and after treatment. One way to summarize this information is to represent the data as event histories and use methods for estimating the cumulative incidence and the prevalence of a particular health state, assuming that health states are coded on an ordinal scale. We will assume that health states can be divided into discrete categories, say 0 (very well), 1 (well), 2 (moderate), 3 (poor) and 4 (very poor). This is true for the QL measure in the QLQ C-30 as well as for any sub-scale score, however the coding is in reverse order ranging from 0 (very poor) to 100 (excellent). For the SOMA/LENT scales, we feel that it is more appropriate to use the maximum score of any item ranging from 0 (none) to 4 (severe) within either the subjective or objective module, rather than a categorized category obtained from an average score of 11 items.

When analyzing this type of data, we will assume that a score of 0 indicates the best or ideal health state of an individual, with increasing integer values up to 4 indicating poorer health states. We label the respective health states S_i, $i = 0, \ldots, 4$. We are interested in estimating two quantities. The first one relates to time until a particular event, where we define an event as the occurrence of a health state of at least grade 3 (corresponding to a mediocre or poor state). Methods relating to survival analysis are appropriate in this setting, since one treatment may delay time to the first occurrence of this event.

However, an analysis of time to the first event will usually not be satisfactory, since health states by nature can be transient lasting for short or long periods of time. They may also be recurrent and reappear in succession and they can be of varying degrees of severity.

Suppose that in a clinical trial, we have QoL scores for patient i, $(i = 1, \ldots, n)$ at J_i time points $(t_{ij}, j = 1, \ldots, J_i)$. Y_{ij} represents the Qol score (0 to 4) for patient i at assessment time t_{ij}. Assessment times can be different for each patient and as a first approach, we will use the method of last value carried forward to handle missing data in the procedures outlined below. This may not be appropriate in all cases, and other imputation-based approaches could be applied (Curran *et al.*, 1996). We will also assume that data are obtained on individuals up until the end of the study or to relapse or death.

2.1 Cumulative Incidence

The time at which a grade 3 or worse health state first occurs is an important summary measure. Cumulative incidence can be estimated and curves can be plotted as a function of time to reflect the cumulative proportion of patients who enter a particular health state for the first time. There are basically two methods for doing this. The first method censors all individuals who do not enter this health state at the time of their last follow-up or relapse or death. The estimates can be obtained from

$$\hat{F}_3(t) = 1 - \hat{S}_3(t),$$

where $\hat{S}_3(t)$ is the usual Kaplan-Meier estimate (Kaplan and Meier, 1958). In this case the event of interest corresponds to a health state of at least grade 3 (S_3 or S_4). Patients who relapse or die or are lost to follow-up before experiencing this health state are considered censored observations. These estimated rates are those that would have been obtained if all other censoring events such as death and relapses were removed. These other events will effect the denominator in the Kaplan-Meier calculations, since the number of patients at risk will decrease over time as patients relapse or die or are lost to follow-up.

Another method estimates the crude cumulative incidence rate using competing risks (Kalbfleisch and Prentice, 1980). The crude cumulative incidence function for S_3, $I_3(t)$, is estimated at time t by :

$$\hat{I}_3(t) = \int_0^t \hat{h}_3(u)\hat{S}(u)du,$$

where $\hat{h}_3(t)$ refers to an estimate of the instantaneous hazard rate for S_3 at time t and $\hat{S}(t)$ refers to an estimate of the event-free survival rate at time t, where an event corresponds to either a grade 3 or worse health state, or relapse or death.

Let us consider the situation of no censoring with 200 patients among whom we observe 10 deaths every year for 4 years and 10 grade 3 or worse health states every year among another 40 patients. Then, the Kaplan-Meier estimate of cumulative incidence at 4 years for S_3 is 22%, but the crude cumulative incidence is 20%. This is due to the difference in the censoring mechanism, since S_3 events do not censor deaths, whereas deaths censor S_3 events.

This illustrates the fact that fewer patients are at risk of experiencing S_3 over time due to early deaths, so in this situation the denominator of the Kaplan-Meier estimator decreases over time faster than for deaths since the appearance of a S_3 event does not remove a patient from the risk set. In this example, however, we may want to conclude that there were 20% deaths ($n = 40$) and 20% patients who had a grade 3 or worse health state ($n = 40$). The 22% rate estimated by the Kaplan-Meier method is an estimate of the rate that we would have observed if there had not been any deaths at all. This is clearly a hypothetical situation.

Both of these methods have their limitations, since they only attach importance to the occurrence of first entry into a particular health state. With longitudinal data, it may be more informative to take into account length of stay as well as other entries into this health state.

2.2 Multi-State Representation

To appreciate the dynamic process of movements into and out of different health states over time, it is useful to conceptualize the process by indicating entries into each health state (S_1, S_2, S_3, S_4) with directional arrows as shown in Figure 1.

Figure 1. Movements between Health States over time. RD denotes "relapse or death."

$$\text{RD} \longleftarrow S_0 \longleftrightarrow [S_1 \text{ or } S_2 \text{ or } S_3 \text{ or } S_4] \longrightarrow \text{RD}$$

All patients start in the initial state S_0. From this initial state, each patient may either stay in this state or move into a worse health state (S_1, S_2, S_3 or S_4) or relapse or die. From S_1, S_2, S_3 or S_4, each patient may remain in the state or move to S_0 or relapse or die. From S_0, each patient may remain in the state, may experience another health state $S_{>0}$ or relapse or die. It is important to note that movements can occur back and forth between a healthy (S_0) and an unhealthy state ($S_{>0}$). Also, once a patient has relapsed or died (or is censored), he is no longer considered at risk. The health states may be composed of as many severity grades as the scoring system allows. Patients can enter a health state of severity grade 1, 2, 3 or 4 and before exiting, they may move between all severity grades by either an increase or decrease in health status. Severity can increase from S_1 to S_2 to S_3 or to S_4, or from S_2 to S_3 or to S_4, or it can decrease by moving from S_2 to S_1, or from S_4 to S_3 to S_2 or to S_1, or from S_3 to S_2 or to S_1.

2.3 Prevalence

The prevalence of a particular health state at time t is defined as the probability of being in that health state among relapse-free surviving patients. This quantity reflects not only entries into the given health state, say S_3, but also provides information as to how many patients are still in S_3 at specific time points.

For the example presented in Section 2.1, let us suppose that 6 patients out of 10 in the grade 3 health state leave this state for a lower grade state after 1.5 years. Then at each time point, we can estimate the proportion of patients who are in the grade 3 health State as the ratio of the proportion of patients in S_3 and the proportion of patients who have not yet died. The ratio of these quantities provides us with an estimate of the prevalence.

In this example, the estimate of prevalence for S_3 at one year is as 5.3% since we have 10 out of 200 patients (0.05) in S_3 and 190 out of 200 patients who are still alive (0.95). The ratio of these quantities gives us our estimate of 5.3%. At two years, 10 patients entered S_3 among 180 patients still alive. This gives us a prevalence estimate of $0.10/0.90 = 11.1\%$. At 2.5 years, 6 of the 10 patients in S_3 left this state, so we have $4 + 10 = 14$ patients in S_3 at 2.5 years (0.07). Also 10 patients died the first year and 10 patients died the second year, so we have 180 patients still at risk of being in S_3 (0.9). The crude estimate of prevalence at 2.5 years is thus 0.07/0.9 or 7.8%.

Altogether out of 40 patients entering S_3, there were 24 exits from this state occurring at half year intervals, with 16 patients still considered in S_3 at 5.5 years. Since there were 40 deaths and all the other patients had sufficient follow-up, the prevalence of 10% at the end of the curve can easily be obtained as the ratio of the number of patients in S_3 ($n = 16$) to those still alive ($n = 160$). The decrease in prevalence can be explicitly seen in a representation such as this one. When no patient is in S_3, the prevalence is zero. Formulas for this example are presented in the following sections. Although this method accounts for duration and possible re-entries, it does not take severity into account. For this situation, we can use weighted prevalence functions.

2.4 Weighted Prevalence

With the above methods, it was necessary to define a particular health state to evaluate prevalence. Since health states are categorized, we can develop these methods by weighting the prevalence functions for each health state. We start by defining separate prevalence functions $Q_s(t)$, for each health state S_s, $s = 1, \ldots, S$ as the probability of occupying Health State s among relapse-free surviving (RFS) individuals.

$$\begin{aligned} Q_s(t) &= Pr(\text{in } S_s \text{ at } t \text{ among RFS subjects at } t) \\ &= \sum_{m=1}^{M} Pr(\text{in } S_s \text{ for the } m\text{-th time at } t \text{ among RFS subjects at } t) \\ &= \frac{\sum_{m=1}^{M} [A_m(t) - B_m(t)]}{[1 - Pr(\text{RD by } t)]}, \end{aligned}$$

where

$$\begin{aligned} A_m(t) &= Pr(\text{enter RD or } S_s \text{ for the } m\text{-th time at } t), \\ B_m(t) &= Pr(\text{enter RD or recovery from } S_s \text{ for the } m\text{-th time at } t), \end{aligned}$$

RD corresponds to a state of relapse or death and S_s can occur a maximum of M times.

The function $Q_s(t)$ is of interest when viewed in conjunction with the survival function itself, its purpose being to describe an aspect of QoL for relapse-free surviving subjects alive at time t (Pepe, Longton and Thornquist, 1991). This function is of particular interest when relapse-free survival rates are similar between groups. Prevalence is a conditional probability function, so that $Q_s(t)$ lies in the range $[0, 1]$. It can be decomposed into separate parts, one for each categorized health state, since all states are considered mutually exclusive. In order to take into account the natural categorical ordering of the health states we propose the use of average weight functions applied to the individual prevalence functions (Lancar, Kramar and Haie-Meder, 1995).

This function can be expressed as a sum of separate prevalence functions for each health state S_s with respective weights w_s :

$$wQ(t) = \sum_{s=1}^{S} w_s Q_s(t),$$

where $w_1 < \cdots < w_s < \cdots < w_S$.

To avoid any ambiguities in the choice of these weights, they need to be fixed in advance. They can of course, be graded as 1, 2, 3 and 4 if it can reasonably be assumed that being in a health state 2 is half as severe as being in a health state 4, for example. Most grading systems should ideally be designed to reflect this.

The event history model presented in Figure 1 can be represented by a nonparametric model with $2SM + 1$ random variables that are uniquely defined, with M representing the maximum of entries into each health state, which again needs to be fixed in advance. This nonparametric setting avoids hypotheses relating to a particular stochastic process and still remains under a general model imposed only by the transition directions. Consider the following $2SM + 1$ random variables :

$X_{(s,2m-1)}$ = time until entry into S_s for the m-th time, or time until entry into RD, for $s = 1, \ldots, S$ and $m = 1, \ldots, M$;

$X_{(s,2m)}$ = time until exit from S_s for the m-th time, or time until entry into RD, for $s = 1, \ldots, S$ and $m = 1, \ldots, M$;

$X_{(\mathrm{RD})}$ = time until entry into RD.

For each one of these variables, it is possible to associate a survival function $S_X(t)$ indexed by the variable name for the $2SM + 1$ random variables. Since censoring only involves relapse-free surviving patients, the censoring mechanism is assumed independent of the $2SM + 1$ survival functions.

2.4.1 Estimation

The prevalence function $Q_s(t)$ can be estimated by the usual Kaplan-Meier survival estimates associated with these variables.

$$\hat{Q}_s(t) = \frac{\sum_{m=1}^{M} [\hat{S}_{X(s,2m)}(t) - \hat{S}_{X(s,2m-1)}(t)]}{\hat{S}_{X(\mathrm{RD})}(t)},$$

with $\hat{S}_X(t)$ the survival estimate at time t of the $2SM + 1$ random variables.

Suppose we are only interested in estimating prevalence for the first event for each graded health state, in which case $M = 1$. Then we need to define the following 7 random variables :

1. $X_{(3,1)}$ = entry into S_3 or RD or the first time;
2. $X_{(3,2)}$ = exit from S_3 or RD for the first time;
3. $X_{(2,1)}$ = entry into S_2 or RD for the first time;
4. $X_{(2,2)}$ = exit from S_2 or RD for the first time;
5. $X_{(1,1)}$ = entry into S_1 or RD for the first time;
6. $X_{(1,2)}$ = exit from S_1 or RD for the first time;
7. $X_{(RD)}$ = entry into RD.

As an example, we consider a subject who enters S_3 at 7 weeks, then enters S_2 at 15 weeks, then relapses at 20 weeks and dies at 29 weeks. For this subject, the random variables take on the following values : $x_{(3,1)} = 7$; $x_{(3,2)} = x_{(2,1)} = 15$. All the other variables are equal to 20. The associated event indicator for each one of these variables is 1 since this patient relapsed.

2.4.2 Example

For the example described in Sections 2.1 and 2.3, we estimated that 7.8% of patients were in S_3 at 2.5 years. Using the nonparametric methods described above, we obtained this estimate using the Kaplan-Meier survival estimates associated with the corresponding variables defined above. In this example, $M = 1$ so we only need to consider first entries. We thus obtain the 2.5-year estimate of 7.8% as before. Details are presented in Table 1 and are shown in Figure 2. We can see from these data that the prevalence estimates of 11.1%, and 14.1% and 17.5% at 2, 3 and 4 years respectively seem to indicate an increasing prevalence of health state 3 although we have the same number of deaths (10 per year) and the same number of individuals occupying S_3 at regular intervals. This is due to the decreasing number of individuals who are at risk of occupying health state 3.

Table 1. Prevalence estimates for the numerical example

t	RD	in S_3	out S_3	$\hat{S}_{X(3,2)}(t)$	$\hat{S}_{X(3,1)}(t)$	$\hat{S}_{X(\mathrm{RD})}(t)$	$\hat{Q}_3(t)$
1.0	10	10	—	0.9	0.95	0.95	0.053
2.0	10	10	—	0.8	0.90	0.90	0.111
2.5	—	—	6	0.8	0.87	0.90	0.078
3.0	10	10	—	0.7	0.82	0.85	0.141
3.5	—	—	6	0.7	0.79	0.85	0.106
4.0	10	10	—	0.6	0.74	0.80	0.175
4.5	—	—	6	0.6	0.71	0.80	0.138
5.0	—	—	—	0.6	0.71	0.80	0.138
5.5	—	—	6	0.6	0.68	0.80	0.100

Figure 2. Prevalence estimates for the numerical example

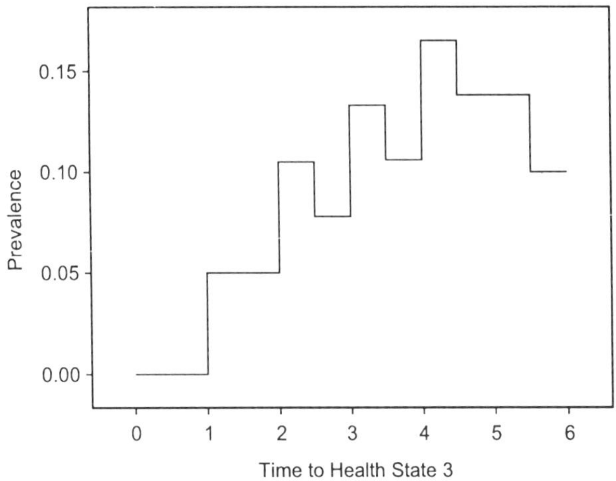

2.4.3 Comparison

Prevalence functions can be estimated for several groups of subjects, and in the case of two groups, the areas under the curves can be compared using a weighted generalized Kaplan-Meier U_Q statistic (Pepe, Longton and Thornquist, 1991). This statistic takes the following form :

$$U_Q = \sqrt{\frac{n_A n_B}{n_A + n_B}} \int_0^T \omega(t)[\hat{Q}_B(t) - \hat{Q}_A(t)]dt,$$

where T is the time frame of the study period and n_A and n_B are the number of subjects in groups A and B respectively. In this comparison, the two prevalence functions are weighted by $\omega(t)$, the left continuous Kaplan-Meier estimate of the censoring distribution. This weight allows a decrease in the importance of the variability in the right hand part of the curve due to the smaller amount of information available. It also guarantees a finite asymptotic variance for the U_Q statistic (Lancar *et al.*, 1994). In the absence of censoring $\omega(t)$ is equal to 1 and the U_Q statistic thus corresponds to the overall difference in the areas under the curves within the selected time frame. Variance calculations are then needed to test for statistical significance (Lancar, Kramar and Haie-Meder, 1995).

3. Application

The second example concerns an updated analysis of 204 patients entered in a single-center, prospective, randomized trial between 1985 and 1988 comparing two preoperative low-dose rates of radiation (0.4 and 0.8 Gy/h) for stage I and limited stage II cervical cancer (Haie-Meder *et al.*, 1994). The objective of this trial was to determine the benefits of the high dose rate in terms of long term complications assuming that local control and survival would be similar between the two groups. In this prospective trial, patients were regularly followed-up and complications of varying nature and severity were observed in succession during follow-up. Complications were evaluated according to a common glossary. At each follow-up visit, information was collected as to the type of complication and its evolution since previous visits. Some data was blindly reviewed retrospectively from hospital records, since the distinction between disease evolution and a severe complication was not always obvious without more follow-up information. The types of complications occurring were numerous and concerned mainly gynecological (38%), urinary (28%), vascular (15%), digestive (10%), nervous (5%), and cutaneous (5%). Each complication was graded according to a severity score ranging from 1 to 4. Each patient was then classified into a severity complication state at each time t according to the maximum complication grade observed at time t among all complication types. Table 2 presents the number of first and total entries into each state for both treatment groups.

Table 2. Number of entries into each state according to treatment group

	First entries		Total entries	
Grade	0.4 Gy/h	0.8 Gy/h	0.4 Gy/h	0.8 Gy/h
1	41	43	44	53
2	24	44	25	49
3	7	13	10	17
Total	72	100	79	119
Relapse/Death	26	35		

Relapse-free survival at 2 years was estimated as 81% and 74% in the two treatment groups respectively. A comparison by the log-rank test yielded a non significant result. The number of first entries into grade 1 was similar between the two treatment groups. However, more total entries were observed in the 0.8Gy/h group. Similar observations can be made for grades 2 and 3. Also, more patients relapsed in the higher-dose-rate group. Using the methods of Sections 2.3 and 2.4, when the first complications and their evolutions were considered, the prevalence of complications was not significantly different between the two groups : 27% versus 38% at 2 years (p = 0.07). When successive entries into and exits from the complication state were taken into account, the prevalence of complications was significantly greater in the higher-dose-rate group : 29% versus 53% at 2 years (p = 0.001). Complication prevalence of grade 2 or worse at 2 years was estimated as 16% and 33% respectively (Figure 3, p = 0.004).

Figure 3. Prevalence estimates for the radiation therapy clinical trial

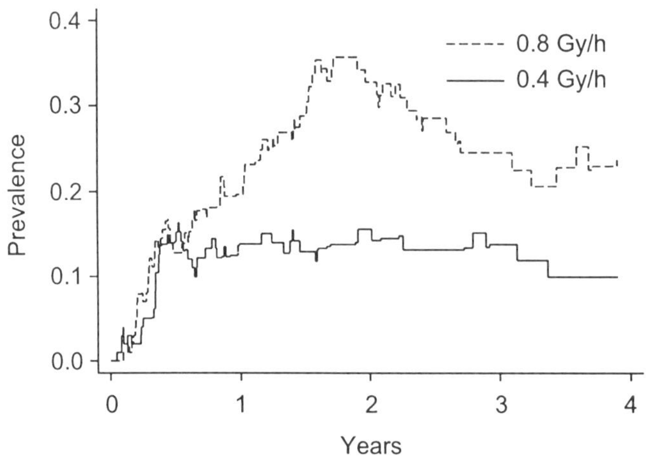

Similar graphs were obtained for weighted prevalence curves. The results of this trial showed that long term effects of treatment, represented by recurrent and transient health states, can use methods of prevalence functions to capture the multi-state nature of this type of data.

4. Discussion

We have presented a way to analyze quality of life data that estimates and compares weighted prevalence functions for categorized health states. The examples presented in this paper clearly show how longitudinal categorized health state data can be represented to reflect the dynamic process of entries into and exits out of different health state categories over time. The summary measures provided with the non parametric prevalence functions give estimates of the proportion of subjects in a particular or worse health state at a particular time point. In public health, this is an important economic measure since it reflects the proportion of patients who may need access to medical treatment depending on the probability of being in a particular health state in the future. Applied to the evaluation of long term recurrent complications, this becomes particularly important, since short term results are usually similar in radiotherapy protocols, and it is only after many years that normal tissue reactions can be seen (Lancar *et al.*, 1994). When we are interested in examining prevalence functions within a particular time frame, then the methods presented here can easily be modified by defining a time frame from t_1 to t_2, with $t_1 > 0$ and $t_2 < T$.

These methods can also be used for situations where patients do not necessarily start in an initial S_0 health state. Examples include categorized scales of depression or anxiety, which can vary in severity over time, but which may already be present at $t = 0$. In this situation, the time frame window can simply be shifted slightly to the left with $t_1 < 0$.

One of the main differences between prevalence functions and quality-adjusted survival methods, such as Q-TWiST, is that the latter methods incorporate components of toxicity, relapse and death to obtain a summary measure depending on utilities associated with each component (Gelber, Gelman and Goldhirsch, 1989; Glasziou, Simes and Gelber, 1990). The interpretation of the results using these methods will depend on the choice of each utility (Cox *et al.*, 1992). Other attempts to incorporate survival information into an analysis of quality of life use trivariate normal modeling approaches (Ribaudo, Thompson and Allen-Mersh, 2000).

Since our methods are conditional on patients being alive, they are more appropriate when relapse-free survival curves are similar between groups. The interpretations of the results of course depends strongly on this assumption. We feel that the point estimates of prevalence at particular time points are nevertheless an important measure since an estimate of the proportion of patients occupying a particular health state is usually only applicable to those patients who are still at risk, that is, alive and relapse-free.

Acknowledgments

Support for this research project was partially provided by the Association pour la Recherche sur le Cancer, Villejuif, France (grant number 9090).

References

Aaronson, N.K., Cull, A.M., Kaasa, S. and Sprangers, M.A.G. (1996). The European Organisation for Research and Treatment of Cancer (EORTC) modular approach to quality of life assessment in oncology : an update. In : Spiker, B. (ed.), *Quality of Life and Pharmacoeconomics in Clinical Trials, 2nd Edition.* New York : Raven Press, pp. 179–189.

Chassagne, D., Sismondi, P., Horiot, J.C., Sinistrero, G., Bey, P., Zola, P., Pernot, M., Gerbaulet, A., Kunkler, I. and Michel, G. (1993). A glossary for reporting complications of treatment in gynaecological cancers. *Radiotherapy and Oncology* **26**, 195–202.

Cox, D.R., Fitzpatrick, R., Fletcher, A.E., Gore, S.M., Spiegelhalter, D.J. and Jones, D.R. (1992). Quality of life assessment : can we keep it simple? *Journal of the Royal Statistical Society, Series A* **155**, 353–393.

Curran, D., Fayers, P., Molenberghs, G. and Machin, D. (1998). Analysis of incomplete quality of life data in clinical trials. In : Staquet, M.J., Hays, R.D. and Fayers, P. (eds.), *Quality of Life Assessment in Clinical Trials. Methods and Practice.* Oxford : Oxford University Press, p. 249–280.

Denekamp, J. (1996). Correction for the use of the SOMA LENT tables. *International Journal of Radiation Oncology Biology Physics* **35**, 417.

Gelber, R.D., Gelman, R.S. and Goldhirsch, A. (1989). A Quality-of-life-oriented endpoint for comparing therapies. *Biometrics* **45**, 781–797.

Glasziou, P.P., Simes, R.J. and Gelber, R.D. (1990). Quality adjusted survival analysis. *Statistics in Medicine* **9**, 1259–1276.

Haie-Meder, C., Kramar, A., Lambin, P., Lancar, R., Scalliet, P., Bouzy, J. and Gerbaulet, A. (1994). Analysis of complications in a prospective randomized trial comparing two brachytherapy low dose rates in cervical carcinoma. *International Journal of Radiation Oncology Biology Physics* **29**, 953–960.

Kalbfleisch, J.D. and Prentice, R.L. (1980). *The Statistical Analysis of Failure Time Data.* New York : Wiley.

Kaplan, E.L. and Meier, P. (1958). Nonparametric estimation from incomplete observations. *Journal of the American Statistical Association* **53**, 457–481.

King, M.T. (1996). The interpretation of scores from the EORTC quality of life questionnaire QLQ C-30. *Quality of Life Research* **5**, 555–567.

Lancar, R., Kramar, A. and Haie-Meder, C. (1995). Non-parametric methods for analyzing recurrent complications of varying severity. *Statistics in Medicine* **14**, 2701–2712.

Lancar, R., Kramar, A., Haie-Meder, C. Lambin, P., Bouzy, J. Scalliet, P. and Chassagne, D. (1994). Méthode d'évaluation des complications tardives. Etude basée sur un essai de phase III comparant deux faibles débits de doses en curiethérapie gynécologique. *Bulletin du Cancer* **81**, 632–637.

Pavy, J.J., Denekamp, J., Letschert, J., Lettbrand, B., Mornex, F., Bernier, J., Gonzales-Gonzales, D., Horiot, J.C., Bolla, M. and Bartelink, H (1995). Late effects toxicity scale : the SOMA scale. EORTC late effects working group. *Radiotherapy and Oncology* **35**, 11–60.

Pepe M.S., Longton G. and Thornquist M. (1991). A qualifier Q for the survivor function to describe the prevalence of a transient condition. *Statistics in Medicine* **10**, 413–421.

Ribaudo, H.J., Thompson, S.G. and Allen-Mersh, T.G. (2000). A joint analysis of quality of life and survival using a random effect selection model. *Statistics in Medicine* **19**, 3237–3250.

MEASURES OF QUALITY ADJUSTED LIFE AND QUALITY OF LIFE DEFICIENCY: STATISTICAL PERSPECTIVES

PRANAB K. SEN

University of North Carolina at Chapel Hill

In the broad range WHO interpretation of Quality of Life, albeit made from an individualistic perspective, there are numerous qualitative factors along with some relatively more quantitative ones which are useful in the context of health related quality of life assessment problems. Though item analysis is commonly used in practice for (quantitative) risk assessment, for drawing valid conclusions, statistical reasoning is essential. Quality of life, survival time and quality adjusted life are important (population-based) measures that need to be appraised in light of statistical and health-related undercurrents. This paper addresses some basic statistical issues prevailing in this context.

1. Introduction

The medical community has been using quality of life (QOL) measures to assess the health status of patients who have undergone specific treatments (e.g., surgery, radiation therapy, etc.) for disease (e.g., cancer, cardiovascular disease, diabetes, etc.). For some patients, their life their physical, mental and functional abilities are likely to be impaired to a greater or lesser extent, perhaps for the rest of their lives. Aside from the question of survival it is also important to assess QOL for remaining life. In the clinical context, some medical diagnostic charts (e.g., Karnofsky performance status) are used to quantify QOL in a way that can be used for risk assessment for making medical decisions. There is widespread use of psychometric and therapeutic item analysis to quantify some of the apparent qualitative states, so that suitable measures can be formulated as a quantitative index of health-related QOL (Cox *et al.*, 1992). Because of extreme variability of human physiological and physical reactions to drugs and virus, as well as mental health behavior, and immense difficulties in the assessment of exact physiological and psychological states, there is a genuine need to have statistical appraisal in assessment of health-related QOL. The health regulatory agencies all over the world also use QOL measurement for guiding health care management decisions; however, their view is predominantly from a population perspective. Thus, there is a need to look at the QOL measure from individual as well as a population perspective.

During the past decade, the World Health Organisation (WHO) has been probing into QOL measures from a broader perspective. The WHOQOL protocol, developed in the early 1990's, came up with the following interpretation: *Quality of life is defined as an individual's perception of their position in life in the context*

M. Mesbah et al. (eds.), Statistical Methods for Quality of Life Studies, 275–286.

of the culture and value system in which they live and in relation to their goals, standard and concerns (WHOQOL, 1994). This interpretation has led to a broad ranging concept of QOL affected in a complex way by the person's physical health, psychological state, level of independence, social relationships, and his or her relationships to salient features of his or her environment. Primarily the WHOQOL instrument is designed to measure QOL related to health and health care.

Two statistical concepts have emerged in QOL assessment. First, the *quality adjusted life* (QAL) concept has often been used by the medical community as a measure of the medical and psychological adjustments that are needed to induce an affordable QOL for patients with health problems. At the same time, QAL results in some deficiency of the normal activities in a broad interpretation, and hence, *quality of life deficiency* (QOLD) measures, introduced by Sen (1996), are also appropriate in this respect. In the WHOQOL interpretation, there is a primary emphasis on individual versus the concerned population. Viewed from a population perspective (as is important for health care and service management), we need to examine the WHOQOL interpretation and assess the QAL/QOLD picture in a more interpretable manner. See Sen (1996) for a broad population complex that underlies health-related QOL assessments in general. The general emphasis is on the intricate network of socio-economic, cultural-religious, physiological, environmental, and mental health impacts, taking the WHOQOL interpretation and extending it to a population-based picture. This population perspective is also evident in quality adjusted survival analysis in clinical trials where Q-TWiST methods have been advocated (Goldhirsch *et al.*, 1989; Glasziou, Simes and Gelber, 1990). This paper emphasizes the statistical aspects that have been disseminated more recently (Sen 1999, Chatterjee and Sen 2000), and appraises the Q-TWiST methodology.

Section 2 presents the QOL picture in a broader perspective. For the QAL and QOLD measures, statistical perspectives are presented in Section 3. Section 4 deals with the main results, and in this context, concepts from socio-economic fields are incorporated to formulate refined QAL and QOLD measures. In spite of the basic difference between socio-economic and QOL measures, they share a common goal: to formulate an interpretable quantitative measure in a context that is dominated by a large number of qualitative or imprecisely defined traits. Section 5 is devoted to general remarks and observations with discussion of Q-TWiST methodology.

2. QOL: The Interface

Like the standard of living in a monetary sense, in socio-economic, cultural-religious, environmental, psychological, and health perspectives, there are numerous measures of QOL. Some of these are specifically geared towards individual health problems, such as a specific disease and disorder, while others are health-related in a broad sense. In this spectrum, there are measures based on an individual's perception and measures based on population perspectives. For medical/clinical decisions, it may be more pertinent to look at QOL from an individual's (e.g., the patient's) point of view. On the other hand, from a health regulatory agency's point of view, it is more appropriate to look at QOL from a much broader perspective, taking into account a variety of diseases and disorders that prevail in the concerned population as well as the relevant cost-benefit issues. For this reason, I examine the QOL interface picture discussed in detail by Sen (1996).

We live in a complex of environments that affect our health, and our modern life style plays a key role. We are increasingly dependent on energy resources (such as gasoline, electricity, coal and other fuels) which are suspected to have carcinogenic effects, environmental pollution and toxicity; and we are experiencing more numerous disruptive social and geo-political activities. Increased stress or tension in life is a significant factor. Hereditary or genetic factors contribute enormously towards the propagation of some major diseases (such as diabetes) over generations. Domestic violence accounts for other problems. Infertility among working couples is on the rise (reproductive toxicity). Given the complex of potential causes, even for a single disease or disorder, it might not be wise to treat a disease in isolation (while assessing its risk).

For the proper assessment of potential causes and possible means to combat the progress of a serious disease or disorder, it may be useful to account for other explanatory factors as auxiliary variables. In this way, we may be better able to conduct statistical modeling and analysis of complex health-related QOL studies. There are roadblocks, however. Unlike in most of other biometric or dosimetric studies, for health-related QOL studies, the subjects are the human beings belonging to a group relevant to the specific study goal. This feature holds for the WHOQOL interpretation. With laboratory animals or tissues, certain types of studies can be made with more flexible dose levels and more controlled experimental settings. On the other hand, with human beings, controlled and truly randomized studies are more difficult to implement. Study designs may be complex because of human-subjects complications such as drop-outs, non-compliance, failure due to reasons other than the target endpoint the need to account for covariates or auxiliary variates. From the statistical modeling and analysis perspectives, there could be challenging problems. In a sense, the situation is comparable to the poverty/affluence study where the standard of living is the main endpoint, though it is usually measured in terms of real income or wealth of the people concerned. A clear-cut demarcation of poor or wealthy people based on a single wage/income variable may not be very rational. Incorporation of other auxiliary variables and pertinent factors, though intuitively more appealing, can lead to more complex study designs and invite more complicated statistical modeling and analysis schemes. In the study of poverty/affluence in a monetary sense, standard of living is interpreted in terms of the deficiency of the usual amenities (nutrition, education, health standards) that constitute an acceptable standard of living in relation to the society and world at large. This assessment is generally based on the notion of real income, and there may be a question on its validity to accommodate fully the less-monetary and more-qualitative factors that pertain to poverty. Likewise, in the health sector, QOL actually addresses the deficiency in the capabilities to perform the normal activities in a relative scale to others who are not inflicted with such a disease or disorder. In this assessment, *item analysis*, with its genesis in psychometry, is often used to quantify the qualitative undercurrents leaving the door open for adequacy of such scores in more complex settings. In that sense, the analogy of poverty in the monetary sense and quality adjusted life in the health-related QOL sense is quite apparent. However, a pertinent question is how far they can be studied or appraised on a common ground incorporating common statistical tools? In this respect, there are some major differences, and I shall discuss some of these points. Section 4 brings out the analogy and dissimilarity of poverty measures and health-related QOL measures, and in that light, formulates suitable QOL measures that are more interpretable. First, in Section 3, I present the basic notion of QAL and QOLD, and quantify them in a rational way.

3. QAL and QOLD Concepts

The assessment of health-related QOL is a quantitative risk assessment of a state with many qualitative factors. The WHOQOL interpretation of QOL is mostly from an individual's perception with special emphasis on health-related problems in the context of culture and value systems. It is quite conceivable that the culture and value system might not be totally quantitative in nature. Moreover, health-related problems (specially in mental health) may have persistent qualitative undercurrents, and we need to account for these in our assessment. More than 50 years ago, Karnofsky and Burchenal (1949) and Steinbrocker, Traeger and Battman (1949) advocated the *Karnofsky scale* in cancer and the *American Rheumatism Association (ARA) scale* in arthritis to go beyond the traditional measures of mortality and morbidity in their assessment of health status. The National Center for Health Services Resources (USA) developed schemes for studying effectiveness and economic costs of health services in the USA, and similar QOL interpretations were adopted by other agencies all over the world. In this sense, the primary focus of these QOL measures has been on alternative uses of resources and their benefits, which in turn, require scrutiny from medical, social end economic points of view. In this context, use of item analysis has led to some quantification of QOL assessments. Because many of the response variables in the questionnaire used for item analysis may be binary, polychotomous or ordinal, there is ample room for misclassification of states. Also, QOL assessments are often made with respect to specific objectives that are usually not precisely formulated prior to data collection. Thus there may be serious questions regarding the validity and reliability of conventional statistical tools that are commonly used. Therefore, statistical planning and designing of a questionnaire is an essential task. Another important aspect of the WHOQOL interpretation is its relevance to an individual, who is already inflicted with a specific disease or disorder, is expected to have a substandard quality of life, and possibly, reduced residual life as well. Therefore, survival time following the occurrence of the disease or disorder is of interest. Also of interest are the adjustments necessary to sustain a minimally acceptable quality of life. In this context, QAL measures have become useful. However, there are multiple issues that merit critical appraisal in such an assessment. There may be multiple response variables covering diverse aspects of the disease or disorder. In fact, there may even be a synergism of diseases or disorders in some cases. A follow-up scheme to trace the developments over time is often used. This results in repeated measurement designs or longitudinal studies. The typical time-effect in this respect may also be of considerable importance (e.g., survival time and relapse times following the detection of cancer). Non-compliance due to drop-outs or withdrawals is common in follow-up studies. Death due to other (unrelated) causes cannot also be ruled out. The response variables as recorded using questionnaires (item analysis) are often binary or polychotomous and hence need considerable care when formulating suitable statistical models. Conventional linear models or log-linear models for categorical data models may not always be suitable. Although generalized linear models are often advocated, they should be judged with respect to their validity and robustness prospects in a given context. Accordingly, consider a four-phase QOL assessment scenario from an individualistic point of view. (1) *Pre-therapy stage*: QOL assessment often lead to a proper therapeutic course. (2) *Ongoing therapy stage*: Watch for toxicity and side effects and emergency options. (3) *Post-therapy stage I*: While being still under medical care, assessment of the therapeutic action on QOL. (4) *Post-therapy stage II*: Long-range standing on QOL. See Sen (1996) and Fayers and Machin (2000) for discussion. It is clear that a measure of QOL (or QAL) may depend on the patient's stage. See Gelber, Gelman and Goldhirsch (1989) for a study on a quality-of-life oriented end-point for comparing therapies that fits with the above scenario. The Q-TWIST methodology (Gelber *et al.*, 1995) has been used to compare treatments in terms of quality adjusted survival time. While I will discuss quality adjusted survival time later, it should be noted that the very interpretation of quality adjusted life time needs a careful appraisal, which is given in this paper. If we look into the QOL prospects from a health services and management point of view, we may need to go to the population perspective instead of the WHOQOL individual perspective. This would typically involve composite disease/disorder models and the various sectors of a population that can be characterized in this manner.

Another important aspect of QOL assessment is to relate the health perspectives to mental health or psychological factors via social, cultural, religious and economic perspectives. Some of these factors when treated as explanatory or auxiliary variables could throw additional light on the QOL picture, and thereby could lead to a more realistic picture. Viewed from this composite perspective, the deficiency-undercurrents in the interpretation and mensuration of QAL and QOLD need to be formulated statistically with care and attention to all extraneous factors. Quality adjusted lifetime has emerged as an important yardstick in many clinical studies. This typically involves the lifetime as the primary endpoint with the incorporation of QAL or QOLD measures through appropriate utility scores that are obtained through appropriate item analysis schemes (Zhao and Tsiatis, 2000; and Chen and Sen 2001). Viewed from this perspective, there is also a genuine interest in defining and interpreting QAL and QOLD in a proper manner. This I bring out in the next section.

4. QAL and QOLD: Statistical Perspectives

From time immemorial, wealth and power have been the key factors in the manifestation of the well-being of a country or community or society, though it might be very difficult to measure or even interpret precisely the real wealth or potential power. From a socio-economic point of view, there has been a systematic attempt to quantify the extent of income inequality with a view to identify the extent of poverty and affluence of a society, as compared to its overall standing. It might be to our advantage to start with a simple outline of the measurement of poverty in a pure monetary sense, and then draw a parallel to the measurement of QAL and QOLD in a most simple setting. This would enable us to appraise more complex situations that arise in actual studies, and to formulate more appropriate statistical measures in such contexts.

A foremost task in the measurement of poverty is the demarcation of a *poverty line*, with people having real income below the poverty line being regarded as poor. The setting of a poverty line is of course based on various socio-economic considerations that may vary considerably from country to country, or even, in a country, from one region to another. Apart from that, the measurement of real income is indeed a very delicate task, and often, there is ample room for misclassification or other types of measurement errors. For simplicity, assume that the documentation of real income can be done fairly accurately and the demarcation of poverty line is also judicious. Then, a very crude measure of poverty is simply the proportion of the poor people in the entire population. But, such a measure is not satisfactory for various obvious reasons. In particular, the measure is insensitive to the income inequality within the class of poor people. We may have two populations with (nearly) identical proportions of poor people, but with one group having a higher concentration of people in the upper part of the income distribution (just below the poverty line) while the other group is closer to the bottom of the income line. Obviously, we need to account for this inequality in the description of poverty.

Let X be the real income variable and $F(x)$ be the corresponding income distribution (for the entire population). Also, let $\rho(>0)$ be the set poverty line, so that $\alpha = F(\rho)$ is the proportion of poor people in the population. Thus, the income distribution of the poor people can be defined as

$$F_P(x) = \alpha^{-1}F(x), \;\; x \leq \rho, \;\; \text{and } 1, x \geq \rho.$$

As in Sen (1999), define the rescaled poor income distribution as

$$F_P^o(y) = F_P(y\rho), \;\; 0 \leq y \leq 1.$$

Define the mean and the Gini coefficient for this rescaled distribution by

$$\mu^o = \int_0^1 y dF_P^o(y), \;\; G^o = (2\mu^o)^{-1} \int_0^1 \int_0^1 |y - z| dF_P^o(y) dF_P^o(z).$$

Then a commonly used poverty index, due to A.K. Sen (1976), and based on a set of axioms, is the following:

$$\pi_S = \alpha\{1 - \mu^o(1 - G^o)\} = \alpha\{G^o + (1 - G^o)(1 - \mu^o)\}.$$

Here, $1 - \mu^o$ is also termed the *income gap ratio* (IGR). Thus this measure reflects the impact of both the income gap ratio and the income inequality through μ^o and G^o. Sen (1986) considered a variant form wherein the arithmetic mean is replaced by the geometric mean, and it has better robustness perspectives. Specifically,

$$\pi_S^* = \alpha\{(1 - \mu^o)^{1-G^o}\}.$$

I now draw a parallel with our QAL and QOLD measures in a most-simplistic model. As the QAL picture relates to the adjusted lifestyle based on the quality of various physical, social, psychological and mental health perspectives following the occurrence of a disorder or prevalence of a disease, it is imaginable that there is some deficiency in the quality of life, and hence the concept of the poverty index may be incorporated to suit the purpose. Note that by definition of the rescaled poor income distribution, the IGR lies in the interval $(0, 1)$, as does the Gini coefficient, G_o. It is conventional to incorporate various item analysis schemes to formulate suitable *utility scores* which are assumed to be in the unit interval $(0, 1)$. I refer to Zhao and Tsiatis (2000) for some useful accounting of related statistical measures, though their emphasis has been mainly on the mean quality adjusted lifetime. Suppose that there are n individuals under study. Let $X_i(t)$ denote the health state of the i-th individual at time t; assume that $X_i(t)$ is nonnegative, and $X_i(t)$ is equal to 0 if a failure occurs, so that the failure time is given by $T_i = \inf\{t \geq 0 : X_i(t) = 0\}$, $i = 1, \dots, n$. Next, contrasted with the acceptable normal health state for the specific population from which the n individuals have been chosen, and taking into account the various explanatory and covariates, consider a utility function $u(.)$ that takes on values in the unit interval $(0, 1)$. The choice of this utility function could be very delicate, and there is a vast literature dealing with it in specific problems (see Staquet, Hays and Fayers, 1998, for discussion and additional references). Considering T_i alone yields the survival time distribution, without any adjustment for QOL. To account for the QOL factor, in the first stage, Gelber and Goldhirsch (1986) introduced the idea of TWiST (time without symptoms of disease and toxicity of treatment) that only partially accentuates the outcome. Subsequently, Gelber, Gelman and Goldhirsch (1989) came up with the (quality adjusted) Q-TWiST concept that is quite relevant in the current context. I formulate this in a slightly more general way. The utility function generally includes the time period where there is possibly a symptom of disease or toxicity but the individual is alive. As such if the utility score at time t is denoted by $u(X_i(t))$, then the quality adjusted survival is

$$U_i = \int_0^{T_i} u(X_i(t))dt, \ i = 1, \dots, n.$$

Zhao and Tsiatis (2000) worked with the U_i, while Chen and Sen (2001) considered a more general case with periodic observations (as is usually the case in clinical trials). With such a quantitative and rescaled utility function, there is no problem in defining the *quality gap ratio* (QGR) and the Gini coefficient in an analogous manner. Thus, assuming that the utility score is a monotone function of the quality level and is rescaled in the unit interval, define, for a given subpopulation characterized by the occurrence of a specific disease or disorder, the mean utility score as $\bar{u}$ and the Gini coefficient by G_u. If the relative size of this subpopulation with respect to a composite population is $\alpha (0 < \alpha < 1)$ then a QOLD index can be taken as

$$QD = \alpha\{1 - \bar{u}(1 - G_u)\} \text{ or } QD^* = \alpha\{(1 - \bar{u})^{1-G_u}\}.$$

On the other hand, if attention is confined only to the afflicted subpopulation then the QOLD is defined as above but with the factor α dropped. Such an index is different from the conventional QOL measures that employ only $\bar{u}$ without any adjustment for the inequality within the class. Note that both π_S and π_S^* are unit-free (as is F_P^o), but they are not invariant under arbitrary increasing transformation on the original income variable (X). Therefore, for the proposed QOLD measures, the same property would hold. However, given the way specific questionnaires are used to quantify QOL status, it could be quite sensitive to the scores derived from them. This naturally puts many constraints on the appraisal of reliability and validity of specific questionnaires in specific contexts. Let me elaborate this point a bit more. Generally, a questionnaire (such as the Karnofsky scale or the ARA scale) has a number of questions, each one having an (often only partially) ordered categorical response. In a typical psychometric fashion, for different categories, suitable scores are introduced (often data-oriented), and these numerical scores are then pooled together (over the set of questions raised) to obtain a composite quantitative score. Statistically speaking, the choice of these scores is a delicate task, and that needs to be done with care. Secondly, different questions may have different levels of perception, and hence, their responses need to be weighed in accordance to some understanding of their relative significance in a specific context. For such (partially-ordered) categorical response models it might be better to put less emphasis on scores and incorporate suitable measures of diversity instead of inequality (Sen, 1999). Such measures of diversity, called *diversity measures*, albeit in the context of income distributions (with visible ordering) were considered by Rao (1982), Nayak (1986), and Nayak and Gastwirth (1989) among others. Motivated by such considerations, Sen (1989) considered some utility-oriented diversity measures which could be used even for other categorical data models with less distinct ordering of the categories. A more unified treatise of this type of measure (covering even partially-ordered categorical data models) is due to Chatterjee and Sen (2000).

One other aspect of QAL and QOLD measures requires a critical appraisal. Generally, such measures are considered for a specific subpopulation and studied over a time period to focus on the changes (if any) over time or to improve the system with more careful planning and management. In that sense, we have a time series model, but not much linearity. It is also the case that such QAL or QOLD measures are considered on a regional basis so as to compare the picture over the regions under review. In this respect, we do have a complex spatio-temporal model with built-in nonlinearity, and possibly without much spatial or temporal homogeneity. Therefore, we need to look into the QAL and QOLD pictures from a broader spatio-temporal perspective, keeping in mind the qualitative undercurrents (that are usually transformed into quantitative ones by the use of item analysis). For this reason, I consider first some categorical models based on measures which can be adopted in the present context. Consider a categorical data model relating to $C(\geq 2)$ categories indexed as $1, \ldots, C$ with respective probabilities $P_1, \ldots, P_C$, so that $\mathbf{P} = (P_1, \ldots, P_C)'$ belongs to the C-simplex $\mathcal{S}_C = \{\mathbf{x} : \mathbf{x} > \mathbf{0}, \mathbf{x}'\mathbf{1} = 1\}$. Consider a set $\mathbf{u} = (u_1, \ldots, u_C)'$ of utility scores associated with the C categories. Then, an utility-oriented Gini-Simpson index can be taken as (Sen, 1999)

$$I_{UGS}(\mathbf{P}) = \sum_{j=1}^{C} u_j P_j (1 - P_j)$$

The classical Gini-Simpson diversity index relates to the special case where all the u_j are equal to 1. Side by side, the Rao (1982) quadratic entropy measure is given by

$$I_R(\mathbf{P}, \mathbf{D}) = \sum_{j=1}^{C} \sum_{k=1}^{c} d_{jk} P_j P_k,$$

where the d_{jk} stand for the distance between the categories j and k; $d_{jj} = 0,\ d_{jk} \geq 0$, for $j \neq k = 1, \ldots, C$. In the context of income distributions, associated with the C categories are suitable class intervals, so that the categories are ordered in a well-defined sense. This makes it possible to use Rao's quadratic entropy measure (which includes the Gini-Simpson index as a particular case where for $j \neq k,\ d_{jk} = 1$). On the other hand, for qualitative data models, it may be difficult to perceive such an ordering in the categories, so that it may be difficult to formulate a suitable distance function, and hence, a quadratic entropy measure may lose its appeal to a greater extent; nevertheless, utility-oriented Gini-Simpson indexes can be worked out more conveniently.

In the context of income inequality there are two commonly used ordering properties, namely, the Lorenz ordering, and the increasing with a left shift of the reduced income distribution (F_P^o), with the latter being advocated by A.K. Sen (1976). These two orderings are not necessarily isomorphic (see Chatterjee and Sen, 2000, for some counterexamples). With more qualitative response variables, it may be harder to seek for Lorenz ordering, but the other one may still be carried out to a certain extent. For this reason, I prefer to use this measure. Suppose now that we have two rescaled poor income distributions F, F^*, such that they are stochastically ordered in the sense that

$$F^*(y) \ \leq \ F(y), \ \forall \ y \ \in \ (0, 1).$$

Then the Sen (1976) monotonicity condition means that under the above stochastic ordering, $\pi(F^*) \leq \pi(F)$. In other words, if the relative income of a poor person is reduced, the degree of poverty in the population goes up, and this is a very natural requirement for any index of poverty. In the context of QOLD (or QAL) we have a similar situation. The more a person becomes physically or mentally incapable of performing the daily necessities of living and communicating with other people the greater would be the extent of QOLD. Thus, as long as a (partial) ordering of the various states can be defined, we could borrow some concepts from diversity measures described before and appraise the monotonicity property so as to characterize an index as appropriate in a specific setup. Chatterjee and Sen (2000) have shown that in general a diversity index may not satisfy this monotonicity property (as can be easily verified with the Gini-Simpson Index). They have introduced an additional condition under which this holds. The matrix $\mathbf{D}$ is said to have *increasing north-westerly trend* (INWT) if

$$\begin{aligned} d_{i'j} &\geq d_{ij}, \forall i' < i, \text{ and all } j; \\ d_{ij'} &\geq d_{ij}, \forall j' < j, \text{ and all } i. \end{aligned}$$

Under this condition, Chatterjee and Sen (2000) show that the A.K. Sen (1976) monotonicity property holds for the corresponding diversity measure. In the context of qualitative traits with some partial ordering one may be able to introduce such a matrix $\mathbf{D}$ that reflects the INWT property, and then construct a suitable index. With that in mind, as in Chatterjee and Sen (2000), I consider the case of C categories, indexed as $1, \ldots, C$, with respective probabilities $P_1, \ldots, P_C$, but only impose a partial ordering on these categories (which need not be linear). Let $i \prec j$ denote that category i is worse-off than j. With that, Chatterjee and Sen (2000) proposed the index

$$T_1 = \alpha\{1 - C^{-1} \sum_{i=1}^{C} (\sum_{j:i \prec j} P_j)^2\}.$$

This measure has a good prospect as a QOLD index in the present context.

I now consider the QAL measure in the light of the above development. Typically, based on suitable scores, a utility function $u(.)$ is attached to depict the quality adjusted state of life. While these scores are based on suitable item analysis and are quantitative in nature, there could be some traits that are essentially qualitative, and can at best be subject to some partial ordering. In this respect, it would be more reasonable to borrow ideas from the QOLD index, presented above, and formulate a utility function that incorporates the qualitative ordering to a greater extent. Typically, if a person under study has the state i (at a given point of time), then we may assign to him or her the utility score $\{1 - (\sum_{j:i \prec j} P_j)^2\}/(CP_i)$, and with this quantification we can proceed as in the conventional case. If instead of an individual person, we consider a concerned subpopulation then this measure would reduce to the QOLD measure considered earlier.

I now address these issues from a population perspective. Instead of a specific disease/disorder, we will have then a collection of such diseases or disorders, and it is also possible that a person may be afflicted by one or more of these health-related factors. Then, we need to stratify the population by the complex of such diseases or disorders. Let $\mathcal{D}$ be the domain of all such health related factors. Following Sen (1996), express

$$\mathcal{D} = \sqcup_{i \in \mathcal{I}} \mathcal{D}_i,$$

where $\mathcal{D}_i$ refers to a more specific subsector, and $\mathcal{I}$ is a finite index set of such subsectors. Denote the proportion of the population belong to the subsector $\mathcal{D}_i$ by α_i, and for each $i \in \mathcal{I}$, and formulate a QOLD or QAL measure as in above. These are denoted these by QD_i, $i \in \mathcal{I}$. Thus, summing over all these subsectors, the overall QOLD measure is

$$QD = \sum_{i \in \mathcal{I}} QD_i.$$

From health management and cost-benefit point of view, such a composite measure can be used for allocation of funds, etc. A natural question arises in this context. If a QOL picture has to be studied over a time period, and/or over different regions or sectors of a composite population, then we may need to express a QOLD measure as

$$QD(s,t), \ s \in \mathcal{S}, \ t \in \mathcal{T},$$

where $\mathcal{S}$ is the spatial domain, and $\mathcal{T}$ is the time-domain. We are then thrown in to spatio-temporal models with complex structures, and lack of spatial or temporal homogeneity may be commonly anticipated.

5. Concluding Remarks

In Sections 2 to 4, I formulated the basic concepts of QAL and QOLD measures, but did not emphasize the quality adjusted lifetime analysis in the light of the proposed measures of QAL and QOLD. This, of course, requires the setting of the survival function based on the primary endpoint, namely, the failure time, in addition to the formulation of quality adjustments that takes into account the complexity due to possible lack of ordering of the various quality states. I intend to study such measures in future communications.

The ideas behind the Q-TWiST methodology, while very appealing in some specific contexts, in more complex situations, where there may be multiple TWiST states following successive relapses, there could be bias in the formulation of utility scores. More-appropriate utility scores that take into account the quality of life during the relapse and treatment phases should be formulated.

In any case, such measures are from a population perspective, and hence, the QOLD measures considered here are very pertinent in such schemes as well. Let me stress the basic point again: a proper choice of the utility function is a very crucial step in any statistical modeling and analysis task. In this respect, medical and psychometric considerations should be most important in statistical formulations.

From statistical analysis point of view, there could be challenging problems stemming from the complex nature of the QAL and QOLD measures in such complex systems. Censoring is quite common in QAL studies (and may arise due to drop-out or non-compliance), and depending on the nature of censoring (Type I, II, random, or progressive censoring), statistical modeling and analysis could be quite complex. Simple linear models may not be appropriate in most of the situations (as the measures are typically nonlinear functions), and generalized linear models, or suitable semiparametric models may fare better. In some cases, there are periodic observations, and suitable Markov models need to be incorporated (Chen and Sen, 2001). There is ample room for development of statistical methodology to suit this purpose, and I intend to be engaged in such studies in a systematic manner in the near future.

REFERENCES

Chatterjee, S.K. and Sen, P.K. (2000). On stochastic ordering and a general class of poverty indexes. *Calcutta Statistical Association Bulletin* **50**, 137–156.

Chen, P.L. and Sen, P.K. (2001). Quality adjusted survival estimation with periodic observations. *Biometrics* **57**, 868–874.

Cox, D.R., Fitzpatrick, R., Fletcher, A.E., Gore, S.M., Spiegelhalter, D.J. and Jones, D.R. (1992). Quality of Life assessment: can we keep it simple? *Journal of the Royal Statistical Society, Series A* **155**, 353–393.

Fayers, P.M. and Machin, D. (2000). *Quality of Life: Assessment, Analysis and Interpretation.* New York: Wiley.

Gelber, R.D. and Goldhirsch, A. (1986). A new endpoint for the assessment of adjuvant therapy in postmenopausal women with operable breast cancer. *Journal of Clinical Oncology* **4**, 1772–1779.

Gelber, R.D., Gelman, R.S. and Goldhirsch, A. (1989). A quality-of-life oriented endpoint for comparing therapies. *Biometrics* **45**, 781–795.

Gelber, R.D., Cole, B.F., Gelber, S. and Goldhirsch, A. (1995). Comparing treatments using quality-adjusted survival: the Q-TWIST method. *The American Statistician* **49**, 161–169.

Glasziou, P.P., Simes, R.J., and Gelber, R.D. (1990). Quality adjusted survival analysis. *Statistics in Medicine* **9**, 1259–1276.

Goldhirsch, A., Gelber, R.D., Simes, R.J., Glasziou, P. and Coates, A. (1989). Ludwig Breast Cancer Study Group: cost and benefit analysis of adjuvant therapy in breast cancer: a quality adjusted survival analysis. *Journal of Clinical Oncology* **7**, 36–44.

Karnofsky, D. and Burchenal, J. (1949). The clinical evaluation of chemotherapeutic agents in cancer. In: McLeod, C. (ed.). *Evaluation of Chemotherapeutic Agents.* New York: Columbia University Press, pp.191–205.

Nayak, T.K. (1986). An analysis of diversity using Rao's quadratic entropy. *Sankhyā, Series B* **48**, 1–9.

Nayak, T.K., and Gastwirth, J.L. (1989). The use of diversity analysis to assess the relative influence of factors affecting the income distribution. *Journal of Business and Economic Statistics* **7**, 453–460.

Rao, C.R. (1982). Diversity: its measurement, decomposition, apportionment and analysis. *Sankhyā, Series A* **44**, 1–21.

Sen, A.K. (1976). The measurement of poverty: an axiomatic approach. *Econometrica* **44**, 219–232.

Sen, P.K. (1986). The Gini coefficient and the poverty indexes: some reconciliation. *Journal of the American Statistical Association* **81**, 1050–1057.

Sen, P.K. (1996). Statistics and quality of life: third world perspectives. *Journal of Applied Statistical Science* **4**, 231–252.

Sen, P.K. (1999). Utility-oriented Gini-Simpson type indexes. *Calcutta Statistical Association Bulletin* **49**, 1–22.

Staquet, M.J., Hays, R.D. and Fayers, P.M. (eds.) (1998). *Quality of Life Assessment in Clinical Trials: Methods and Practice.* New York: Oxford University Press.

Steinbrocker, O., Traeger, C. and Battman, S. (1949). Therapeutic criteria in rheumatoid arthritis. *Journal of the American Medical Association* **140**, 659–662.

WHOQOL Group (1994). The development of the World Health Organization quality of life assessment instrument (the WHOQOL). In: Orley, J. and Kuyken, W. (eds.). *Quality of Life Assessment in Health Care Setting.* Heidelberg: Springer-Verlag.

Zhao, H. and Tsiatis, A.A. (2000). Estimating mean quality of lifetime with censored data. *Sankhyā, Series B* **62**, 175–188.

QUALITY-ADJUSTED SURVIVAL ANALYSIS IN CANCER CLINICAL TRIALS

BERNARD F. COLE[1] AND KERRY L. KILBRIDGE[2]

[1]*Dartmouth Medical School and* [2]*University of Virginia*

The quality of life of patients is an important component for the evaluation of therapies in clinical trials, especially in cancer. The Quality-adjusted Time Without Symptoms and Toxicity (Q-TWiST) method evaluates treatment trade-offs in clinical trials using an endpoint based on both quantity and quality of life. The methodology has been most useful for evaluating the trade-off between increased toxic side effects of treatment and improved clinical outcome. This paper provides an overview of the Q-TWiST method, brief descriptions of related statistical tools for regression analysis and meta-analysis, and examples illustrating the techniques using data from cancer clinical trials.

1. Introduction

Quality-of-life-adjusted survival time is a complementary outcome that is increasingly being used in cancer clinical research. It represents a patient's survival time weighted by the quality of life experienced, where the weightings are based on utility values. Utility is measured on the unit interval (0,1), where 0 denotes "as bad as death," 1 denotes "as good as best possible health" and values between 0 and 1 represent degrees between these extremes. As a result, Quality-adjusted survival time is in the same time units as overall survival. This allows comparisons of treatments that differ in their quality-of-life effects and their effects on survival using a metric that simultaneously accounts for both of these differences.

The Quality-adjusted Time Without Symptoms of disease or Toxicity of treatment method (Q-TWiST) [1,2] is a technique for evaluating quality-adjusted survival in clinical trials. Q-TWiST compares treatments by computing the time spent in a series of clinical health states that may impact a patient's quality of life. Each health state is then weighted by a utility value, and the Q TWiST outcome is defined by the sum of the weighted health state durations. The method is especially useful when there is a trade-off between increased treatment toxicity and improved response. For example, a new therapeutic regimen may significantly delay disease recurrence, disease progression or death but may also have undesirable side effects as compared to standard treatment. A quality-adjusted endpoint in this case may be useful in helping patients and physicians interpret the results of a clinical trial and make treatment decisions. This paper provides an overview of the Q-TWiST method. First, the three steps for conducting a standard Q-TWiST analysis are described, followed by brief descriptions of several extensions of the methodology. The standard procedure is then illustrated in an analysis of high-dose interferon therapy for malignant melanoma. One of the methodological extensions, meta-analysis using Q-TWiST, is illustrated using data from almost 17,000 women who participated in 47 clinical trials of adjuvant chemotherapy for breast cancer. Finally,

M. Mesbah et al. (eds.), Statistical Methods for Quality of Life Studies, 287–300.

other applications of Q-TWiST are summarized and guidelines for applying the method are outlined.

2. The Q-TWiST Technique

The first step in the analysis is to define quality-of-life-oriented health states that are relevant for the disease setting and the treatments being studied. The health states should reflect changes in clinical status that may be associated with changes in quality of life (e.g., treatment-related adverse events, disease progression, late sequelae), and they should be progressive. That is, patients must move through the health states in order, although health states may be skipped. For example, we may define a k-state model with health states $S_1,\ldots,S_k$ where the only possible transitions are from S_i to S_j, $1 \leq i \leq j \leq k$. For example, in the adjuvant chemotherapy setting health states may be defined as follows: S_1 = time to the end of treatment-related toxicity; S_2 = time without toxicity and without disease recurrence; and S_3 = time with disease recurrence until death.

The second step is to estimate the mean health state durations using the clinical trial data. This is accomplished by partitioning the overall survival time into the health states for each treatment group separately. The Kaplan-Meier method [3] can be used for this purpose; however, in practice, censoring precludes one from estimating the entire survival curve. In this case, the partitioning is done up to a restriction time L. A common choice for L is the median follow-up duration. For each patient, the clinical trial data are used to define the exiting time for each health state. For the k-state model, let t_i denote the exiting time (measured from study entry or randomization time) from health state S_i, $i = 1,\ldots,k$. If a state S_j is skipped then $t_j = t_{j-1}$. If S_1 is skipped then $t_1 = 0$. The exiting time from state S_k will be the time of death. For example, in the adjuvant chemotherapy setting, the health state exiting times may be defined as follows: t_1 = time from randomization until the end of treatment-related toxicity, disease progression or death, whichever occurs first; t_2 = time from randomization until disease progression or death, whichever occurs first; and t_3 = time from randomization until death. If any of the exiting times are censored, then the exiting times for all subsequent states will be similarly censored.

Multiple visits to a single health state can be accommodated by defining states for the model based on the timing of the visits. For example, in the case of intermittent toxicity, S_1 may represent any initial toxicity, S_2 may represent a state of no toxicity, and S_3 may represent a second occurrence of toxicity. Additional toxicity states may be defined as needed. The mean durations of the individual toxicity states may then be summed as appropriate to provide a single estimate of the total toxicity duration.

Let $K_i(\cdot)$ denote the Kaplan-Meier estimate corresponding to t_i, $i = 1,\ldots,k$. Then the mean health state duration, restricted to L for health state S_1 is

$$\hat{\tau}_1 = \int_0^L K_1(u)du$$

and the mean health state duration for health state S_i $(2 \leq i \leq k)$ is

$$\hat{\tau}_i = \int_0^L \left(K_i(u) - K_{i-1}(u)\right)du.$$

This approach to the estimation of the health state durations provides consistent estimates, whereas averaging individual health state durations when censoring is present leads to biased results [4].

The third step is to compare the treatments using a weighted sum of the mean health state durations. For example, if $u_1,\ldots,u_k$ denote the utility weights for the respective health states $S_1,\ldots,S_k$, the Q-TWiST endpoint is given by

$$\text{Q-TWiST} = \sum_{i=1}^{k} u_i \hat{\tau}_i .$$

Each utility weight is measured on a scale from 0 to 1, where 0 denotes a state as bad as death, and 1 denotes a state as good as best possible health. Values between 0 and 1 denote degrees between these extremes. Note that if all of the utility weights equal 1, Q-TWiST is equivalent to the mean survival time restricted to L. Note also that the analysis may be repeated using different choices for L. By allowing L to range from 0 to the median follow-up duration, one can describe the evolution of the Q-TWiST treatment effect over time using a Q-TWiST gain function [2].

Q-TWiST is calculated separately for each treatment group, and the treatment effects are obtained by subtracting the Q-TWiST estimates corresponding to two treatment groups (e.g., experimental drug group versus control group). Standard errors for the treatment effects can be obtained using the bootstrap method [5] or recently derived closed-form estimators [5–7]. If data are available for estimating $u_1,\ldots,u_k$, then these data can be incorporated directly into the analysis. When utility data are not available, the treatment comparison can be evaluated by computing the treatment effect for varying values of the utility weights in a sensitivity analysis. When two utility weights are unknown and two treatments are being compared, the treatment comparison can be plotted for all possible values of the unknown utility weights in a two-dimensional graph called a threshold utility analysis. Contour lines can be used to indicate the magnitude of the Q-TWiST treatment effect associated with different pairs of utility values. The contour line corresponding to a treatment effect of zero is called the threshold line. The threshold line indicates all utility value pairs for which the treatment effects are equal in terms of Q-TWiST. Confidence bounds for the threshold line can also be plotted to define regions of utility weight values for which the treatment effect is statistically significant.

For example, in the case where $k = 3$ and $u_2 = 1$ the contour lines for the threshold utility plot are defined by

$$u_3 = (c - u_1\Delta_1 - \Delta_2)/\Delta_3 \quad \text{or} \quad u_1 = (c - u_3\Delta_3 - \Delta_2)/\Delta_1,$$

where c represents the Q-TWiST treatment effect and Δ_i is the treatment group difference for the duration of health state S_i. Note that if $c = 0$, the above equations represent the threshold line. Contour lines can be obtained by setting appropriate values for c and plotting the resulting equations (e.g., c =-3,-2,-1,0,1,2,3 months). When 3 utility weights are unknown, the threshold utility analysis can be displayed for selected values of one of the weights. For example, in the case where $k = 3$, and all utility weights are unknown, the threshold utility analysis can be displayed for $u_2 = 0.4$, 0.6, 0.8 and 1.0.

3. Additional Statistical Tools

Quality-of-life adjusted survival in clinical trials is an area of active methodological research. Parametric [8] and semi-parametric [9] regression models have been developed for quality-adjusted survival. In addition, methods have been developed for forecasting treatment effects [10] and performing meta-analyses [11]. A number of recently published papers hold promise for an increasing array of statistical tools. In particular, Glasziou et al. [12] describe methods for combining longitudinal quality-of-life data with survival data using an integration-based approach. Zhao and Tsiatis [5] present a consistent estimator for the distribution of quality-adjusted survival time and, in a second paper [6], describe techniques for estimating mean quality-adjusted lifetime based on their consistent estimator. On-going research focuses on developing statistical tools for the analysis of utility data in conjunction with quality-adjusted survival analysis.

4. Analysis of Adjuvant Interferon for Melanoma

The Eastern Cooperative Oncology Group (ECOG) clinical trial EST1684 compared high-dose interferon alfa-2b therapy versus clinical observation for the adjuvant treatment of high-risk resected malignant melanoma in 280 patients [13–16]. The health states defined for the Q-TWiST analysis were: Tox = all time with toxicity due to high-dose interferon; TWiST = all time without interferon toxicity and without symptoms of disease relapse; and Rel = all time following disease relapse. These health states reflect the major clinical changes in quality of life that are important for evaluating the impact of high-dose interferon. To improve readability, we label the states Tox, TWiST and Rel (rather than S_1, S_2 and S_3), and the respective utility weights u_{Tox}, u_{TWiST}, and u_{Rel}.

Figure 1 shows the partitioning of overall survival into the health states according to treatment group based on the product limit method and restricted to the median follow-up interval of 84 months. For each graph, the area beneath the overall survival curve (OS) is partitioned into the health states Tox, TWiST and Rel. This was accomplished by plotting, on the same graph as OS, a survival curve for the duration of interferon toxicity (Tox) and a survival curve for the time until disease relapse or death (RFS).

Table 1 shows the mean health state durations, the mean overall survival time (OS) and the mean relapse-free survival time (RFS) within the first 84 months from randomization in the study. The results indicate that there was a tendency for patients in the interferon group to experience more time in TWiST and less time in Rel as compared with the observation group, but the differences were not statistically significant. The interferon group experienced more time with severe or life-threatening toxicity. Table 2 shows the computation of Q-TWiST for two possible selections of the utility weights u_{Tox} and u_{Rel} applied to Tox and Rel, respectively. The utility weight for TWiST in this analysis was assumed to be unity because TWiST represents a state of best possible quality of life. The utility weights shown in Table 2 represent two scenarios. The first is a patient who values time with interferon side effects and time with disease recurrence half as much as time in best possible health (u_{Tox} = 0.5, u_{Rel} =0.5). In this case, one month spent with interferon side effects is valued the same as one half month spent in best possible health. The second is a patient having fairly high tolerance for side effects of interferon but low valuation for disease recurrence (u_{Tox} = 0.9, u_{Rel} =0.4).

Figure 2 illustrates the threshold plot for the treatment comparison. Note that in this case, the interferon group experienced more quality-adjusted time than the control group for almost all utility values used. The threshold line appears in the lower right corner of the graph. The contour lines indicate that the Q-TWiST benefit for interferon ranges from 0 to 8 months depending on the selection of utility weight values. In addition, the upper 95 percent confidence band for the threshold line appears as a dashed line. Values of the utility weights above the dashed line correspond to a significant ($P < 0.05$) benefit for interferon in terms of Q-TWiST, and values below the dashed line indicate utility coefficient value pairs for which the comparison favored the interferon group but did not reach statistical significance.

Figure 1. Partitioning of overall survival into the health states Tox, TWiST and Rel in the ECOG trial EST1684 (source: Ref. 14)

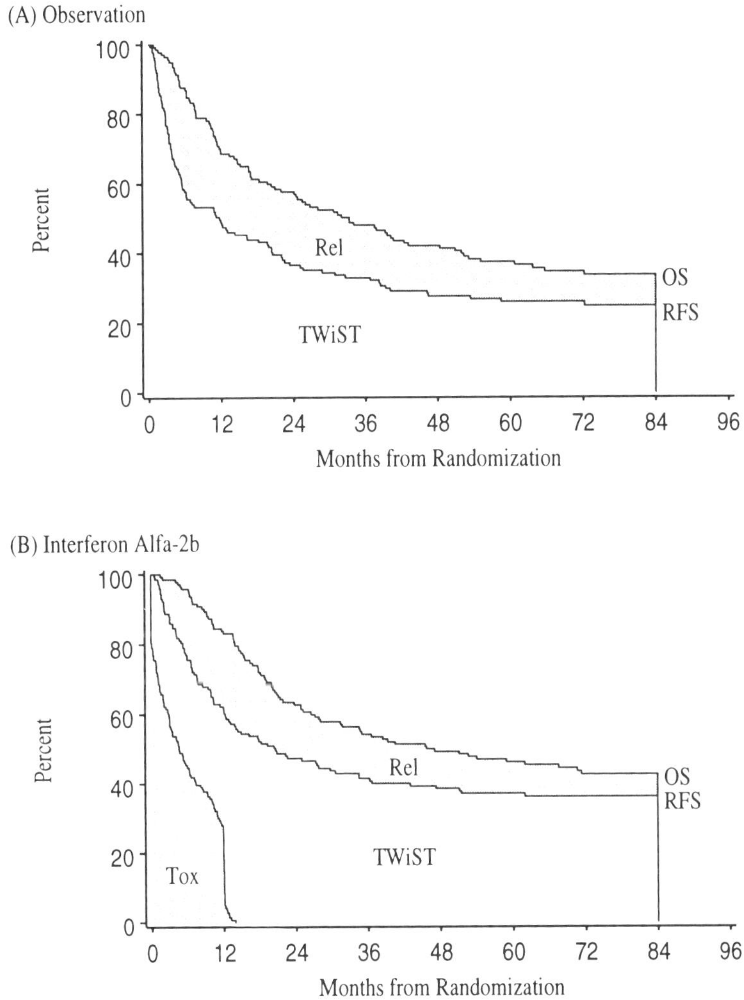

Table 1. Mean time in months for the components of Q-TWiST restricted to 84 months of median follow up in the ECOG trial EST1684 (source: Ref. 14,16)

Outcome	Treatment Group: Observation	Treatment Group: Interferon Alfa-2b	Difference	95% CI	*P* (2-sided)
Tox	0.0	7.4	7.4	6.7 to 8.1	< 0.001
TWiST	30.0	31.5	1.5	−6.3 to 9.3	0.7
Rel	12.4	10.4	−2.0	−6.2 to 2.3	0.4
OS	42.4	49.3	7.0	−0.6 to 14.5	0.07
RFS	30.0	38.9	8.9	0.8 to 17.0	0.03

Table 2. Mean Q-TWiST in months within 84 months of median follow-up in the ECOG trial EST1684 for two hypothetical sets of utility weight values

Utility Values: u_{Tox}	Utility Values: u_{Rel}	Treatment Group: Observation	Treatment Group: Interferon Alfa-2b	Difference	95% CI	*P* (2-sided)
0.5	0.5	36.2	40.4	4.2	−3.2 to 11.6	0.3
0.9	0.4	34.9	42.3	7.4	−0.1 to 15.0	0.05

Figure 2. Threshold utility analysis for the ECOG trial EST1684 (source: Ref. 16)

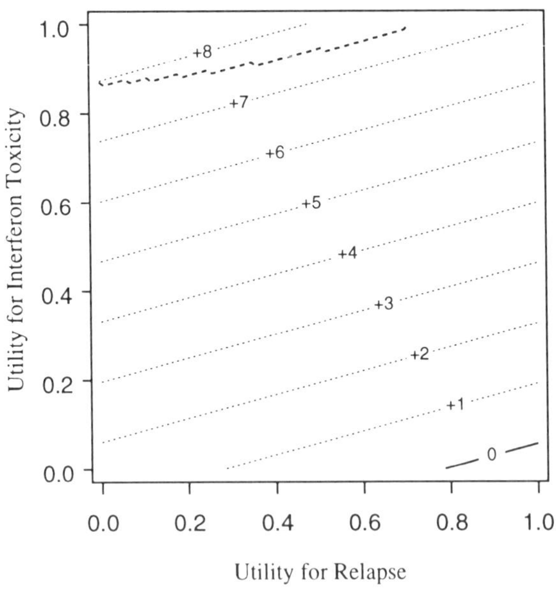

5. Incorporating Patient-Derived Utility Values

The utility weights for a Q-TWiST analysis may be obtained either directly from the patients in the clinical trial, or a separate cross-sectional study may be used. To further evaluate high-dose interferon, utility data were obtained from 95 melanoma patients enrolled in a cross-sectional study [15,16]. These patients were interviewed using the standard gamble technique to elicit their utilities for health states associated with adjuvant interferon treatment and disease relapse. Figure 3 shows the Q-TWiST threshold analysis for EST1684 superimposed with the resulting utility data. Each point on the graph represents the (u_{Tox}, u_{Rel}) utility pair of one of the 95 melanoma patients interviewed in the cross-sectional utility study. The results indicate that all patients had utility pairs falling above the Q-TWiST threshold represented by the solid line, suggesting that interferon would provide an improvement in quality-adjusted survival. A subset of 15 (16%) patients had utility pairs that fell above the 95% confidence interval represented by the dashed line, suggesting that these patients would experience a statistically significant improvement in quality-adjusted survival. Figure 3 also illustrates that patient-derived utility data can be highly variable, and a single summary measure may be inadequate. Therefore, possibly the most useful way to summarize utility data in the context of Q-TWiST is to display the threshold analysis overlaid with the scatter of utility weights, as in Figure 3. In this way, one can view the range of the quality-adjusted treatment effect while also seeing where most patients place their utility values.

Figure 3. ECOG trial EST1684 threshold utility analysis with patient-derived utility data (source: Ref. 16)

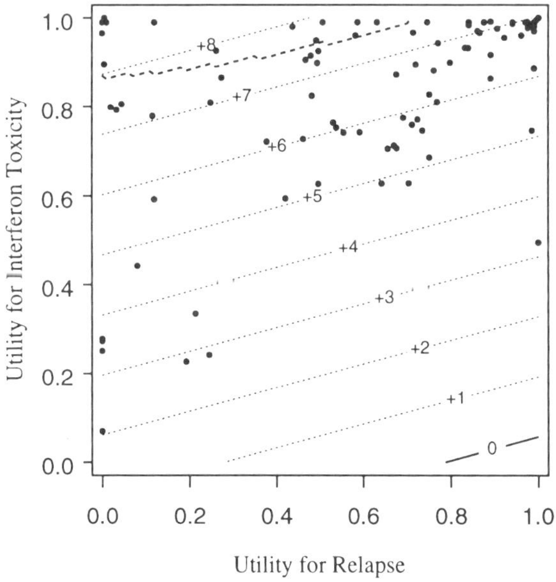

6. Meta Analysis of Polychemotherapy for Breast Cancer

Adjuvant polychemotherapy has been shown to increase relapse-free survival (RFS) and overall survival (OS) for women with resectable breast cancer [17,18]. Despite this finding, it is important to determine whether the magnitude of the gains achievable with adjuvant chemotherapy justifies its use [19,20]. This is particularly true considering the toxic effects of chemotherapy and the associated decrease in quality of life for a population of patients who following primary surgery would otherwise enjoy a relatively good quality of life. The Q-TWiST method was used to evaluate data from the Early Breast Cancer Trialists' Collaborative Group (EBCTCG) overview database of 1995, which includes patient-level follow-up data from a total of 17,723 women enrolled in the 47 trials of polychemotherapy.

The 581 women over the age of 69 years were excluded from the analysis. In addition, within each age group (under 50 years and 50-69 years) any trial with fewer than 10 women in each treatment group was excluded to reduce the chance that small trials with little variation among outcomes might disproportionately affect the Q-TWiST overview estimates. A total of 250 women were excluded based on this criterion. Following these exclusions, 4,337 women aged less than 50 years at study entry and 12,555 women aged 50–69 years at study entry were available for the Q-TWiST overview analysis [21]. For brevity, only results for women aged 50-69 years are shown. The Q-TWiST method was used to analyse each clinical trial individually using health states defined similarly to those used in the melanoma analysis described above. Tox was time with toxicity due to polychemotherapy treatment, TWiST was time without toxicity and without symptoms of disease relapse, and Rel was time following disease relapse. The trial-specific results were then combined in a meta-analysis to provide overall estimates of quality-adjusted survival. The technical details of the meta-analysis methodology are reported elsewhere [11]. Briefly, the individual trial results were combined using a regression model. The dependent variable was the treatment effect (chemotherapy-group mean minus control-group mean) in terms of RFS and OS. The independent variable was median follow-up duration (and the square of median follow-up duration to allow for a curvilinear relationship). This approach allowed the meta-analysis to accommodate the varying median follow-up intervals among the trials. The regression parameters were estimated by generalized least squares to weight the trials inversely according to their respective variance estimates.

The estimated regression models were used to predict the treatment effects in terms of the clinical health state durations at a fixed follow-up time of 120 months. The resulting predictions were the overview estimates of the health state duration treatment effects. Covariation among these estimates was also derived from the regression model. The results were substituted into the equation for Q-TWiST, and the Q-TWiST treatment effect was determined for all possible values of the unknown utility weights in a threshold utility analysis. Comparisons were performed on subgroups of patients defined by nodal status, oestrogen receptor (ER) status.

The Q-TWiST overview analyses for women aged 50-69 years of age at study entry are summarized in Table 3 according to prognostic group. Table 3 shows the treatment effect (polychemotherapy minus control) within 10 years of median follow-up for each clinical health state based on the overview analysis. Among all women in this age group, polychemotherapy provided on average 6.8 additional relapse-free months and 2.9

Table 3. Q-TWiST meta-analysis of polychemotherapy for breast cancer. Number of months gained with chemotherapy (chemotherapy minus control) within the first 10 years of follow-up for each of the Q-TWiST clinical health states for women aged 50-69 years (source: Ref. 21)

Category	Trials	Number of Patients	Average Months of Follow-up (range)*	Number of months gained with chemotherapy (95% CI) TWiST	Rel	RFS	OS
All patients	45	12555	118 (32–248)	0.8 (–0.9,2.5)	–3.9 (–4.8,–3.0)	6.8 (5.1,8.5)	2.9 (1.4,4.4)
Node negative	17	2488	108 (35–182)	2.1 (–2.0,6.2)	–4.0 (–6.4,–1.6)	8.1 (4.0,12.2)	4.1 (0.8,7.3)
Node positive	37	9964	120 (30–248)	0.3 (–1.6,2.2)	–4.0 (–5.0,–2.9)	6.3 (4.4,8.2)	2.3 (0.7,4.0)
ER poor	22	2697	108 (33–176)	6.9 (2.4,11.3)	–5.2 (–7.5,–3.0)	12.9 (8.4,17.3)	7.6 (3.6,11.7)
ER positive	24	6072	109 (33–216)	–0.7 (–3.5,2.2)	–3.8 (–5.3,–2.2)	5.3 (2.5,8.2)	1.6 (–0.8,4.0)
ER unknown	22	3443	131 (25–248)	–1.0 (–3.6,1.6)	–2.2 (–3.6,–0.8)	5.0 (2.4,7.6)	2.9 (0.6,5.1)
Age 50–59	44	6200	112 (29–241)	2.8 (0.4,5.1)	–4.7 (–6.0,–3.4)	8.8 (6.4,11.1)	4.1 (2.1,6.1)
Age 60–69	38	6110	112 (33–240)	–1.4 (–4.1,1.4)	–3.2 (–4.7,–1.2)	4.6 (1.9,7.4)	1.4 (–1.0,3.9)

* The average follow-up was obtained by first determining the median follow-up duration for each trial. These results were then averaged across the trials considered. The range of median follow-up (minimum and maximum) is given in parentheses. Median follow-up within each trial was recomputed for each subject of patients.

Figure 4. Threshold utility meta-analysis of polychemotherapy for breast cancer among women aged 50-69 years (source: Ref. 21)

(A) Node Negative

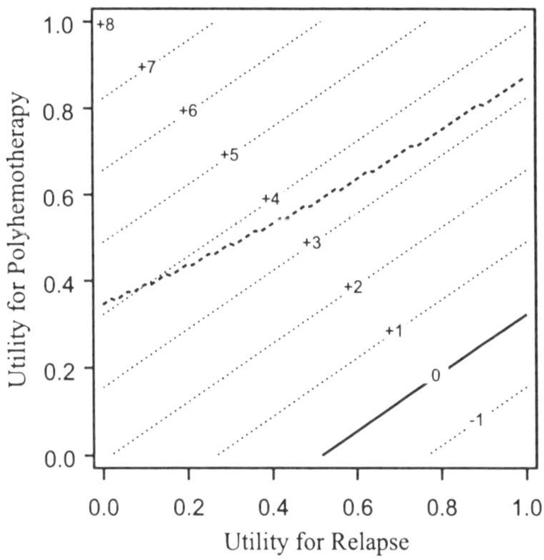

(B) Node Positive

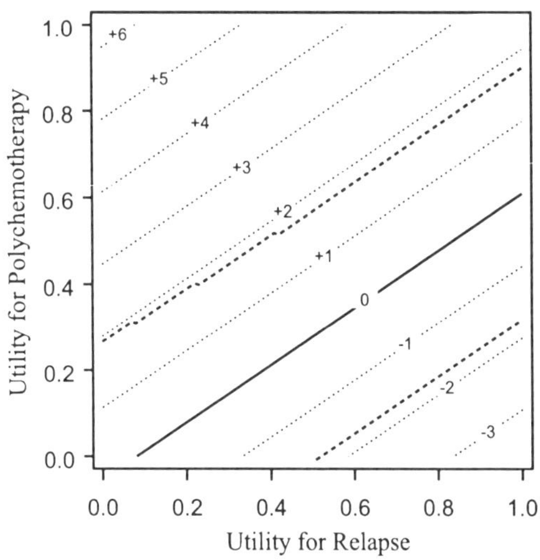

additional months of overall survival time compared with control within a maximum follow-up of 10 years. Treatment effects were larger in the node-negative subgroup compared with the node positive subgroup. Among node-negative patients, polychemotherapy resulted in gains of 8.1 months for RFS and 4.1 months for OS, while among node-positive patients, respective gains of 6.3 months and 2.3 months were observed. Figure 4 uses threshold utility analysis to illustrate the Q-TWiST comparisons among older women according to nodal status. Other breakdowns are omitted for brevity. Dotted contour lines in Figure 4 indicate the range of quality-adjusted benefit for chemotherapy. The threshold line, indicating equal quality-adjusted time for chemotherapy and control, is represented by a solid line. The heavy dashed lines represent 95% confidence bands for the threshold line.

7. Conclusion

This brief paper provides an overview of quality-of-life-adjusted survival analysis (Q-TWiST) in clinical research. The main advantage of the Q-TWiST method is that it quantifies the trade-off between possible decreases in quality of life due to treatment side effects and possible benefits in terms of delayed disease progression and death. The threshold utility analysis provides a convenient illustration of the treatment comparison in terms of quality-adjusted time. In particular, the display may be used to aid in the interpretation of a clinical trial result in light of an individual patient's utility values.

The Q-TWiST analysis of the ECOG trial EST 1684 improved the clinical usefulness of the information obtained from the clinical trial by explicitly accounting for the toxicity of interferon. The inclusion of patient-derived utility data provides an even stronger result allowing one to interpret the clinical trial data across the spectrum of utility weight values while being able to see where individual patients tend to cluster.

The quality-adjusted meta-analysis evaluated the potential benefits of polychemotherapy for breast cancer after surgery in terms of gains in relapse-free time and overall survival time taking into account the undesired subjective side effects that are typically associated with the use of cytotoxics. Although patient-derived utility data were not available for this comparison, the strength of the analysis is the ability to combine data from a large number of trials to arrive at a summary display describing the risks and benefits of polychemotherapy.

Q-TWiST has also been applied in a number of other cancer settings. These include rectal cancer [22], multiple myeloma [23], leukemia [24], lymphoma [25], and prostate cancer [26]. A non-cancer setting in which it has been useful is AIDS [27,28].

As illustrated by the melanoma and breast cancer examples in this paper, the Q-TWiST method may be applied retrospectively. Alternatively, such an analysis may be prospectively designed for a clinical trial. This enables a more precise definition of the clinical health states and ensures that the data necessary for estimating the durations of these health states are collected. It also provides the possibility of collecting utility weight data from the trial participants.

The Q-TWiST methodology provides population-based estimates of the treatment effect in terms of quality-adjusted survival. These estimates are in the form of mean time gained. However, the technique is also useful from an individual perspective. The threshold utility analysis allows one to interpret the clinical trial data with respect to an individual patient's valuations of quality of life in the health states considered. For example, the threshold utility analyses shown for breast cancer chemotherapy allow one to interpret the quality-adjusted benefit of chemotherapy, as measured from the worldwide trial data, for any specific set of valuations placed on chemotherapy toxicity and disease relapse. Such an interpretation is important because the choice to use any therapy with side effects depends on the trade-off between it's risks and benefits. The main strength of the Q-TWiST analysis is that it allows this type of interpretation.

ACKNOWLEDGEMENTS

We thank the patients, physicians, nurses and data managers who participated in the clinical trials described in this paper. We thank the Eastern Cooperative Oncology Group (ECOG) for providing data from the melanoma clinical trial and the Early Breast Cancer Trialists' Collaborative Group (EBCTCG) for providing access to the breast cancer clinical trials of chemotherapy. We thank Richard D. Gelber, Aron Goldhirsch, Alan Coates and Shari Gelber for their help in conducting the Q-TWiST analyses and interpreting the results. We finally thank John Kirkwood, Frank Haluska, Michael Atkins, John Ruckdeschel, Dana Sock, Robert Nease, Jr., Craig Slingluff and Jane Weeks for their collaboration in evaluating utility weights relevant to interferon treatment of melanoma.

REFERENCES

1. Glasziou, P.P., Simes, R.J. and Gelber, R.D. (1990). Quality adjusted survival analysis. *Statistics in Medicine* **9**, 1259–1276.
2. Gelber, R.D., Cole, B.F., Gelber, S. and Goldhirsch, A. (1996). The Q-TWiST method. In: Spilker, B. (ed.), *Quality of Life and Pharmacoeconomics in Clinical Trials, 2nd Edition*. Philadelphia: Lippincott-Raven.
3. Kaplan, E.L. and Meier, P. (1958). Nonparametric estimation from incomplete observations. *Journal of the American Statistical Association* **53**, 457–481.
4. Gelber, R.D., Gelman, R.S. and Goldhirsch, A. (1989). A quality-of-life oriented endpoint for comparing therapies. *Biometrics* **45**, 781–795.
5. Zhao, H. and Tsiatis, A.A. (1997). A consistent estimator for the distribution of quality adjusted survival time. *Biometrika* **84**, 339–348.
6. Zhao, H. and Tsiatis, A.A. (2000). Estimating mean quality adjusted lifetime with censored data. *Sankhya (Series B, Part 1)* **62**, 175–188.
7. Murray, S. and Cole, B.F. (2000). Variance and sample size calculations in quality-of-life adjusted survival analysis (Q-TWiST). *Biometrics* **56**, 173–182.
8. Cole, B.F., Gelber, R.D. and Anderson, K.M. (1994). Parametric approaches to quality-adjusted survival analysis. *Biometrics* **50**, 621–631.
9. Cole, B.F., Gelber, R.D. and Goldhirsch, A. (1993). Cox regression models for quality adjusted survival analysis. *Statistics in Medicine* **12**, 975–987.
10. Gelber, R.D., Goldhirsch, A. and Cole, B.F. (1993). Parametric extrapolation of survival estimates with applications to quality of life evaluation of treatments. *Controlled Clinical Trials* **14**, 485–499.
11. Cole, B.F., Gelber, R.D. and Goldhirsch, A. (1995). A quality-adjusted survival meta-analysis of adjuvant chemotherapy for premenopausal breast cancer. *Statistics in Medicine* **14**, 1771–1784.
12. Glasziou, P., Cole, B.F., Gelber, R.D., Hilden, J. and Simes, R.J. (1998). Quality-adjusted survival analysis with repeated quality-of-life measures. *Statistics in Medicine* **17**, 1215–1229.
13. Kirkwood, J.M., Strawderman, M.H., Ernstoff, M.S., Smith, T.J., Borden, E.C. and Blum, R.H. (1996). Interferon alpha-2b adjuvant therapy of high-risk resected cutaneous melanoma: The Eastern Cooperative Oncology Group Trial EST 1684. *Journal of Clinical Oncology* **14**, 7–17.
14. Cole, B.F., Gelber, R.D., Kirkwood, J.M., Goldhirsch, A., Barylak, E. and Borden, E. (1996). Quality-of-life-adjusted survival analysis of interferon alfa-2b adjuvant

treatment of high-risk resected cutaneous melanoma: an Eastern Cooperative Oncology Group Study. *Journal of Clinical Oncology* **14**, 2666–2673.

15. Kilbridge, K.L., Weeks, J.C., Haluska, F.G., Slingluff, C.L., Atkins, M.B., Sock, D.E., Kirkwood, J.M. and Nease, R.F. Patient preferences for adjuvant interferon alfa-2b treatment. *Journal of Clinical Oncology* **19**, 812–823.
16. Kilbridge, K.L., Cole, B.F., Kirkwood, J.M., Haluska, F.G., Atkins, M.A., Ruckdeschel, J.C., Sock, D.E., Nease, R.F. and Weeks, J.C. Quality-of-life adjusted survival analysis of high-dose adjuvant interferon alfa-2b for high-risk melanoma patients using intergroup clinical trial data. *Journal of Clinical Oncology* **20**, 1311–1318.
17. Early Breast Cancer Trialists' Collaborative Group (1992). Systemic treatment of early breast cancer by hormonal, cytotoxic or immune therapy: 133 randomised trials involving 31,000 relapses and 24,000 deaths among 75,000 women. *Lancet* **339**, 1–15; 71–85.
18. Early Breast Cancer Trialists' Collaborative Group (1998). Polychemotherapy for early breast cancer: an overview of the randomised trials. *Lancet* **352**, 930–942.
19. Gelber, R.D., Cole, B.F., Goldhirsch, A., Bonadonna, G., Howell, A., McArdle, C.S., Mouridsen, H.T., Rubens, R.D. and Welvaart, K. (1995). Adjuvant chemotherapy for premenopausal breast cancer: a meta-analysis using quality-adjusted survival. *The Cancer Journal from Scientific American* **1**, 114–121.
20. Gelber, R.D., Cole, B.F., Goldhirsch, A., Rose, C., Fisher, B., Osborne, C.K., Boccardo, F., Gray, R., Gordon, N.H., Bengtsson, N.-O. and Sevelda, P. (1996). Adjuvant chemotherapy plus tamoxifen compared with tamoxifen alone for postmenopausal breast cancer: a meta-analysis using quality-adjusted survival. *Lancet* **347**, 1066–1071.
21. Cole, B.F., Gelber, R.D., Gelber, S., Coates, A.S. and Goldhirsch, A. (2001). Polychemotherapy for early breast cancer: an overview of the randomized trials with quality-adjusted survival analysis. *Lancet* **358**, 277–286.
22. Gelber, R.D., Goldhirsch, A., Cole, B.F., Wieand, H.S., Schroeder, G. and Krook, J.E. (1996). A quality-adjusted time without symptoms or toxicity (Q-TWiST) analysis of adjuvant radiation therapy and chemotherapy for resectable rectal cancer. *Journal of the National Cancer Institute* **88**, 1039–1045.
23. Zee, B., Cole, B.F., Li, T., Browman, G., James, K., Johnston, D., Sugano D. and Pater, J. (1998). Quality-adjusted time without symptoms or toxicity analysis of interferon maintenance in multiple myeloma. *Journal of Clinical Oncology* **16**, 2834–2839.
24. Parsons, S.K., Gelber, S., Cole, B.F., Ravindranath, Y., Ogden, A., Yeager, A.M., Chung, M., Shuster, J., Weinstein, H.J. and Gelber, R.D. (1999). Quality-adjusted survival after treatment for acute myeloid leukemia in childhood: a Q-TWiST analysis of the pediatric oncology group study 8821. *Journal of Clinical Oncology* **17**, 2144–2152.
25. Cole, B.F., Solal-Céligny, P., Gelber, R.D., Lepage, E., Gisselbrecht, C., Reyes, F., Sebban, C., Sugano, D., Tendler, C. and Goldhirsch, A. (1998). Quality-of-life-adjusted survival analysis of interferon alfa-2b treatment for advanced follicular lymphoma: an aid to clinical decision making. *Journal of Clinical Oncology* **16**, 2339–2344.
26. Rosendahl, I., Kiebert, G.M., Curran, D., Cole, B.F., Weeks, J.C., Denis, L.J. and Hall, R.R. (1999). Quality-adjusted survival (Q-TWiST) analysis of EORTC trial

30853: comparing goserelin acetate and flutamide with bilateral orchiectomy in patients with metastatic prostate cancer. *The Prostate* **38**, 100–109.

27. Gelber, R.D., Lenderking, W.R., Cotton, D.J., Cole, B.F., Fischl, M.A., Goldhirsch, A. and Testa, M.A. (1992). Quality-of-life evaluation in a clinical trial of zidovudine therapy in patients with mildly symptomatic HIV infection. *Annals of Internal Medicine* **116**, 961–966.
28. Lenderking, W.R., Gelber, R.D., Cotton, D.J., Cole, B.F., Goldhirsch, A., Volberding, P.A. and Testa, M.A. (1994). Evaluation of the quality of life associated with zidovudine treatment in asymptomatic human immunodeficiency virus infection. *New England Journal of Medicine* **330**, 738–743.

Chapter 6

Methods for Informatively Missing Longitudinal Quality-of-Life Data

HANDLING OF MISSING DATA

MICHEL CHAVANCE

INSERM U472

A number of the chapters in this volume deal with incomplete observations, offering a broad view of the issues surrounding missing data and of the main strategies proposed to deal with them. I provide some brief comments on these chapters.

1. Classification of Incomplete Observations and Statistical Issues

The classification of missing data mechanisms proposed by Little and Rubin (1987) is used by most authors. When missingness is independent of both observed and unobserved data, the missing data are said to be missing completely at random (CAR). When missing data depend only on completely observed variables, they are said to be missing at random (AR). When missing data depend on the incompletely observed variables, they are said to be missing not at random (NAR). CAR is a particular case of AR. Clearly, incomplete observations carry the risk of biased estimates and are associated with increased variances. The most common strategy of analysis, complete case analysis, ignores all incomplete observations. It ranks among the worst strategies. For longitudinal data, statisticians from the pharmaceutical industry often carry forward the last observed value. This is also a bad strategy due to the bias it generates (Revicki, 2002). If the data are misssing AR and if the vectors of coefficients that define the observation mechanism differ from the parameters that define the evolution of the response, then it is possible to obtain proper estimates of the latter by maximizing the likelihood of the full data. Since this can be done without specifying the observation process, this process is said to be ignorable. When the observation process is not ignorable it is said to be informative. However, the transposition of these concepts to longitudinal data has led to different definitions.

Let us assume that individual evolutions can be modeled using a mixed model. Some authors, such as Molenberghs *et al.* (2002) for example, stick to the original definition and consider a dropout to be CAR if it does not depend on any variable, AR if it depends only on known quantities (totally observed variables or observed values of the incomplete outcome), and NAR if it depends also on unobserved values. Others like Diggle and Kenward (1994), Wu, Borkowf and Albert (2002), or Revicki (2002), have their definitions depending mainly on the relation between the observation process and the outcome, so that when dropout depends on other variables (e.g., baseline values or time), it is CAR; but while Diggle and Kenward (1994) consider the direct effect of the observed and unobserved outcomes, Wu, Borkowf and Albert (2002) and Revicki (2002) consider the influence of the unknown random parameters. Although different, all these definitions lead to the same concept of informative dropout, which means that dropout depends on unobserved values. Note that if dropouts depend on the individual rates of

M. Mesbah et al. (eds.), Statistical Methods for Quality of Life Studies, 303–305.

change of the outcomes, they depend on all the missing measures following dropout because each of these missing measures contains some information regarding the slope.

For the analysis of real data, we would like to know, as in the simulations presented by Wu, Borkowf and Albert (2002), whether the dropouts are informative or not. Unfortunately, it is only possible to check whether dropouts depend on the observed measurements. Thus, it is impossible to know which estimates are biased. With medical data, like longitudinal measures of quality of life (QoL), missingness CAR is the least and NAR is the most likely mechanism. One has to look for variables related to the observation process (time, age, side effects of the treatment, etc., and of course, the observed values of QoL). In many situations, an analysis of the dropout under the AR assumption will help to understand how subjects dropout, and it will help to reduce some possible bias, for instance through multiple imputation (Fairclough, 2002). But as stated by Gnecco and Lachenbruch (2002) one should also perform sensitivity analyses to evaluate to what extent informative dropout could modify the conclusions of the study. Sensitivity analyses can be simple, as with the worst case method (Gnecco and Lachenbruch, 2002), or require elaborate modeling as in the pattern mixture models illustrated by Molenberghs *et al.* (2002) or in selection models (Diggle and Kenward, 1994) as illustrated by Dupuy (2002).

2. What is a Dropout ?

Asking for a definition of a dropout is not as naive as it seems because not all authors used the same definition. Two authors (Fairclough and Revicki} simulated data to illustrate how they could impute QoL scores that were missing due to death, while others firmly stated that QoL scores cannot be missing due to death as death is a poor outcome in its own right. When speaking of QoL, it seems clear to me that imputing a predefined score to the dead is preferable to wondering what the score would have been had the patient survived. An alternative would be to separately study survival and QoL scores conditional on survival. But what about other outcomes such as CD4 counts or blood pressure measurements? Concepts of explanatory or pragmatic attitudes (Schwartz and Lellouch, 1967; Armitage, 1998) in clinical trials can help to define dropouts.

The explanatory attitude concerns trying to understand precisely the biological effects of treatments when administered under ideal conditions. The pragmatic attitude concerns comparing treatments under less rigorous conditions (i.e., those likely to be found in practice). These different attitudes have different consequences on the design and the analysis of a clinical trial and may affect the definition of treatment regimens, choice of subjects, assessment of results and the method of comparison. For instance the explanatory approach will emphasize outcome measures of biological significance, while the pragmatic approach will emphasize practical measures. It already appears that QoL scores are typically used in pragmatic studies. As stated by Armitage, (1998), "The current practice [in clinical trials], leans very heavily in the pragmatic direction." Another difference between these two attitudes regards the handling of patients who do not adhere to the treatment initially allocated. In an explanatory prospect, one is expecting that each patient will follow the strictly defined treatment regimen, leading to exclusion criteria often more rigorous than in a pragmatic prospect. However, there may be some departures from the initial treatment, either because of the patient's desires or because of a medical decision. These will be considered as dropouts. One wonders what would have been the final outcome for these patients, had they adhered to the initial treatment. The situation is not different if a patient dies before the end of the trial for some cause not related to the treatment. However if the patient dies because of treatment toxicity or lack of efficacy, attempting to guess what the outcome would have been, had the patient survived, amounts to guessing what the effect of the treatment would be if the toxicity did not occur. This is not quite a scientific question. Now, from a pragmatic point of view, the study protocol may allow patients to have their treatment modified because of side effects or lack of efficacy, just as would happen in current practice, anu the problem is not to find what the final outcome could have been otherwise but to measure what it is (i.e., to follow up all the patients). If one wants to know whether the introduction of a new medical strategy will improve the well being of a population of patients, one needs to observe what happens to the whole sample, including those who did not like or could not stand this strategy. There will be some dropouts (i.e., patients lost to follow up who cannot be measured) but from a pragmatic point of view, a change of treatment should not be considered a cause of dropout by itself.

REFRENCES

Armitage, P. (1998). Attitudes in clinical trials. *Statistics in Medicine* **17**, 2675–2683.

Diggle, P. and Kenward, M.G. (1994). Informative drop-out in longitudinal data analysis. *Applied Statistics* **43**, 49–93.

Dupuy, J.F. (2002). Joint modeling of survival and nonignorable missing longitudinal quality of life data. In: Mesbah, M., Cole, B.F. and Lee, M.-L. (eds.), *Statistical Methods for Quality of Life Studies. Design, Measurements and Analysis.* Boston: Kluwer Academic Publishers.

Fairclough, D.L. (2002). Multiple imputation for non-random missing data. In: Mesbah, M., Cole, B.F. and Lee, M.-L. (eds.), *Statistical Methods for Quality of Life Studies. Design, Measurements and Analysis.* Boston: Kluwer Academic Publishers.

Gnecco, C. and Lachenbruch, P.A. (2002). Regulatory aspects of quality of life. In: Mesbah, M., Cole, B.F. and Lee, M.-L. (eds.), *Statistical Methods for Quality of Life Studies. Design, Measurements and Analysis.* Boston: Kluwer Academic Publishers.

Little, R.J.A. and Rubin, D.B. (1987). *Statistical Analysis with missing data.* New York: Wiley.

Molenberghs, G., Thijs, H., Verberke, G., Michiels, B. and Kenward, M. (2002) Strategies to fit pattern-mixture models. In: Mesbah, M., Cole, B.F. and Lee, M.-L. (eds.), *Statistical Methods for Quality of Life Studies. Design, Measurements and Analysis.* Boston: Kluwer Academic Publishers.

Revicki, D.A. (2002). Analyzing longitudinal health-related quality of life data: missing data and multiplicity issues. In: Mesbah, M., Cole, B.F. and Lee, M.-L. (eds.), *Statistical Methods for Quality of Life Studies. Design, Measurements and Analysis.* Boston: Kluwer Academic Publishers.

Schwartz. D. and Lellouch, J. (1967). Explanatory and pragmatic attitudes in clinical trials. *Journal of Chronic Diseases* **20**, 637–648.

Wu, M.C., Borkowf, C.B. and Albert P.S. (2002). Analysis of longitudinal quality of life data with informative dropout. In: Mesbah, M., Cole, B.F. and Lee, M.-L. (eds.), *Statistical Methods for Quality of Life Studies. Design, Measurements and Analysis.* Boston: Kluwer Academic Publishers.

GUIDELINES FOR ADMINISTRATION OF SELF-REPORTED HEALTH-RELATED QUALITY OF QUESTIONNAIRES: HOW TO MINIMIZE AVOIDABLE MISSING DATA?

DOMINIQUE DUBOIS

Janssen Pharmaceutica

Missing health-related quality of life (HRQL) data represent a potential source of bias in randomized clinical trials. HRQL data may be missing because of mortality, disease progression, treatment-related adverse events, poor subject compliance, or variations in implementing the research protocol. Regarding the latter, we suggest that the best approach to address missing HRQL data is to implement rigorous HRQL administration guidelines.

At my company, we developed a set of standardized guidelines for administering self-reported HRQL questionnaires alongside clinical trials. The purpose of these guidelines is to reduce as much as possible the variance due to measurement error by standardizing the HRQL administration procedures across all countries, centers, and subjects participating in a clinical trial. We suggest that the systematic use of these simple guidelines may substantially reduce the amount of avoidable missing data, and increase the ability of the questionnaire to pick-up meaningful changes, if present. Below I list the 10 guidelines.

1. Confidentiality

Emphasize that absolute confidentiality will be maintained at all times. The subject should be viewed as an active participant in research. Tell the subject he/she is a valuable source of information about disease and treatment. To be helpful, the subject needs to supply high quality information.

2. Describe the Purpose

Describe the purpose of the assessment to the subject. The HRQL questionnaire is an important measure to help evaluate the impact of treatment. Specifically, it provides the subject's own viewpoint on the disease and changes due to therapy.

3. Schedule-Setting and Timing.

Questionnaire completion and review will usually require up to 20 or 30 minutes. The subject and the investigator/staff need to plan for sufficient time. Subjects should be provided a quiet semi-private location with easy access to study coordinator. All subjects are to complete HRQL questionnaire at the same time (i.e., at the beginning of the visit, prior to any clinical examination, medical tests or procedures).

M. Mesbah et al. (eds.), Statistical Methods for Quality of Life Studies, 307–308.

4. Recall Period.

Explain to the subject what time period the questionnaire is referring to.

5. No Incorrect Answers.

Explain that the questions ask for the subject's opinions about how he or she feels. There are no incorrect answers. It is not an exam!

6. No Rush.

There is no need to complete the assessment rapidly. The assessment is not timed. Two to three items per minute is a reasonable pace.

7. Remind Subjects to Provide Only One Answer Per Question.

8. Re-reading Only.

Do not provide paraphrasing of the items when a subject asks to clarify a question or item. Questions about the items should be answered by re-reading the items aloud, followed by asking the subject to respond according to what he or she thinks is appropriate.

9. Check for Completeness.

When the subject has completed the questionnaire, and before continuing with the study visit assessments, make sure the subject has answered each question.

10. Thank You.

Ask if there are any questions or issues, and thank the subject for his/her participation.

JOINT MODELING OF SURVIVAL AND NONIGNORABLE MISSING LONGITUDINAL QUALITY-OF-LIFE DATA

JEAN-FRANÇOIS DUPUY

University of South-Brittany

A problem that frequently arises in clinical trials where quality-of-life values are repeatedly measured on each individual under study, is that of dropout. In some settings, dropout may depend on unobserved components of the longitudinal process. Dropout is then termed nonignorable. Recently, several approaches have been proposed that accommodate nonignorable dropout in the modeling of a longitudinal process. However, most of these approaches rest upon the assumption that dropout can only occur at one of the pre-specified measurement times of quality-of-life. In this paper, we review some of these approaches and we propose a new joint model for longitudinal data with nonignorable dropout and time to dropout, which allows dropout to occur at any point in time. This model combines a first-order Markov model for the longitudinal quality-of-life data with a time-dependent Cox model for the dropout process. We discuss nonparametric maximum likelihood estimation in the suggested joint model and rely on an EM algorithm to calculate estimates of the parameters. The method is illustrated through analysis of quality-of-life data among patients involved in a cancer clinical trial. Comparison of its results to the ones obtained by fitting Diggle and Kenward's model for nonignorable dropout to the same data is provided.

1. Introduction

In clinical trials involving repeated assessment of quality-of-life measures, it is usual that some sequences of measurements terminate prematurely. Such a phenomenon is called a *dropout* (Diggle and Kenward, 1994; Little, 1995) and raises specific problems since one has to take account of the fact that dropout may occur for reasons directly or indirectly connected to the longitudinal measurement process. to accommodate dropout in the modeling of a longitudinal process, Little and Rubin (1987) hence distinguish between three types of dropout processes. A dropout process is termed *completely random* when the dropout is independent of both observed and unobserved measurements of the longitudinal process. It is called *random* when dropout is independent of the unobserved measurements but depends on the observed ones. Finally, when dropout depends on unobserved values of the longitudinal process, the dropout is termed *nonignorable*.

It turns out that completely random and random dropouts are *ignorable* for likelihood-based inference. That is under these dropout mechanisms, valid likelihood-based inference about the measurement process can be obtained without

M. Mesbah et al. (eds.), Statistical Methods for Quality of Life Studies, 309–322.

explicitly modeling the dropout mechanism. This holds under the additional *separability* condition that there are no parameters in common between the dropout and longitudinal measurements models. It turns out that under these dropout mechanisms and the separability condition, the measurement process itself is ignorable for the purpose of making likelihood-based inference about the dropout model. Under nonignorable dropout, a model which relates dropout to the longitudinal measurements is required.

Models for nonignorable dropout in longitudinal studies have received considerable attention over the past few years. These models are classified into two classes, called selection and pattern-mixture model classes, depending on the factorization chosen to describe the joint density of the longitudinally-measured variable and of the dropout time. In a selection model, this density is factored as the conditional density of dropout given the longitudinal outcomes multiplied by the marginal density of the longitudinal outcomes. Pattern-mixture models are obtained via the converse factorization. Several approaches from both classes have recently been suggested and detailed reviews of this literature are provided by Little (1995), Hogan and Laird (1997a, 1997b) and Verbeke and Molenberghs (2000).

However, most of these approaches rest upon the assumption that dropout only occurs at one of the pre-specified measurement times of the longitudinal variable, and only a few of them allow for censoring of the dropout times. In this paper, we consider situations where dropout may occur at any point in time, and where the dropout times may also be censored.

The data set motivating our work consists of repeated measurements of quality-of-life values on patients involved in a cancer clinical trial. Measures of the patients' own perception of their well-being were scheduled to be obtained until death, using a questionnaire self-administered by each patient. Some of the patients dropped out of the longitudinal study. Since dropout and quality-of-life are likely to be closely related, modeling of the quality-of-life response needs to account for the dropout process. All other patients were removed from the study following a disease progression. We let such a removal be censoring of the dropout time. Difficulty comes from the fact that quality-of-life values at dropout and at time of removal due to disease progression are not observed.

Obviously, pattern-mixture models cannot accommodate continuous-in-time dropout since they require large numbers of dropouts at each dropout timepoint to estimate a usually large number of parameters (Hogan and Laird, 1997a, 1997b; Verbeke and Molenberghs, 2000). Hence we propose a selection-model based approach to this situation. The suggested model combines a first-order Markov model for the longitudinal quality-of-life data with a Cox model (Cox, 1972) for the dropout process, where the longitudinally-observed variable appears as a time-dependent covariate. The hazard of dropout is assumed to depend on the longitudinal measurements through the last observed response prior to dropout and through the unobserved response value at the time of dropout.

Section 2 reviews some selection-modeling approaches to nonignorable dropout in longitudinal data. Section 3 defines notation and presents the model. In Section 4, we discuss estimation in the suggested joint model, and we investigate the existence of nonparametric maximum likelihood estimators. In Section 5, the model is applied to the example data set and the results are compared to those obtained by fitting the model of Diggle and Kenward (1994) for nonignorable dropout. We discuss the results in Section 6.

2. Some Selection Models for Nonignorable Dropout in Longitudinal Data

In a selection model, the joint distribution of the dropout time and the longitudinal outcomes is factorized as the conditional distribution of dropout given the outcomes and the marginal distribution of the outcomes.

Diggle and Kenward (1994) propose a model for *continuous* longitudinal data with nonignorable dropout. It combines a multivariate linear model for the longitudinal response with a logistic regression model for the dropout process. This logistic model allows dependence of dropout on one missing observation, thus introducing nonignorable dropout. Letting z_j denote the observation of the longitudinally measured variable Z to be made at time t_j ($j = 0, 1, \dots$), T be the time of the first missing measurement and V be some additional vector of covariates, Diggle and Kenward (1994) model the probability that an individual drops out at time t_j, given this individual is still under study at time t_{j-1} as:

$$\text{logit}[P(T = t_j | T \geq t_j, z_0, \dots, z_j, V)] = \beta_0 + \beta_1 z_j + \sum_{k=1}^{j} \beta_{k+1} z_{j-k} + \gamma^T V. \quad (1)$$

Letting $\beta_1 = 0$ in (1) specifies a random dropout model. Letting each parameter β, except β_0, be 0 specifies a completely random dropout model.

The likelihood is then obtained by combining a multivariate Gaussian distribution for the longitudinal outcomes with the dropout model (1), and by integrating over the unobserved data. Under completely random and random dropouts, the likelihood partitions into two components, one involving parameters of the dropout model only, the other involving parameters of the longitudinal response model only. Estimation then proceeds by separate maximization of these two components. On the other hand, under nonignorable dropout, the likelihood does not separate and its maximization is more complicated. It requires numerical integration and is achieved by Diggle and Kenward (1994) using the simplex algorithm (Nelder and Mead, 1965), implemented for Diggle and Kenward's model in the Splus suite of functions called OSWALD (Smith, Robertson and Diggle, 1996).

Some extensions of Diggle and Kenward's work have then been proposed. Molenberghs, Kenward and Lesaffre (1997) suggest a model for longitudinal *categorical* data with nonignorable dropout. They combine a multivariate Dale model for the outcomes with a logistic regression model similar to that of Diggle and Kenward's for the dropout mechanism. They maximize the resulting likelihood using an EM algorithm.

Troxel, Harrington and Lipsitz (1998) and Troxel, Lipsitz and Harrington (1998) extend the work of Diggle and Kenward (1994) to nonignorable *non-monotone* continuous missing data. Non-monotone patterns of missing data arise when patients move *in* and *out* the studied population. The authors assume a logistic model for the dropout mechanism, which allows the missingness probabilities to depend on current potentially unobserved values of the response. They introduce missingness indicators R_j, equal to 1 if z_j is observed and 0 otherwise, assume that $R_j \sim \text{Ber}(1 - P(R_j = 0|z_j))$ with $\text{logit}[P(R_j = 0|z_j)] = \beta_0 + \beta_1 z_j$, and assume a univariate normal density for the response at time t_j. They then derive the likelihood by assuming that the longitudinal measurements are independent over time and by integrating over the range of unobserved measurements. However, the computations required by the numerical integrations are intensive and become especially cumbersome with more than three or four assessments of the longitudinal process per patient.

Following Little (1995), such models can be classified as *outcome-based* selection models since dropout depends directly on the repeated measures. In some situations however, dropout may be more related to an underlying trend over time. For example, one might suppose that dropout is related to the underlying level of quality-of-life, rather than to the values as measured by the questionnaire. One solution consists in directly modeling the underlying trend, using a random effects model. Allowing both the longitudinal response and the dropout models to depend on the random effects yields to so-called *random-coefficient-based* selection models (Little, 1995).

Wu and Carroll (1988) combine a linear random effects model for the longitudinal outcomes with a probit model for time to dropout. The probit model relates time to dropout to the individual random intercept and slope. Schluchter (1992) and DeGruttola and Tu (1994) propose random-coefficient-based models that assume a multivariate normal distribution for the event time and the random effects of the response process.

For example, Schluchter (1992) assumes a linear random effects model for the longitudinal response. Letting $\mathbf{z}_i = (z_{i,0}, \ldots, z_{i,n_i})^T$ be the vector of measurements of the response variable obtained at times $t_0, \ldots, t_{n_i}$ on the ith individual, V_i be a matrix of fixed-effect covariates, W_i be a an $n_i \times 2$ matrix with all elements in the first column equal to 1 and second column containing the measurement times, Schluchter (1992) assumes that $\mathbf{z}_i|\beta_i = \gamma V_i + W_i\beta_i + e_i$, where $e_{i,j} \sim N(0, \sigma^2)$ are errors terms such that $e_{i,j}$ are independent from β_i. Schluchter then assumes that β_i is normally distributed with mean $\beta = (\beta_0, \beta_1)^T$ and covariance matrix Σ.

A joint model for the random parameters β_i and the logarithm of the survival time $\log T_i$ is finally specified as

$$\begin{bmatrix} \beta_i \\ \log T_i \end{bmatrix} \sim N\left(\begin{bmatrix} \beta \\ \mu \end{bmatrix}, \begin{bmatrix} \Sigma & \sigma_{\beta T} \\ \sigma_{\beta T}^T & \sigma_T^2 \end{bmatrix} \right),$$

where μ and σ_T^2 are the mean and variance respectively of $\log T_i$, and $\sigma_{\beta T}$ is a 2×1 vector with elements the covariances of the log survival time with the elements of β_i.

Schluchter (1992) and DeGruttola and Tu (1994) use an EM algorithm to obtain maximum likelihood estimates of all model parameters. Ribaudo, Thompson and Allen-Mersh (2000) discuss the use of the model described above for the joint analysis of quality-of-life and log survival time.

An other approach deserves attention although it was developed in a context different from that of longitudinal studies. It relies on the use of a semiparametric model for the dropout and has been proposed by Scharfstein, Rotnitzky and Robins (1999). They consider a study designed to end at a fixed time T, at which an outcome of interest Y is measured on each individual. Denoting by $\bar{V}(t)$ the history up to time t of some time-dependent variables V, they propose to model the hazard of dropout by

$$\lambda(t|\bar{V}(t), Y) = \lambda_0(t|\bar{V}(t)) \exp(\alpha_0 Y), \tag{2}$$

thus introducing nonignorable dropout through the term $\exp(\alpha_0 Y)$. Letting $\alpha_0 = 0$ in (2) specifies a random dropout model.

Scharfstein, Rotnitzky and Robins (1999) then propose regarding the parameter α_0 as known, rather than estimating it from the data. To make inference about the marginal distribution of Y, they perform a sensitivity analysis, to see how inference about Y changes as α_0 varies over a plausible range of values.

In the next section, we suggest a new outcome-based selection model for longitudinal quality-of-life data with nonignorable dropout. This model combines a first-order Markov model for the longitudinal quality-of-life measurements and a time-dependent Cox model (Cox, 1972) for the dropout process.

3. The Model

3.1 Notation

In a longitudinal study, suppose that n subjects are to be observed until death at a set of common fixed times t_j $(j = 0, 1, \dots)$, such that $\Delta_t = t_{j+1} - t_j$ $(j = 0, 1, \dots)$ for some constant Δ_t. For the i-th individual $(i = 1, \dots, n)$, let T_i denote the time to dropout.

We assume that the quality-of-life is piecewise constant on the intervals $[t_j, t_{j+1}]$, with values z_j. We assume that z_j is unobserved until t_{j+1}. That is, the current value of quality-of-life for an individual in the interval $[t_j, t_{j+1}]$ is known at the end of the interval, when the individual returns the questionnaire. Let z_{ij} denote the value of z_j for the i-th individual. We assume that Z_{ij}, $j = 0, 1, \dots$ are defined by the following: $Z_{ij} = \alpha Z_{i,j-1} + u_j$ and $u_j \sim N(0, \sigma^2)$.

If $t \in [t_j, t_{j+1}]$ $(j = 0, 1, \dots)$, let $[t] = j$. Let $z_{(t)} = (z_{[t]-1}, z(t))'$ and $z_{i,(t)} = (z_{i,[t]-1}, z_i(t))'$, $i = 1, \dots, n$. With this notation and study design, $z_{i,[t]-1}$ is the last observed quality-of-life value before t on the ith individual.

3.2 Model

The distribution of a survival time (here, time to "survival" is time to dropout) conditional given a time-dependent covariate is characterized by the hazard function

$$\lambda(t|z(u), 0 \leq u \leq t) = \lim_{h \to 0} \frac{1}{h} \Pr[t \leq T \leq t + h | T \geq t; z(u), 0 \leq u \leq t]$$

We assume that T can be modeled via a time-dependent Cox model (Cox, 1972) where the hazard rate is given by:

$$\lambda_0(t)\exp(\beta^T z_{(t)}) = \lambda_0(t)\exp(\beta_0 z_{[t]-1} + \beta_1 z(t)), \tag{3}$$

where $\beta = (\beta_0, \beta_1)'$ is a vector of unknown regression coefficients and λ_0 is an unspecified baseline hazard function.

Formula (3) states that the hazard of dropout at time t depends on quality-of-life through the last observed value before t, $z_{[t]-1}$, and the current *unobserved* quality-of-life value $z(t)$. This way of relating the dropout process to longitudinal quality-of-life specifies an outcome-based nonignorable model.

In most clinical trials, the event time of interest (here dropout from the longitudinal study of quality of life) is subject to right-censoring. Hence for each subject i ($i = 1, \ldots, n$), instead of T_i, we actually observe $S_i = \min(T_i, C_i)$ and a failure indicator $\delta_i = 1_{\{T_i \le C_i\}}$, where C_i is a random censoring time for the i-th subject.

We assume that conditional on $(z_0, z_1, \ldots)$, censoring is independent of dropout. We also assume that the distribution of the censoring time does not depend on $(\beta, \lambda_0, \alpha, \sigma^2)$, nor on $z(s)$. This last hypothesis could be relaxed to allow censoring to depend also on unobserved value of the longitudinal process. However, in our application, this is not the case: censoring of the true dropout time of an individual occurs when doctors diagnose disease progression. Removal of a patient from the longitudinal study of quality-of-life is then decided on the basis of clinical criteria, hence independently of the current value of quality-of-life of the corresponding individual.

4. Nonparametric Likelihood Estimation

4.1 Nonparametric Likelihood Function

We observe n vectors $\mathbf{y}_i = (s_i, \delta_i, z_{i,0}, \ldots, z_{i,[s_i]-1})$, $i = 1, \ldots, n$. We wish to estimate the parameters of the suggested joint model via maximum likelihood, using these observations. We obtain the likelihood for the observed data by first writing the likelihood for $(\mathbf{y}_i, z_i(s_i))$ and then by integrating over $z_i(s_i)$.

Assuming independence between individuals, the likelihood for the observed data is obtained by multiplying over subjects the following individual contribution:

$$\begin{aligned} L_i\left(\beta, \alpha, \sigma^2, \lambda_0(\cdot)\right) &= \int_{\mathbb{R}} \lambda_0\left(s_i\right)^{\delta_i} \exp\left[\delta_i \beta^T z_{i,(s_i)} - \int_0^{s_i} \lambda_0\left(u\right) e^{\beta^T z_{i,(u)}}\, du\right] \\ &\times\ f_{\alpha,\sigma^2}\left(z_{i,0}, \ldots, z_{i,[s_i]-1}, z_i(s_i)\right) dz_i(s_i). \end{aligned} \tag{4}$$

Working on model (2), Scharfstein, Rotnitzky and Robins (1999) have shown that the parameter α_0 can not be identified, when no assumptions are placed on the joint distribution of the observed $\bar{V}(t)$ and the potentially unobserved Y. Non-identifiability of parameters has been discussed by many authors as a potential drawback of selection models for nonignorable dropout (Little, 1995; Scharfstein, Rotnitzky and Robins 1999; Verbeke and Molenberghs, 2000).

Identifiability of model (3) has been proved by Dupuy, Grama and Mesbah (2001) under mild conditions, namely that the parametric distribution $f_{\alpha,\sigma^2}(\cdot)$ of Z is identifiable and that each subject included in the study provides at least one measurement of Z.

Under random dropout (i.e., assuming that the hazard of dropout depends only on the observed quality-of-life measurements, and not on the current unobserved value), the likelihood $\prod_{i=1}^n L_i\left(\beta_0, \alpha, \sigma^2, \lambda_0(\cdot)\right)$ separates into one component for the dropout process, involving the parameters β_0 and $\lambda_0(\cdot)$, and another component for the longitudinal process involving α and σ^2. Estimation of the parameters can then proceed by standard techniques within each component. In particular, one may obtain a consistent and asymptotically normal estimator of β_0 by maximizing the following partial likelihood $L(\beta_0)$, where the baseline hazard does not appear:

$$\prod_{i=1}^{n}\left[\frac{e^{\beta_0 z_{i,[s_i]-1}}}{\sum_{j=1}^{n} e^{\beta_0 z_{j,[s_i]-1}} 1_{\{s_i \le s_j\}}}\right]^{\delta_i}.$$

Under nonignorable dropout, maximization of the integrated likelihood (4) is complicated by the unobserved $z_i(s_i)$ and the presence of the unspecified baseline hazard. There is no maximizer of the likelihood for λ_0 ranging over the class of all positive functions on $[0, +\infty)$. Hence, we suggest making use of nonparametric maximum likelihood estimation in this model. To this end, we restrict the cumulative baseline hazard function $\Lambda_0(t) = \int_0^t \lambda_0(u)\, du$ to be a discrete function with jumps at the observed distinct dropout times $u_1, \ldots, u_{p(n)}$ $(p(n) \le n)$. We replace in (4) $\lambda_0(\cdot)$ by the jumps $\lambda_1, \ldots, \lambda_{p(n)}$ of Λ_0 at $u_{(1)}, \ldots, u_{(p(n))}$, where $u_{(1)} \le \ldots \le u_{(p(n))}$ are the order statistics corresponding to $u_1, \ldots, u_{p(n)}$.

Nonparametric maximum likelihood estimation has recently been used in the contexts of frailty models (Nielsen *et al.*, 1992) and of covariate measurement error in the Cox (Hu, Tsiatis and Davidian, 1998) and frailty models (Li and Lin, 2000). Chen and Little (1999) rely on this approach in the context of missing values in time-independent covariates in the Cox model. The nonparametric likelihood function of $\psi = (\beta, \alpha, \sigma^2, \lambda_1, \ldots, \lambda_{p(n)})$, $L_{(n)}(\psi)$, is obtained by multiplying the following contributions over subjects

$$\begin{aligned} L_i(\psi) &= \int_{\mathbb{R}} \left[\prod_{l=1}^{p(n)} \lambda_l^{\delta_i 1_{\{s_i=u_l\}}}\right] \exp\left[\delta_i \beta^T z_{i,(s_i)} - \sum_{l=1}^{p(n)} \lambda_l e^{\beta^T z_{i,(u_l)}} 1_{\{u_l \le s_i\}}\right] \\ &\quad \times f_{\alpha,\sigma^2}(z_{i,0}, \ldots, z_{i,[s_i]-1}, z_i(s_i))\, dz_i(s_i). \end{aligned} \tag{5}$$

We may obtain an estimator of ψ by maximizing $L_{(n)}(\psi)$. The following proposition shows that such an estimator exists (proof is given in appendix).

Proposition: *A maximizer of $L_{(n)}(\psi)$ exists and is finite.*

Because direct maximization of $L_{(n)}(\psi)$ is cumbersome, an EM algorithm (Dempster, Laird and Rubin, 1977) is proposed for calculating nonparametric maximum likelihood estimates of the parameters.

4.2 Estimation via the EM Algorithm

The EM algorithm (Dempster, Laird and Rubin, 1977) consists of two steps, expectation and maximization, which are repeated in an iterative manner until a convergence criterion is satisfied. Each iteration evaluate and then maximize the expectation of the complete data log-likelihood for $S, \delta, Z_0, \ldots, Z_{[s]-1}, Z(s)$, where the expectation is taken with respect to the unobserved data given the observed data and the current estimates of the parameters.

There exist closed-form formulas for updating the estimates of $(\alpha, \sigma^2, \lambda_1, \ldots, \lambda_{p(n)})$ at each iteration of the EM algorithm. Such a closed-form does not exist for updating β. We use a Newton-Raphson algorithm for that purpose: at the $(m+1)$-th iteration of the EM algorithm, the $(k+1)$-th iteration of the Newton-Raphson algorithm computes an updated estimate of β as

$$\beta^{(k+1)} = \beta^{(k)} + (I^{(m)}(\beta^{(k)}))^{-1} U^{(m)}(\beta^{(k)}),$$

where $U^{(m)}(\beta)$ and $I^{(m)}(\beta)$ are respectively the score and information for β.

Closed-form solutions for updating the estimates of $(\alpha, \sigma^2, \lambda_1, \ldots, \lambda_{p(n)})$ and expressions for $U^{(m)}(\beta)$ and $I^{(m)}(\beta)$ can be found in Dupuy and Mesbah (2002). Moreover, numerical integration is needed for evaluating the conditional expectations in the E-step. We use Gauss-Hermite quadrature for that purpose and detailed calculations are given by Dupuy and Mesbah (2002).

Computations for the example of Section 5 have been carried out in the programming language Scilab (Scilab Group, 1998). This program is available from the author's homepage at http://www.univ-ubs.fr/sabres/dupuyj/index.html. The EM algorithm was stopped and considered to have converged when change in $L_{(n)}(\psi)$ between two consecutive iterations was less than 10^{-4}.

Asymptotic variance of maximum likelihood estimators is usually estimated by inverting the observed Fisher information matrix. However, in the case of non-parametric maximum likelihood estimation, the number of parameters may be very large, implying that one has to invert a high-dimensional matrix. Hence, we estimate the asymptotic variance of the estimators of β, α, σ^2 via the profile likelihood method. More details on this can be found in Dupuy and Mesbah (2002).

5. Application

The studied data set comes from a clinical trial designed to evaluate a new therapy against cancer, and where quality-of-life measures were scheduled to be repeatedly obtained on each patient until death, using a questionnaire. Some of the patients dropped out from the longitudinal study before death. All the other were removed of the study because of disease progression. We wish to investigate the relationship between the longitudinal outcomes and time to dropout. Dropout time is considered as being censored for those individuals who are removed from the quality-of-life study because of disease progression.

Since the current values z_{ij} of quality-of-life in the interval $[t_j, t_{j+1}]$ are known at the end of the interval when the patients give back their questionnaire, values

z_{ij} are not observed for the individuals who leave the longitudinal study (because of dropout or disease progression) within the interval.

The studied data set involves 107 patients, each having between 2 and 13 measures of quality-of-life. Among these individuals, 79 dropped out from the study and 28 were removed following disease progression. Sex and a measure of gravity of illness at beginning of the study were also recorded for each patient. Since none of these covariates had a significant effect when included in the model, we do not include them in the analysis presented below. Table 1 gives the EM algorithm estimates and estimates of standard errors for the parameters in the joint model described in Section 3, along with the estimates resulting from a random dropout analysis (obtained by setting $\beta_1 = 0$ in (3)).

Table 1. Maximum likelihood estimates (standard errors) from random and nonignorable dropout analysis

Parameter	Random dropout	Nonignorable dropout
β_0	-0.221 (0.083)	0.048 (0.085)
β_1	0.000	-0.335 (0.093)
α	0.955 (0.009)	0.948 (0.009)
σ^2	0.589 (0.041)	0.593 (0.042)

The negative value for the regression parameter β_0 obtained from a random dropout analysis implies that individuals with low values of the quality-of-life measurements are more likely to dropout. This is natural as high values obtained from the questionnaire used in this study indicate a better overall quality-of-life. Hence we would expect that a patient feeling pretty well is more likely to complete the questionnaire. Moreover, the results obtained from a nonignorable dropout analysis ($\beta_1 = -0.335$) seem to support the hypothesis of nonignorable dropout over the hypothesis of random dropout (a proof of asymptotic normality of the estimator of β is under progress, in order to allow us to derive formal test of the hypothesis of nonignorable dropout within the postulated model).

The estimated hazard function resulting from a nonignorable analysis is given by

$$\hat{\lambda}_0(t) \exp\left[0.048 z_{[t]-1} - 0.335 z(t)\right].$$

Following Diggle and Kenward (1994) and Verbeke and Molenberghs (2000), we might reparameterize the model (3) as a function of the increment $(z(t) - z_{[t]-1})$ and the level $z_{[t]-1}$ of the outcome variable. The estimated hazard rate can then be written as

$$\hat{\lambda}_0(t) \exp\left[-0.335(z(t) - z_{[t]-1}) - 0.287 z_{[t]-1}\right], \tag{6}$$

which confirms that low levels of quality-of-life are associated with higher rates of dropout. Moreover, this suggests that the hazard of dropout is also associated with a change in the level of quality-of-life. More precisely, the hazard of dropout increases as the level of quality-of-life decreases. Finally, Z_{ij} has density (given

$z_{i,j-1}$) a Gaussian density with estimated mean $0.948 z_{i,j-1}$ (suggesting an overall slow decrease of quality-of-life over time) and estimated variance 0.593.

We now provide comparison of our results to the ones obtained by fitting Diggle and Kenward's model to the same data set. Such a comparison may be interesting since the suggested model, described in Section 3, may be viewed as a generalization of Diggle and Kenward's approach to situations where dropout may occur at any point in time and where dropout times are allowed to be censored. Diggle and Kenward's model (1994) assumes that dropout occurs at one of the fixed measurement times of Z. Hence, when fitting their model to our data set, dropout is set to occur at the time of the first missing measurement. Moreover, we stated that quality-of-life value at time of removal of the study because of disease progression was not observed. Since Diggle and Kenward's approach, implemented in the OSWALD software (Smith, Robertson and Diggle, 1996) does not accommodate censoring, we also treat such events as nonignorable dropouts for this approach. No covariates were included in the model. The resulting fitted model is

$$\text{logit}[P(T = t_j | T \geq t_j, z_0, \dots, z_j)] = -0.006 z_{j-1} - 0.23 z_j,$$

which may be reparameterized as

$$\text{logit}[P(T = t_j | T \geq t_j, z_0, \dots, z_j)] = -0.23(z_j - z_{j-1}) - 0.236 z_{j-1}. \tag{7}$$

From this model, we also conclude that lower values of quality-of-life and a decreasing evolution in quality-of-life are associated with higher probabilities of dropout.

A mere comparison of the estimates of the regression parameters between models (6) and (7) may not be useful since model (6) specifies a hazard function for dropout and model (7) is the logit of probability of dropout. Hence we suggest comparing instead estimated relative risks of dropout between two individuals, obtained from both models. Let two individuals have the same value of quality-of-life z at t_j. This value remains constant for one individual and evolves in time (from a quantity denoted by *incr* in the following) for the other one. We compare relative risks of dropout between these two individuals, as estimated by both models. Estimated relative risks versus *incr* are represented on Figure 1 by the solid and dotted lines.

We have also fitted the suggested joint model under the same two conditions that we used for fitting Diggle and Kenward's model, namely (a) that dropout is set to occur at the time of the first missing measurement and (b) by ignoring censoring. Representation of estimated relative risk of dropout resulting from this analysis lies on Figure 1 close to the one obtained from Diggle and Kenward's model. If we fit the proposed selection model under the intermediate set of conditions of (a) discrete dropout times and (b) permission of censoring, and then, on the other hand, under the conditions of (a) continuous dropout time and (b) no censoring, we obtain two intermediate curves, shown on Figure 1. In these last two cases, estimated relative risk of dropout is underestimated for individuals with large negative values of *incr*. Under the conditions for application of Diggle and Kenward's model, both this model and the model we suggested in Section 3 underestimate, but both to the same extent, the relative risk of dropout for individuals with decreasing evolution of Z.

Figure 1. Relative risk of dropout versus *incr* for the joint model (JM) and Diggle and Kenward's model. *incr* quantifies the evolution of the quality of life score.

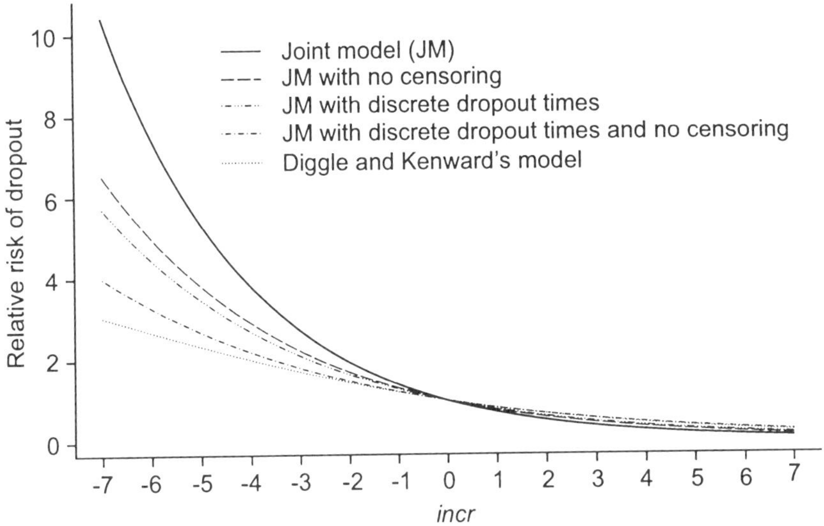

6. Discussion

We have proposed a new model for longitudinal data with nonignorable dropout, which falls into the class of outcome-based selection models. It combines a model for the longitudinal measures of quality-of-life with a time-dependent Cox model for dropout. This model relaxes a usual assumption underlying existing selection-models (Diggle and Kenward, 1994; Molenberghs, Kenward and Lesaffre, 1997; Troxel, Harrington and Lipsitz 1998; Troxel, Lipsitz and Harrington, 1998) and pattern-mixture models (Hogan and Laird, 1997a, 1997b). That is, that dropout only occurs at one of the fixed times at which the longitudinal variable is measured. Moreover, this model allows for censoring of the dropout times.

The longitudinal variable appears as a time dependent covariate in the Cox model used for the dropout process. Maximum likelihood estimation of the parameters in the suggested joint model is complicated by the presence of the unspecified baseline hazard function. We show existence of nonparametric maximum likelihood estimators of the parameters of this model and we compute estimates by maximizing a so-called nonparametric likelihood function, obtained by discretizing the cumulative baseline hazard function as a step function with jumps at the distinct observed dropout times. An EM algorithm is used for obtaining these estimates.

We have applied the suggested model to a longitudinal study of quality-of-life. It appeared from a random dropout analysis that high hazard of dropout is associated with low levels of quality-of-life. A nonignorable dropout analysis allowed us to show that high hazard of dropout is also associated with an unfavorable change in the level of quality-of-life. Similar conclusions were drawn when fitting Diggle and

Kenward's model for nonignorable dropout to the same data set. We compared results obtained from the suggested joint model and Diggle and Kenward's model on our data set.

However, there still remain some unresolved issues. Several authors have pointed out the fact that selection models make distributional assumptions which cannot easily be checked from the available data (discussants of Diggle and Kenward, 1994; Hogan and Laird, 1997b; Scharfstein, Rotnitzky and Robins, 1999). Dupuy and Mesbah (2002) make some suggestions to assess validity of the model described in Section 3. An alternative approach to the problem of nonignorable dropout in longitudinal data may be sensitivity analysis. Verbeke and Molenberghs (2000) provide a detailed review of the work done in this area, and obtain promising results by adapting Diggle and Kenward's selection model to a form tractable for sensitivity analysis.

Asymptotic properties of the nonparametric maximum likelihood estimators are subject of current work. Formal results on say, asymptotic normality of the estimator of β, would provide us a method of comparison of treatments with regard to their impact on quality-of-life. It may then be interesting to compare results obtained, with the ones obtained from other approaches (for example semi-Markov models for quality-of-life (Heutte and Huber-Carol, 2002).

REFERENCES

Chen, H.Y. and Little, R.J.A. (1999). Proportional hazards regression with missing covariates. *Journal of the American Statistical Association* **94**, 896–908.

Cox, D.R. (1972). Regression models and life-tables (with discussion). *Journal of the Royal Statistical Society, Series B* **34**, 187–220.

DeGruttola, V. and Tu, X.M. (1994). Modeling the progression of CD4-lymphocyte count and its relationship to survival time. *Biometrics* **50**, 1003–1014.

Dempster, A.P., Laird, N.M. and Rubin, D.B. (1977). Maximum likelihood from incomplete data via the EM algorithm (with discussion). *Journal of the Royal Statistical Society, Series B* **39**, 1–38.

Diggle, P.J. and Kenward, M.G. (1994). Informative dropout in longitudinal data analysis (with discussion). *Applied Statistics* **43**, 49–93.

Dupuy, J.-F., Grama, I. and Mesbah, M. (2001). Identifiability in a Cox model with nonignorable missing time-dependent covariate. Technical Report SABRES/ University of South-Brittany, France.

Dupuy, J.-F. and Mesbah, M. (2002). Joint modelling of event time and nonignorable missing longitudinal data. *Lifetime Data Analysis* (to appear).

Heutte, N. and Huber-Carol, C. (2002). Semi-Markov models for quality of life data with censoring. In: Mesbah, M., Cole, B.F. and Lee, M.-L. (eds.), *Statistical Methods for Quality of Life Studies: Design, Methods and Analysis.* Boston: Kluwer.

Hogan, J.W. and Laird, N.M. (1997a). Mixture models for the joint distribution of repeated measures and event times. *Statistics in Medicine* **16**, 239–257.

Hogan, J.W. and Laird, N.M. (1997b). Model-based approaches to analysing incomplete longitudinal and failure time data. *Statistics in Medicine* **16**, 259–272.

Hu, P., Tsiatis, A.A. and Davidian, M. (1998). Estimating the parameters in the Cox model when covariate variables are measured with error. *Biometrics* **54**, 1407–1419.

Li, Y. and Lin, X. (2000). Covariate measurement errors in frailty models for clustered survival data. *Biometrika* **87**, 849–866.

Little, R.J.A. and Rubin, D.B. (1987). *Statistical Analysis with Missing Data.* New York: Wiley.

Little, R.J.A. (1995). Modeling the dropout mechanism in repeated-measures studies. *Journal of the American Statistical Association* **90**, 1112–1121.

Molenberghs, G., Kenward, M.G. and Lesaffre, E. (1997). The analysis of longitudinal ordinal data with nonrandom dropout. *Biometrika* **84**, 33–44.

Nelder, J.A. and Mead, R. (1965). A simplex method for function minimisation. *The Computer Journal* **7**, 303–313.

Nielsen, G.G., Gill, R.D., Andersen, P.K. and Sørensen, T.I.A. (1992). A counting process approach to maximum likelihood estimation in frailty models. *Scandinavian Journal of Statistics* **19**, 25–43.

Ribaudo, H.J., Thompson, S.G. and Allen-Mersh, T.G. (2000). A joint analysis of quality of life and survival using a random effect selection model, *Statistics in Medicine* **19**, 3237–3250.

Scharfstein, D.O., Rotnitzky, A. and Robins, J.M. (1999). Adjusting for nonignorable drop-out using semiparametric nonresponse models. *Journal of the American Statistical Association* **94**, 1096–1120.

Schluchter, M.D. (1992). Methods for the analysis of informatively censored longitudinal data. *Statistics in Medicine* **11**, 1861–1870.

Scilab Group (1998). *Introduction to Scilab, User's Guide.* INRIA Meta2 Project/ENPC Cergrene.

Smith, D.M., Robertson, W.H. and Diggle, P.J. (1996). Oswald: object-oriented software for the analysis of longitudinal data in S. Technical Report MA 96/192, Department of Mathematics and Statistics, University of Lancaster, LA1 4YF, United Kingdom.

Troxel, A.B., Harrington, D.P. and Lipsitz, S.R. (1998). Analysis of longitudinal data with non-ignorable non-monotone missing values. *Applied Statistics* **47**, 425–438.

Troxel, A.B., Lipsitz, S.R. and Harrington, D.P. (1998). Marginal models for the analysis of longitudinal measurements with nonignorable non-monotone missing data. *Biometrika* **85**, 671–672.

Verbeke G. and Molenberghs, G. (2000). *Linear Mixed Models for Longitudinal Data.* New York: Springer-Verlag.

Wu, M.C. and Carroll, R.J. (1988). Estimation and comparison of changes in the presence of informative right censoring by modeling the censoring process. *Biometrics* **44**, 175–188.

APPENDIX

In this appendix, we prove the existence of the nonparametric likelihood estimator. Let us assume that $\theta = (\alpha, \sigma^2)$ and β belong respectively to some compact sets $\mathcal{A}$

and $\mathcal{B}$. Suppose first that $\lambda_i \leq U$ $(i = 1, \ldots, p(n))$ for some finite U. Since $L_{(n)}$ is a continuous function of θ, β and of the jump sizes λ_i $(i = 1, \ldots, p(n))$ on the compact set $\mathcal{A} \times \mathcal{B} \times [0, U]^{p(n)}$, $L_{(n)}$ achieves its maximum on this set.

To show that a maximum of $L_{(n)}$ exists on $\mathcal{A} \times \mathcal{B} \times [0, \infty)^{p(n)}$, we show that there exists a finite U such that for all $\psi_U = (\theta_U, \beta_U, \lambda_{1,U}, \ldots, \lambda_{p(n),U}) \in \{\mathcal{A} \times \mathcal{B} \times [0, \infty)^{p(n)}\} \setminus \{\mathcal{A} \times \mathcal{B} \times [0, U]^{p(n)}\}$, there exists a $\psi = (\theta, \beta, \lambda_1, \ldots, \lambda_{p(n)}) \in \mathcal{A} \times \mathcal{B} \times [0, U]^{p(n)}$ such that $L_{(n)}(\psi) > L_{(n)}(\psi_U)$. A proof by contradiction is adopted for this purpose.

Assume that for all U, there exists $\psi_U = (\theta_U, \beta_U, \lambda_{1,U}, \ldots, \lambda_{p(n),U}) \in \{\mathcal{A} \times \mathcal{B} \times [0, \infty)^{p(n)}\} \setminus \{\mathcal{A} \times \mathcal{B} \times [0, U]^{p(n)}\}$ such that for all $\psi = (\theta, \beta, \lambda_1, \ldots, \lambda_{p(n)}) \in \mathcal{A} \times \mathcal{B} \times [0, U]^{p(n)}$, $L_{(n)}(\psi) < L_{(n)}(\psi_U)$.

Let $m = \min_{\mathcal{B},i,l} e^{\beta^T z_{i,(u_l)}}$ and $M = \max_{\mathcal{B},i,l} e^{\beta^T z_{i,(u_l)}}$. Then,

$$\sum_{l=1}^{p(n)} \lambda_l e^{\beta^T z_{(u_l)}} 1_{\{u_{(l)} \leq x\}} \geq m \sum_{l=1}^{p(n)} \lambda_l 1_{\{u_{(l)} \leq x\}},$$

and the likelihood $L_{(n)}(\psi)$ is bounded above by

$$\prod_{i=1}^{n} \left[M \lambda_0(s_i) \exp(-m \sum_{l=1}^{p(n)} \lambda_l 1_{\{u_{(l)} \leq s_i\}}) f_{\alpha,\sigma^2}(z_{i,0}, \ldots, z_{i,[s_i]-1}) \right]$$

where $\lambda_0(s_i)$ denotes the jump λ_l at s_i.

If $\psi_U = (\theta_U, \beta_U, \lambda_{1,U}, \ldots, \lambda_{p(n),U}) \in \{\mathcal{A} \times \mathcal{B} \times [0, \infty)^{p(n)}\} \setminus \{\mathcal{A} \times \mathcal{B} \times [0, U]^{p(n)}\}$, then there exists j $(j \in \{1, \ldots, p(n)\})$ such that $\lambda_{j,U} > U$. Hence there exists at least one i_U $(i_U \in \{1, \ldots, n\})$ such that $\sum_{l=1}^{p(n)} \lambda_l 1_{\{u_{(l)} \leq s_{i_U}\}} > U$. Hence $\sum_{l=1}^{p(n)} \lambda_l 1_{\{u_{(l)} \leq s_{i_U}\}} \longrightarrow +\infty$ as $U \longrightarrow +\infty$. It follows that the upper bound of $L_{(n)}(\psi_U)$ (and hence $L_{(n)}(\psi_U)$) can be made as close to 0 as desired by increasing U. This is the desired contradiction.

MULTIPLE IMPUTATION FOR NON-RANDOM MISSING DATA IN LONGITUDINAL STUDIES OF HEALTH-RELATED QUALITY OF LIFE

DIANE L. FAIRCLOUGH

AMC Cancer Research Center

Missing health-related quality of life (QOL) data in longitudinal studies rarely occur for a single reason. Some individuals drop out of the study as a result of mortality or morbidity of the disease or its treatment, others because their disease symptoms have disappeared. Individuals may have intermittent missing assessments for reasons both unrelated and related to treatment. Most methods for analysis focus on a single mechanism, such as informative dropout, and do not address multiple causes and patterns of missing data. These methods are generally based on strong assumptions that cannot be tested because of the missing data. Further, the estimates are often sensitive to the assumptions underlying the methods. The concepts of multiple imputation can be extended to longitudinal studies of QOL allowing 1) the incorporation of a mixture of models reflecting the variety of causes of missing data that occurs in these studies and 2) the uncertainty associated with the underlying assumptions of the models. However, the assumptions underlying the methods for imputing the missing data should be carefully examined in settings where the missing assessments are nonignorable.

1. Introduction

In longitudinal studies involving self-assessment of health-related quality of life (QOL), missing assessments occur for many reasons. In some cases data may be missing for reasons clearly unrelated to the outcome being measured. For example, assessments may be missing due to administrative errors, as when research staff forgets to administer the questionnaire. In this case the data analyst would be comfortable ignoring the missing data. In contrast, assessments may be missing for reasons clearly related to the outcome. When the subject "feels too ill," or drops out of the study because the intervention failed to work or was too toxic, ignoring the missing data is likely to lead to biased estimates of QOL. In most studies, missing data are often due to a mixture of causes unrelated and related to the outcome of interest. Many analytic approaches assume a single mechanism for the process that results in missing data. There may be documentation of the reasons for missing assessments that allows their classification as to whether the missing assessment is likely to be unrelated or related to the outcome. Incorporating this information into a single model may be technically challenging if not impossible. This is especially true of selection models [1–7] where the dropout process is modeled as if it arises from a single mechanism. It is one of the objectives of this paper to illustrate how

M. Mesbah et al. (eds.), Statistical Methods for Quality of Life Studies, 323–337.

multiple imputation techniques provide flexible approaches to address the mixture of reasons for missing data and incorporate into the analysis additional information about the reasons for missing data. For example, one might use one model to impute the QOL observations that were documented to be missing due to "staff oversight" while using an entirely different method to handle missing data occurring when the subject "feels too ill."

Traditional use of imputation was motivated by the desire to avoid bias due to missing data and the advantages of analysis using methods appropriate for complete data. The advantages of complete data analysis have diminished with the accessibility of estimation procedures [8,9] for longitudinal studies with ignorable missing data (MAR). However, the issue of bias when the data are not missing at random (MNAR) still remains. The challenge is how to implement multiple imputation techniques in settings with non-random missing data. Because multiple imputation is relatively easy to implement, at least in a naive way, it is possible to overlook the implicit assumptions about the missing data mechanism in these methods.

2. Example

In 1993, a multicenter phase III clinical trial was activated by the Eastern Cooperative Oncology Group (ECOG) to compare two new Paclitaxel-cisplatin regimens with a traditional etoposide cisplatin regimen for the treatment of stage IIIB-IV non-small-cell lung cancer (NSCLC) [10]. All treatment arms included cisplatin at the same dose (75 mg/m^2 IV over 1 hour). The traditional treatment arm contained VP-16 (100 mg/m^2 IV $\times$ 3) in addition to the cisplatin. The other two arms contained low dose Paclitaxel (135 mg/m^2 IV) or high dose Paclitaxel (250 mg/m^2 IV) with G-CSF (5 g/kg/day). Three hundred thirty-two patients (58%) started four or more cycles of therapy and 210 (36%) started six or more cycles. In addition to traditional endpoints, such as time to disease progression and death, health related QOL was included in this trial.

The stated objective of the QOL component of this study was "To compare quality of life for the three treatment arms and correlate quality of life to toxicity." Four QOL assessments were scheduled for each patient. The assessment times were carefully selected after balancing a number of considerations. These included (1) concern for excessive burden to this often debilitated group of patients, (2) the relatively short median time to progression and death expected in these patients, and (3) practical matters related to feasibility of the study at multiple clinical treatment sites. These issues contributed to the decision to have relatively few assessments (four) over a fairly brief period of time (6 months from initiation of treatment). Thus, the four assessments were scheduled to be prior to the start of treatment, before the start of the third and fifth courses of chemotherapy, and at 6 months (Week 26). If patients were off treatment, then the second and third assessments were to be scheduled 6 and 12 weeks after the initiation of therapy. The Functional Assessment of Cancer Therapy, Lung Cancer Version 2 (FACT-L) was used to measure QOL in this trial [11]. It is a 43-item questionnaire, 33 items of which are general questions relevant to all cancer patients and 10 of which are items relevant to lung cancer. It provides reliable scores for subscales measuring

Table 1. Summary of missing FACT-L assessments

	Follow-up Number[1]				
	1	2	3	4	All
	Number (%)				
Completed[2]	538 (94)	382 (72)	290 (60)	192 (50)	1,402 (71)
Missed due to:[2]					
Language	0 (0)	2 (0)	0 (0)	0 (0)	2 (0)
Staff unavailable	0 (0)	5 (1)	2 (0)	1 (0)	8 (0)
Staff oversight	9 (2)	35 (7)	66 (14)	57 (15)	167 (8)
Patient feels too ill	0 (0)	4 (1)	3 (1)	3 (1)	10 (1)
Staff felt pt too ill	1 (0)	19 (4)	15 (3)	11 (3)	46 (2)
Refusal	9 (2)	40 (8)	53 (11)	69 (18)	171 (8)
Other	9 (2)	12 (2)	23 (5)	19 (5)	63 (3)
Unknown	9 (2)	30 (6)	28 (6)	32 (8)	99 (5)
Total Expected	575	529	480	384	1,968
Patient Expired[3]	0 (0)	46 (8)	95 (17)	191 (33)	332 (14)
All Patients	575	575	575	575	2,300

[1]Follow-up number 1 = baseline (prior to 1st cycle), 2 = 6 weeks (prior to 3rd cycle), 3 = 12 weeks (prior to 5th cycle), 4 = 6 months post randomization.
[2]% of expected assessments (i.e., patient still alive).
[3]% of all possible assessments.

physical well-being, social/family well-being, emotional well-being, functional well-being and lung cancer symptoms [11,12]. Three of the scales, physical well-being, functional well-being and lung cancer symptoms, are combined to form the Trial Outcome Index (FACT-TOI Lung). Higher scores on all the FACT-L scales imply better quality of life.

A total of 1,402 QOL assessments were obtained in this study. This represents 94%, 72%, 60% and 50% of the expected assessments in surviving patients at each of the four planned assessment times (Table 1). The most common documented reason for missing assessments was patient refusal (8%) and staff oversight (8%). A detailed listing of the reasons for missing assessments is presented in Table 1. Factors associated with missing assessments in surviving patients include older age, lower QOL scores (FACT-TOI) at previous assessment, early removal from therapy due to progressive disease and proximity to death (Table 2). Unexpectedly, patients with more toxicity were less likely to have a missing assessment. This is possibly due to additional visits scheduled to resolve the toxicity. These results and previous sensitivity analyses [13] suggested that dropout in this study was likely to be related to QOL at the time of the missing assessment.

Table 2. Characteristics associated with missing QOL assessments among survivors. Odds ratios were obtained from stepwise logistic regression analyses of the probability of a missing FACT-L assessment with age and previous FACT-TOI score forced into model

Assessment	Characteristic	Odds Ratio	(95% CI)
Baseline	≥5% weight loss prior 6 months	0.62	(0.42 to 0.92)
6 weeks	Age (decades)[1]	1.44	(1.13 to 1.84)
	Prior FACT-TOI[2]	0.86	(0.75 to 0.99)
	Neurotoxcity[3]	0.74	(0.61 to 0.91)
	PD[4] within 6 cycles	1.23	(1.23 to 3.07)
	Death within 2 months	4.40	(2.45 to 7.93)
12 weeks	Age (decades)[1]	1.19	(0.90 to 1.57)
	Prior FACT-TOI[2]	0.80	(0.68 to 0.95)
	PD[4] within 6 cycles	2.84	(1.66 to 4.87)
	Death within 2 months	5.34	(2.20 to 12.9)
6 months	Age (decades)[1]	1.31	(0.96 to 1.77)
	Prior FACT-TOI[2]	0.76	(0.63 to 0.92)
	Other Toxicity[3]	0.74	(0.61 to 0.91)
	Death within 2 months	2.70	(1.25 to 5.84)

[1]Age at date of randomization
[2]10 point difference on FACT-TOI
[3]Maximum NCI Common Toxicity Criteria (CTC) grade
[4]Early discontinuation of therapy (before 6 cycles) due to progressive disease

3. Multiple Imputation

3.1 Definitions and Notation

Let Y_i be a vector of possible measurements of the response (QOL) for the ith patient where Y_i can be partitioned into the observed measurements, Y_i^{obs}, and the missing measurements, Y_i^{mis}. It is assumed that the complete data follow a multivariate distribution $Y_i \sim N[X_i\beta, \Sigma_i]$ in which X_i is the design matrix containing treatment indicators and covariates and β is the corresponding vector of parameters. The covariance of the measurements, Σ_i, is a known function of the vector of unknown variance parameters.

Let R_i be a vector corresponding to Y_i where $r_{ij} = 1$ if the jth possible measurement, y_{ij}, is observed and $r_{ij} = 0$ otherwise. If all observations are missing after the first occurrence of a missing observation, the missing data pattern is described as *monotone*.

The missing data is *missing completely at random* (MCAR) if the probability that an observation is missing depends only on covariates,

$$Pr[R_i|X_i, Y_i^{obs}, Y_i^{mis}] = Pr[R_i|X_i].$$

The missing data is *missing at random* (MAR) if the probability of missingness depends on the observed data (Y_i^{obs}) but is independent of the missing observations (Y_i^{mis}),

$$Pr[R_i|X_i, Y_i^{obs}, Y_i^{mis}] = Pr[R_i|X_i, Y_i^{obs}].$$

If the probability of a missing observation depends on the missing value, then the data are *not missing at random* (MNAR),

$$Pr[R_i|X_i, Y_i^{obs}, Y_i^{mis}] = Pr[R_i|X_i, Y_i^{obs}, Y_i^{mis}].$$

Finally, if the data are MCAR or MAR and the parameters of the response model (Θ) are distinct from the parameters of the dropout model (Φ), then the missing data are *ignorable.*

3.2 General Strategy of Multiple Imputation

There are four steps common to all multiple imputation methods. The general procedure is to (1) select an appropriate strategy for imputing the missing values, (2) generate M datasets of imputed values of the missing values, (3) estimate the primary parameters ($\hat{\beta}^{(m)}$) and their variance (Var[$\hat{\beta}^{(m)}$]) for each of the M "complete" datasets using either complete data or maximum likelihood methods, and (4) compute the final combined parameter estimates ($\hat{\beta}$) and their variance (Var[$\hat{\beta}$]) from the results of the M analyses. Details for Step 4 are provided in the next section.

Though the least technical, the most difficult step is the first. There are many implicit and explicit methods that can be used for multiple imputation [14–18]. Explicit methods generally utilize regression models whereas implicit methods rely on sampling techniques. Two examples will be described in the subsequent sections.

3.3 Analysis of the M Imputed Data Sets

For each of the M imputed data sets, the parameter estimates ($\hat{\beta}^{(m)}$) and their variance ($Var[\hat{\beta}^{(m)}]$) are computed using an appropriate analytic method. In the NSCLC example, maximum likelihood estimation was used to estimate the parameters of a mixed effects model allowing for mistimed observations and time-varying covariates [8,19]. In addition, linear combinations of the parameters ($\theta^{(m)} = C\beta^{(m)}$) and their variance, which will be used to test specific hypotheses (e.g., $H_0 : \theta = 0$), are also estimated for each of the M data sets.

Rubin [20, Chapter 3], Rubin and Schenker [15] and Schafer [16, Chapter 4] give the rules for combining the estimates and test statistics from the M analyses. The parameter estimates are obtained by averaging the estimates from the analyses of the M imputed data sets: $\hat{\beta} = (\sum \hat{\beta}^{(m)})/M$. The total variance is computed by the sum of the within-imputation component ($\bar{W}_\beta$) and the between-imputation component (B_β) weighted by a correction for a finite number of imputations (1 +

M^{-1}). The same procedure can be used for the secondary parameters ($\theta = C\beta$). The computations are summarized in Table 3.

Table 3. Computations for combining the analyses of the M data sets

Within Imputation	
Parameter estimates	$\hat{\beta}^{(m)}$
Within imputation variance of estimates	$W_\beta^{(m)} = Var(\hat{\beta}^{(m)})$
Between Imputation	
Between imputation variance of estimates	$B_\beta = \frac{1}{M-1}\sum_{m=1}^{M}(\hat{\beta}^{(m)} - \bar{\beta})^2$
Pooled Analyses	
Pooled parameter estimates	$\bar{\beta} = \sum_{m=1}^{M}\hat{\beta}^{(m)}/M$
Pooled within imputation variance	$\bar{W}_\beta = \sum_{m=1}^{M} W_\beta^{(m)})/M$
Total variance	$V_\beta = \bar{W}_\beta + (1 + \frac{1}{M})B_\beta$
Miscellaneous	
Between to within variance ratio	$r_\beta = (1 + M^{-1})B_\beta/W_\beta$
Fraction of missing information about β that is missing due to nonresponse	$\gamma_\beta = r_\beta/(1 + r_\beta) = (1 + M^{-1})B_\beta/V_\beta$

Table 4. Example of between and within imputation variation in estimated treatment group means over time

Time	Taxol	Within imputation variance	Between imputation variance	Between-to-within ratio	Fraction information lost due to non-response	Proportion missing assessments
Baseline	No	1.76	0.10	0.06	0.05	0.11
	Yes	0.89	0.09	0.11	0.10	0.10
6 weeks	No	2.01	0.81	0.44	0.31	0.44
	Yes	1.01	0.20	0.22	0.18	0.31
12 weeks	No	2.16	1.83	0.93	0.48	0.56
	Yes	1.09	0.46	0.47	0.32	0.49
6 months	No	2.92	3.20	1.20	0.55	0.71
	Yes	1.48	1.48	1.10	0.52	0.66

The fraction of information about the parameters that is missing due to non-response (γ) for each parameter can be estimated from the ratio of the between imputation variance to the total variance [14]. As the amount of missing data increases, γ increases. In contrast, as the amount of information about the missing data in the covariates of the imputation model increases, γ decreases. The estimated fraction of missing information is accurate only if the model used to impute the missing observations is correct and does not reflect our ignorance of the true missing data mechanism. Table 4 provides one example of these computations.

4. Implicit Sampling Based Imputation

Implicit sampling procedures for imputation include hot deck imputation [21] and approximate Bayesian Bootstrap (ABB) [14,15]. The basic idea is to draw random values from subjects with similar characteristics and substitute them for the missing observations. Simple hot deck procedures underestimate the variance of the estimates because they ignore the uncertainty about the stratification. ABB remedies this problem. The procedure is to draw random repeated imputations from the posterior predictive distribution by first creating a *possible* distribution of values and then drawing randomly from that distribution.

4.1 ABB Procedure

The first step is to identify strata where subjects have the same characteristics. These strata could be defined by one or two dichotomous patient characteristics. In the NSCLC study presented here, initial stage of disease, best tumor response, and progressive disease during therapy are possible candidates. As the number of characteristics increase or if the characteristics are continuous (e.g., length of response or number of cycles of therapy), the number of strata becomes unmanageable and many strata will not contain enough observations to provide an adequate sampling frame. Lavori et al. [18] proposed an extension of this approach to a longitudinal trial with a monotone missing data pattern. In this approach, the strata were formed based on *propensity scores* for the probability of missing observations at each follow-up. A logistic model is used to estimate the probability of a missing assessment as a function of multiple covariates and previously observed or imputed QOL scores. Strata are then formed on the basis of quintiles or quartiles of the predicted probability of a missing observation.

Once the strata have been identified, the sampling procedure is as follows. In each stratum, there will be a total of N_s possible observations with n_s^{obs} values observed and n_s^{mis} values missing ($N_s = n_s^{obs} + n_s^{mis}$). The next step is to create the potential distribution of values by randomly drawing with replacement a set of n_s^{obs} observations with replacement from the original n_s^{obs} values. The third step is to choose n_s^{mis} observations at random from this potential set of observations, again with replacement and with equal probability. The entire procedure is repeated M times. This is basically the procedure that is implemented in "Solas for Missing Data Analysis, Version 1" by Statistical Solutions Ltd. [22] and the new experimental SAS procedure [23].

4.2 Assumptions

While the procedure sounds straightforward, it is important to understand the underlying assumptions and limitations. First note that the ABB procedure was originally developed for a simple random sample with ignorable missing data. There is a strong assumption that within strata the missing data are completely random and come from exactly the same distribution as the observed data. However, in the NSCLC trial, it seems likely that the individuals with missing assessments are experiencing poorer QOL than those who completed the assessment. Thus, even within strata based on the propensity scores, this assumption may not be justified for QOL measures. A related disadvantage of the propensity scores is that potentially different subgroups of patients are lumped together based on similar propensities for missing data. This could potentially group individuals who are dropping out of a study due to lack of efficacy or excessive toxicity with those that are dropping out when they become asymptomatic as a result of effective treatment.

There are several proposed modifications of the ABB procedure when one believes that subjects within a stratum with missing assessments may have poorer responses. The first approach is to modify the sampling so that values are sampled from the available observations with probability dependent on Y [14]. Another approach is to randomly draw k (usually 2 or 3) observations and take the minimum of the k draws. VanBuuren *et al.* [24] suggest a δ-adjustment where a predetermined constant is subtracted from the imputed value. The difficulty is that all these methods are ad hoc and there is no way to empirically validate a particular choice. For example, there is no way to determine what probability function to use or what is the appropriate constant to subtract from the sample value. These approaches may, however, have considerable value in sensitivity analyses. For example, one might select specific values of δ from a range of reasonable choices and examine the impact on the conclusions of the analysis.

Another limitation occurs when estimates of longitudinal change are of interest. The ABB procedure with propensity scores uses only the information about the association between patient characteristics or previous QOL with missingness. The procedure does not use any information about the correlation of the outcome over time and the correlation among the repeated measures is likely to be underestimated. Thus ABB may be useful when the intent of the analysis is to make cross-sectional comparisons among groups, but is not appropriate for the estimation of change over time. Similarly, if missing values of covariates are imputed with this approach, then the relationship between the covariate and the outcome may be underestimated.

4.3 Practical Considerations

There are two competing goals that impact the implementation of the ABB procedure. The first goal motivates a larger number of strata, while the second goal motivates a smaller number of strata. The first goal is the need to define strata in which the MCAR assumption is valid. Increasing the number of strata will create more homogeneous groups where the assumption may become more reasonable.

The second goal is to have sufficient subjects with observed data in each stratum for the sampling procedure. The better the predictive model for missingness, the more likely the stratum with the highest propensity for missingness will be close to empty. As the number of strata is increased, the likelihood that some strata will be close to empty increases. This is less likely in large sample surveys (the context for which ABB was originally developed) involving thousands of subjects, but will occur in the typically smaller clinical trials. Even when there are 200 subjects per arm, it is very easy to find strata in which there are less than 10 observed values.

Other challenges associated with this approach come from the longitudinal structure of the data. In the NSCLC study, approximately 15% of the cases have a missing assessment followed by a observed assessment. Thus, the missing data pattern is not solely monotone as was the case for the study described by Lavori *et al.* [18].

4.4 NSCLC Example

In the NSCLC example, missing QOL data were imputed using a series of univariate regression models. Three variations were considered, differing in the selection of covariates. In the first procedure, the models used to form the propensity scores were based on only two strong predictors of dropout, proximity to death and the previous QOL score. Imputation of the missing baseline assessments used the pooled data and an indicator of the proximity to death. Then missing values at 6 weeks where imputed separately in each of the treatment arms, using both covariates and baseline scores. When baseline QOL was missing, the imputed values generated in the previous step were used in the imputation model. Imputation of the 12 week and 6 month observations followed in a sequential fashion, again separately in each arm.

In the second procedure, variables used to predict dropout were selected in a stepwise procedure with the selection criterion set at $\alpha = 0.05$. This resulted in the inclusion of more covariates in the imputation models and a small increase in the estimated rate of decline by 12 weeks in the patients not receiving Taxol (Figure 1). In the third procedure, the consequence of omitting an important covariate is illustrated. For this illustration, indicators of the closeness to death were omitted. Again, the estimates in the smaller treatment group were sensitive to this omission. In all of the procedures, the number of strata was reduced from 5 to 4 at 12 weeks and from 5 to 3 at 6 months in the smaller of the two treatment arms.

Figure 1. Estimates for FACT-TOI scores using ABB procedures.

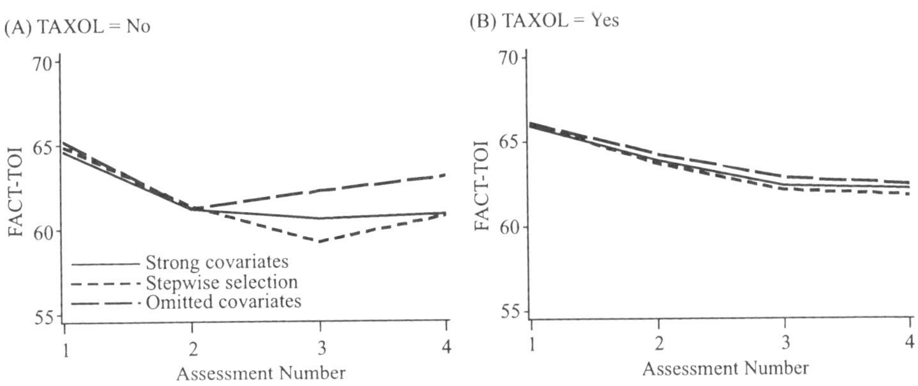

5. Explicit Imputation Models

Explicit methods of imputation employ regression models to generate the imputed values of the missing observations. In longitudinal studies, this will either be a series of simple regression models [25] or a multivariate model such as a mixed effects model for incomplete longitudinal data [16]. Choosing a good imputation model is the hardest part of the imputation procedure. Knowledge of the disease, side effects of treatment and the clinical course of the disease, whether the therapy succeeds or fails, as well as available auxiliary data, is essential.

When there is concern that the data may not be missing at random, it will be desirable to include additional covariates that are not appropriate for the analytic model. The objective is to identify covariates for the imputation model that both explain variation in observed QOL and are related to the reasons for the missing data. If, conditional on these additional covariates and the observed data, missing data in the imputation model is ignorable then the imputed values will be unbiased. In the NSCLC patients in our example, candidates include the tumor response, measures of side-effects and toxicity, number of cycles of therapy completed, early removal from therapy due to progressive disease and proximity to death (Table 2). These covariates would generally not be included in the analytic model used to test the effect of the interventions because the covariates would explain variability in the response that should be attributed to the intervention. Thus, it would be appropriate to include indicators of response to therapy and toxicity as covariates in the imputation model but not in the analytic model.

5.1 The Procedure

Unlike simple imputation methods, which generally utilize mean or predicted values from the imputation, multiple imputation methods incorporate both the uncertainty associated with the parameter estimates ($\text{Var}[\tilde{\beta}^*]$) and the variability of individual observations ($\text{Var}[Y_{ij}]$) into the imputed values. Given the chosen model for imputation, the first step is to estimate the imputation model parameters ($\tilde{\beta}^*$ and $\tilde{\Sigma}_i^*$) and their variance (note that an asterisk has been added to differentiate these parameters from those that will be obtained for the analytic model),

$$Y_i = X_i^* \beta^* + e_i^*, \quad \text{Var}[Y_i] = \Sigma_i^*.$$

The second step is to draw M random sets of the model parameters, $\beta^{(m)}$ and $\sigma^{2(m)}$ from their estimated distributions. The third step is to generate the imputed values of y_{ij}^{mis} by adding random error corresponding to the between and within subject variability of the outcome ($\text{Var}[y_{ij}] = \sigma^{*2}$):

$$y_{ij}^{mis(m)} = X_{ij}^{mis} \beta^{(m)} + \sigma^{*(m)} r_Y^{(m)},$$

where $r_Y^{(m)}$ is a random number drawn from a standard normal distribution.

This procedure and minor variations for monotone missing data patterns are described by Rubin [20], Crawford [17], and Little and Yau [25]. Schafer [16] reviews a Markov chain Monte Carlo (MCMC) procedure that assumes multivariate normality. The MCMC procedure is implemented in the new experimental SAS procedure [23].

5.2 Assumptions

When the imputation procedure uses a regression approach as described above, the primary assumption is that the missingness is MCAR conditional on covariates included in the imputation model. When Bayesian methods such as MCMC are used or the imputation model includes the observed data, the assumption is relaxed to MAR. When there is the potential for non-random missing data, the model used for imputing the missing observations (the *imputation model*) will generally differ from the model that will be used to test the primary hypotheses of the study (the *analytic model*). This is in contrast to the setting where the data can be considered to be MAR for the analytic model, as discussed by Schafer in Chapter 4 of his book [16].

The primary implication is that the relationship between observed QOL and covariates in the imputation model predicts the relationship between unobserved QOL and the same covariates. While it is possible that these covariates may be different than the covariates that predict changes in QOL when it is measured, in practice, the analyst will need to assume that they are the same.

5.3 Practical Considerations

Just as there were competing considerations in the implicit models, there are also similar considerations in the explicit models. The addition of more predictors of the outcome will increase the variation in the outcome explained by the imputation model (R^2). However, when the precision of the associated parameter estimates ($\tilde{\beta}^*$) decreases, this will result in a wide range of potential parameter values of ($\beta^{(m)}$) across the M imputations, thus the imputed values may only add noise to the observed data. Thus, explicit models will not be very useful when the size of the study is small or there is a lack of strong predictors of the QOL measure.

5.4 NSCLC Example

As previously mentioned, missing data may arise from a variety of mechanisms. In the NSCLC study, one would expect that during the early part of the study missingness would be more closely related to toxicity and the initial response of the disease to treatment. However, after disease progression, the proximity to death may be a better predictor of missing QOL assessments. In the following illustration, we use different models to impute missing data that occurs early and just prior to death. The first step is to impute values for missing assessments that are more than 2 months prior to death relying on baseline characteristics, the previous QOL scores and clinical indicators of toxicity, best tumor response and early disease progression. Missing values were imputed using a series of univariate regression models [25] in which the R^2 was 0.18 for the first assessment and ranged from 0.30–0.43 for the remaining time points.

Missing values that are within two months of the date of death were then imputed using previous QOL measures (including those imputed in the first step) and the observed change over time in subjects whose QOL was observed during the relevant period. In contrast to the previous step, this was a single step using a repeated measure model with a piecewise linear regression model for the time to death [26]. This was motivated by the small number of observed QOL scores within two months of death at each of the four assessments. The resulting estimates of change over time are displayed in Figure 2A. Missing scores were not imputed after the time of death. The assumption is then that the observations after death are MAR. Basically, conditional on the previously observed scores, the QOL after death follows the same pattern as the survivors. The result is that by default, we are assuming that the QOL improves slightly after death. Estimates were obtained using restricted maximum likelihood for a repeated measures model [8,19].

In the second analysis, observations scheduled to occur after death were imputed as if they occurred at the time to death. In this analysis, we are assuming that QOL declines as the patient approaches death and then levels off after death. The resulting overall estimates are displayed in Figure 2B. While the differences between the two treatments remained constant for the two approaches, the estimated change over time is dramatically different. Other approaches are possible, all of which require strong value judgements about *quality of life* after death. With scales that are anchored at zero for death, substituting zero for observations occurring after death is a possible strategy. However, when a substantial proportion of the subjects expire during the study, the results will approximate the traditional survival analysis.

Figure 2. FACT-L scores as a function of time from randomization and number of treatment cycles started. Panel (A) displays results when QOL scores after death are not imputed. Panel (B) displays results when QOL scores after death are imputed.

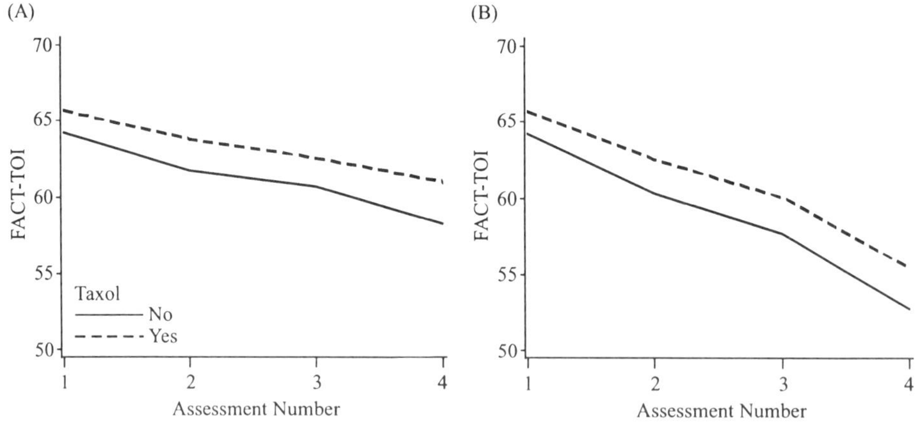

6. Discussion

In longitudinal studies of patients who experience considerable morbidity and/or mortality, it is likely that morbidity and poorer QOL are associated with missing observations over the course of the study. In these studies, the possibility of nonignorable missing data must be considered. While there has been extensive theoretical work on analytic techniques for nonignorable missing data, the usefulness of these methods across a variety of settings has yet to be demonstrated. In this paper we have suggested that multiple imputation techniques may be useful in the analysis of missing QOL data in this NSCLC trial for several reasons. The most compelling reason, in my opinion, is the ease with which different models can be used to impute observations that are missing for different reasons. The second reason is that the techniques are relatively straightforward and can be implemented with combinations of available software. SAS Proc Mixed [8] and Proc IML were the primary tools used in the analyses presented here. Finally, these techniques lend themselves readily to sensitivity analyses of the results across different models for the missing data mechanism.

However, there are also limitations to imputation. One of the arguments that Rubin and colleagues have made over time for imputation in public-use datasets is that a team of individuals or an individual who is intimately familiar with the study can incorporate that unique knowledge into the imputation procedures. In the same context, I would suggest that imputation techniques based on a thorough knowledge of the disease, its treatment and the conduct of the study will enhance the quality of the analysis of these studies. The converse is also true; naive implementation can result in disaster. Moreover, the analyst must understand the implications of the underlying assumptions in the methods used to generate the missing observations. With the availability of more statistical analysis software that can be used by almost anyone, there is increasing danger that individuals will not stop to consider these assumptions carefully and may have a false sense of security about the results of their analysis. I am not advocating that we limit the availability of software. On the contrary, it is only when techniques become widely accessible and are applied in a wide variety of settings that we begin to understand the true strengths and weaknesses of any analytic approach.

In summary, multiple imputation techniques provide considerable flexibility for handling missing data, which occur for a variety of reasons. It is, however, critical to understand the assumptions underlying the imputation methods, especially in studies with extensive non-random missing observations. We acknowledge that the conclusions drawn from a study with as much missing data as is present in this example should be made cautiously. However, this NSCLC example very clearly illustrates the sensitivity of estimates to the underlying assumptions of the multiple imputation procedures and the need for a thorough knowledge of the study, the underlying disease and the reasons for missing data before application of these techniques.

ACKNOWLEDGEMENTS

The NSCLC study was coordinated by the Eastern Cooperative Oncology Group and supported by Grant CA-23318, awarded by the National Cancer Institute, DHHS. I would especially like to thank the patients that participated in this study. Finally, I would like to thank Ms. Pam Wolfe, Monika Baier, Julie Maloy, Dr. Richard Jones and two anonymous reviewers for their suggestions and comments.

REFERENCES

1. Wu, M.C. and Bailey, K.R. (1988). Analyzing changes in the presence of informative right censoring caused by death and withdrawal. *Statistics in Medicine* **7**, 337–346.
2. Wu, M.C. and Bailey, K.R. (1989). Estimation and comparison of changes in the presence of informative right censoring: conditional linear model. *Biometrics* **45**, 939–955.
3. Wu, M.C. and Carroll, R.J. (1988). Estimation and comparison of changes in the presence of informative right censoring by modeling the censoring process. *Biometrics* **44**, 175–188.
4. Mori, M., Woodworth, G.G. and Woolson, R.F. (1992). Application of empirical Bayes inference to estimation of rate of change in the presence of informative right censoring. *Statistics in Medicine* **11**, 621–631.
5. Schluchter, M.D. (1992). Methods for the analysis of informatively censored longitudinal data. *Statistics in Medicine* **11**, 1861–1870.
6. Diggle, P. and Kenward, M.G. (1994). Informative drop-out in longitudinal analysis (with discussion). *Applied Statistics* **43**, 49–93.
7. Troxel, A.B., Harrington, D.P. and Lipsitz, S.R. (1998). Analysis of Longitudinal Data with Nonignorable non-monotone missing values. *Applied Statistics* **47**, 425–438.
8. SAS Institute (1996). *The MIXED procedure. SAS/STAT Software. Changes and Enhancements (through Release 6.11).* Cary, NC: SAS Institute.
9. Schluchter, M.D. (1990). 5V: unbalanced repeated measures models with structured covariance matrices. In: *BMDP Statistical Software Manual Part 2.* Berkley, CA: University of California Press.
10. Bonomi, P., Kim, K.M., Fairclough, D., Cella, D., Kugler, J., Rowinsky, E., Jiroutek, M. and Johnson, D. (2000). Comparison of survival and quality of life in advanced non-small cell lung cancer patients treated with two dose levels of paclitaxel combined with cisplatin versus etoposide-cisplatin: results of an Eastern Cooperative Oncology Group trial. *Journal of Clinical Oncology* **18**, 623–631.
11. Cella, D.F., Bonomi, A.E., Lloyd, S.R., Tulsky, D.S., Kaplan, E. and Bonomi, P. (1995). Reliability and validity of the Functional Assessment of Cancer Therapy – Lung (FACT-L) quality of life instrument. *Lung Cancer* **12**, 199–220.
12. Cella, D.F., Tulsky, D.S., Gray, G., Sarafian, B., Linn, E., Bonomi, A., Silberman, M., Yellen, S.B., Winicour, P. and Brannon J. (1993). The Functional Assessment of Cancer Therapy (FACT) scales: development and validation of

the general measure. *Journal of Clinical Oncology* **11**, 570–579.
13. Fairclough, D.L., Peterson, H., Bonomi, P. and Cella, D.F. (1998). Comparison of model based methods dependent of the missing data mechanism in two clinical trials of cancer therapy. *Statistics in Medicine* **17**, 781–796.
14. Rubin, D.B. and Schenker, N. (1991). Multiple imputation in health-care data bases: an overview and some applications. *Statistics in Medicine* **10**, 585–598.
15. Rubin, D.B. and Schenker, N. (1985) Multiple imputation for interval estimation from simple random samples with ignorable nonresponse. *Journal of the American Statistical Association* **81**, 366–374.
16. Schafer, J.L. (1997). *Analysis of Incomplete Multivariate Data.* London: Chapman and Hall.
17. Crawford, S.L., Tennstedt, S.L. and McKinlay, J.B. (1995). A comparison of analytic methods for non-random missingness of outcome data. *Journal of Clinical Epidemiology* **48**, 209–219.
18. Lavori, P.W., Dawson, R. and Shera, D. (1995). A multiple imputation strategy for clinical trials with truncation of patient data. *Statistics in Medicine* **14**, 1912–1925.
19. Jennrich, R.I. and Schluchter, M.D. (1986). Unbalanced repeated-measures models with structured covariance matrices. *Biometrics* **42**, 805–820.
20. Rubin, D.B. (1987). *Multiple Imputation for Nonresponse in Surveys.* New York: John Wiley and Sons.
21. Little, R.J. and Rubin, D.B. (1987). *Statistical Analysis with Missing Data.* New York: John Wiley and Sons.
22. Statistical Solutions (1997). *Solas for Missing Data Analysis 1.0 User Reference.*
23. Yuan, Y.C. (2000). *Multiple Imputation for Missing Data: Concepts and New Development.* Rockville, MD: SAS Institue Inc. Cork, Ireland: Statistical Solutions Ltd.
24. VanBuuren, S., Boshuizen, H.C. and Knook, D.L. (1999). Multiple imputation of missing blood pressure covariates in survival analysis. *Statistics in Medicine* **18**, 681–694.
25. Little, R. and Yau, L. (1996). Intent-to-treat analysis for longitudinal studies with drop-outs. *Biometrics* **52**, 1324–1333.
26. Neter, J. and Wasserman, W (1974). *Applied Linear Statistical Models.* Homewood, IL: Richard Irwin, Inc.

STRATEGIES TO FIT PATTERN-MIXTURE MODELS

GEERT MOLENBERGHS, HERBERT THIJS, GEERT VERBEKE, BART MICHIELS AND MICHAEL G. KENWARD

Universiteit Limburg, Katholieke Universiteit Leuven, Janssen Research Foundation, London School of Hygiene and Tropical Medicine

Whereas most models for incomplete longitudinal data are formulated within the selection model framework, pattern-mixture models have gained considerable interest in recent years. In this chapter, we outline several strategies to fit pattern-mixture models, including the so-called identifying-restrictions strategy. Multiple imputation is used to apply this strategy to realistic settings, such as quality-of-life data from a longitudinal study on metastatic breast cancer patients.

1. Introduction

It is not unusual in practice for some sequences of measurements to terminate early for reasons outside the control of the investigator, and any unit so affected is often called a dropout. It might therefore be necessary to accommodate dropout in the modeling process, either to obtain correct inference, or because this process can itself be of scientific interest. In this paper, we will restrict attention to dropout, i.e., monotone missingness.

Rubin (1976) and Little and Rubin (1987, Chapter 6) make important distinctions between different missing values processes. A dropout process is said to be completely random (MCAR) if the dropout is independent of both unobserved and observed data and random (MAR) if, conditional on the observed data, the dropout is independent of the unobserved measurements; otherwise the dropout process is termed non-random (MNAR). If a dropout process is random then a valid analysis can be obtained through a likelihood-based analysis that ignores the dropout mechanism, provided the parameter describing the measurement process is functionally independent of the parameter describing the dropout process, the so-called parameter distinctness condition. This situation is termed ignorable by Little and Rubin (1987). This leads to considerable simplification in the analysis. In many examples, however, the reasons for dropout are many and varied and it is therefore difficult to justify on a priori grounds the assumption of random dropout. Arguably, in the presence of non-random dropout, a wholly satisfactory analysis of the data is not feasible. Several approaches have been proposed in the literature (Little, 1995; Kenward and Molenberghs, 1999).

Most methods are formulated within the selection modeling frame (Little and Rubin, 1987) as opposed to pattern-mixture modeling (PMM; Little, 1993, 1994).

M. Mesbah et al. (eds.), Statistical Methods for Quality of Life Studies, 339–351.

A selection model factors the joint distribution of the measurement and response mechanisms into the marginal measurement distribution and the response distribution, conditional on the measurements. This is intuitively appealing since the marginal measurement distribution would be of interest also with complete data. Further, Little and Rubin's taxonomy is most easily developed in the selection setting. However, it is often argued that, especially in the context of non-random missingness models, selection models, although identifiable, should be approached with caution (Glynn, Laird and Rubin, 1986). Therefore, pattern-mixture models, employing the reverse factorization, have gained renewed interest in recent years (Little, 1993, 1994; Hogan and Laird, 1997). Note that a further framework consists of shared random-effects models (e.g., Wu and Carroll, 1988).

An important issue is that pattern-mixture models are by construction under-identified. Little (1993, 1994) solves this problem through the use of identifying restrictions: inestimable parameters of the incomplete patterns are set equal to (functions of) the parameters describing the distribution of the completers. Identifying restrictions are not the only way to overcome under-identification and we will discuss alternative approaches as well.

All in all, while some authors perceive this under-identification as a drawback, we believe it is an asset since it forces one to reflect on the assumptions made. We will indicate in this paper how it can serve as a starting point for sensitivity analysis. In Section 2 we will introduce the vorozole study, to which our methods will be applied. Section 3 sketches modeling approaches for incomplete data. Sensitivity analysis strategies in a pattern-mixture context is the topic of Section 4, while in Section 5 the strategy of identifying restrictions is considered in detail. Finally, in Section 6 we discuss the results of all methods applied to the vorozole set of data.

2. The Vorozole Study

This study was an open-label, multicenter, parallel group design conducted at 67 North American centers (29 Canadian, 38 US). Patients were randomized to either vorozole (2.5 mg taken once daily) or megestrol acetate (40 mg four times daily). The patient population consisted of postmenopausal patients with histologically confirmed estrogen-receptor positive metastatic breast carcinoma. To expedite enrollment, patients with nonmeasurable/nonassessable disease were entered and eligible patients were stratified into three groups according to whether they had measurable, assessable, or nonmeasurable/nonassessable disease. All 452 randomized patients were followed until disease progression or death. The main objective was to compare the treatment group with respect to response rate while secondary objectives included a comparison relative to duration of response, time to progression, survival, safety, pain relief, performance status and quality of life. Full details of this study are reported in Goss *et al.* (1999). This paper focuses on overall quality of life, measured by the total Functional Living Index: Cancer (FLIC; Schipper *et al.*, 1984). Precisely, a higher FLIC score is the more desirable outcome.

Patients underwent screening, and for those deemed eligible, a detailed examination at baseline (occasion 0) took place. Further measurement occasions were months 1, then from months 2 at bi-monthly intervals until month 44. Goss *et al.* (1999) analyzed the FLIC scores using a two-way ANOVA model with effects for treatment, disease status, as well as their interaction. No significant treatment difference was found. The main conclusion from the primary analysis was that vorozole is well tolerated and as effective as megestrol acetate in the treatment of postmenopausal advanced breast cancer patients with disease progression after tamoxifen treatment. In this paper, we will, apart from treatment, correct for dominant site of the disease as well as clinical stage.

3. Modeling Approach

In modeling missing data one is interested in $f(\boldsymbol{y}_i, d_i|\boldsymbol{\theta}, \boldsymbol{\psi})$, which is the joint distribution of the measurements Y_i, and the dropout indicators D_i defined by adding 1 to the time of the last measurement. A first and most popular approach uses selection models based on the factorization $f(\boldsymbol{y}_i, d_i|\boldsymbol{\theta}, \boldsymbol{\psi}) = f(\boldsymbol{y}_i|\boldsymbol{\theta})f(d_i|\boldsymbol{y}_i, \boldsymbol{\psi})$. In this framework, standard missing data concepts such as MCAR, MAR, MNAR (Rubin, 1976; Little and Rubin, 1987) can be constructed. Recently, there has been interest in using the opposite factorization, $f(\boldsymbol{y}_i, d_i|\boldsymbol{\theta}, \boldsymbol{\psi}) = f(\boldsymbol{y}_i|d_i, \boldsymbol{\theta})f(d_i|\boldsymbol{\psi})$, as the basis for pattern-mixture models. Molenberghs, *et al.* (1998) showed that pattern-mixture models allow for a natural analog of MAR, hence enabling a similar classification of missing data mechanisms. We will use a popular model for repeated measurements, incorporating random effects and serial correlation. Assuming $\boldsymbol{\beta}$ as the p-dimensional vector containing the fixed effects, and $\boldsymbol{\varepsilon}_i \sim N(\mathbf{0}, \Sigma)$ as the vector of correlated error terms, we can write this model

$$\boldsymbol{Y}_i = X_i\boldsymbol{\beta} + \boldsymbol{\varepsilon}_i.$$

For a detailed description we refer to Diggle, Liang, and Zeger (1994) and Verbeke and Molenberghs (2000). In the pattern-mixture case, the parameters involved in this model can depend on the dropout pattern.

Sensitivity analysis for pattern-mixture models can be conceived in many different ways. Crucial aspects are whether pattern-mixture and selection modeling are to be contrasted with one another or rather the pattern-mixture modeling is the central focus of interest.

In the latter case, it is natural to conduct sensitivity analysis *within* the pattern-mixture family. The key area where sensitivity analysis should be focused is on the unidentified components of the model and the way(s) in which this is handled. We will explicitly consider three strategies to deal with under-identification.

<u>Strategy 1:</u> Little (1993, 1994) advocated the use of identifying restrictions and presented a number of examples. We will outline a general framework for identifying restrictions in Section 4. One of those, *available case missing values* (ACMV), will be the natural counterpart of MAR in the pattern-mixture-model framework. This provides a way to compare ignorable selection models with their counterpart in the pattern-mixture setting.

<u>Strategy 2:</u> As opposed to identifying restrictions, model simplification can be done in order to identify the parameters. The advantage is that the number of parameters

decreases, which is desirable since the length of the parameter vector is a general issue with pattern-mixture models. Indeed, Hogan and Laird (1997) noted that in order to estimate the large number of parameters in general pattern-mixture models, one has to make the awkward requirement that each dropout pattern occurs sufficiently often. Broadly, we distinguish between two types of simplifications.

Strategy 2a: Trends can be restricted to functional forms supported by the information available within a pattern. For example, a linear or quadratic time trend is easily extrapolated beyond the last obtained measurement. An *ad hoc* solution might be necessary for the first few patterns. For example, if a linear trend is to be extrapolated, one needs at least two observed measurements. For the first pattern (with only one measurement), one can then borrow the slope from the second pattern. In order to fit such models, one simply has to carry out a model building exercise within each of the patterns separately.

Strategy 2b: Next, one can let the parameters vary across patterns in a controlled parametric way. Thus, rather than estimating a separate time trend within each pattern, one could for example assume that the time evolution within a pattern is unstructured, but parallel across patterns. This is effectuated by treating pattern as a covariate. The available data can be used to assess whether such simplifications are supported within the time ranges for which there is information.

While the second strategy is computationally simple, it is important to note that there is a price to pay. Indeed, simplified models, qualified as "assumption rich" by Sheiner, Beale and Dunne (1997), are also making untestable assumptions, just as in the selection model case. In the identifying restrictions setting on the other hand, the assumptions are clear from the start.

A final observation, applying to both strategies, is that pattern-mixture models do not always automatically provide estimates and standard errors of marginal quantities of interest, such as overall treatment effect or overall time trend. Hogan and Laird (1997) provided a way to derive selection model quantities from the pattern-mixture model. Several authors have followed this idea to formally compare the conclusions from a selection model with the selection model parameters in a pattern-mixture model (Molenberghs, Michiels, and Lipsitz, 1999). An example of such a marginalization is given in Section 5.

4. Identifying Restriction Strategies

In line with the results obtained by Molenberghs *et al.* (1998), we restrict attention to monotone patterns. In general, let us assume we have $t = 1, \ldots, T$ dropout patterns where the dropout indicator is $d = t + 1$. For pattern t, the complete data density is given by

$$f_t(y_1, \ldots, y_T) = f_t(y_1, \ldots, y_t) f_t(y_{t+1}, \ldots, y_T | y_1, \ldots, y_t). \tag{1}$$

The first factor is clearly identified from the observed data, while the second factor is not. It is assumed that the first factor is known or, more realistically, modeled using the observed data. Then, identifying restrictions are applied in order to identify the second component.

While, in principle, completely arbitrary restrictions can be used by means of any valid density function over the appropriate support, strategies which relate back to the observed data deserve privileged interest. One can base identification on all patterns for which a given component, y_s say, is identified. A general expression for this is

$$f_t(y_s|y_1,\dots y_{s-1}) = \sum_{j=s}^{T} \omega_{sj} f_j(y_s|y_1,\dots y_{s-1}), \quad s = t+1,\dots,T. \tag{2}$$

We will use $\boldsymbol{\omega}_s$ as shorthand for the set of ω_{sj}'s used. Every $\boldsymbol{\omega}_s$ which sums to one provides a valid identification scheme.

Let us incorporate (2) into (1):

$$f_t(y_1,\dots,y_T) = f_t(y_1,\dots,y_t) \prod_{s=0}^{T-t-1} \left[\sum_{j=T-s}^{T} \omega_{T-s,j} f_j(y_{T-s}|y_1,\dots,y_{T-s-1}) \right]. \tag{3}$$

Expression (3) clearly shows which information is used to complement the observed data density in pattern t in order to establish the complete data density.

Let us consider three special but important cases. Little (1993) proposes *complete case missing values* (CCMV) which uses the following identification:

$$f_t(y_s|y_1,\dots y_{s-1}) = f_T(y_s|y_1,\dots y_{s-1}), \quad s = t+1,\dots,T. \tag{4}$$

In other words, information which is unavailable is always borrowed from the completers. This strategy can be defended in cases where the bulk of the subjects are complete and only small proportions are assigned to the various dropout patterns. Also, extension of this approach to non-monotone patterns is particularly easy.

Alternatively, the nearest identified pattern can be used:

$$f_t(y_s|y_1,\dots y_{s-1}) = f_s(y_s|y_1,\dots y_{s-1}), \qquad s = t+1,\dots,T.$$

We will refer to those restrictions as *neighboring case missing values* or NCMV.

The third special case of (2) will be ACMV. Thus, ACMV is reserved for the counterpart of MAR in the PMM context. The corresponding $\boldsymbol{\omega}_s$ vectors can be shown to have components:

$$\omega_{sj} = \frac{\alpha_j f_j(y_1,\dots,y_{s-1})}{\sum_{\ell=s}^{T} \alpha_\ell f_\ell(y_1,\dots,y_{s-1})}, \tag{5}$$

where α_j is the fraction of observations in pattern j.

4.1 Strategy Outline

We will briefly outline a general strategy. Several points which require further specification will be discussed in subsequent sections. (1) Fit a model to the pattern-specific identifiable densities: $f_t(y_1,\dots,y_t)$. This results in a parameter estimate,

$\hat{\gamma}_t$. (2) Select an identification method of choice. (3) Using this identification method, determine the conditional distributions of the unobserved outcomes, given the observed ones:

$$f_t(y_{t+1}, \ldots, y_T | y_1, \ldots, y_t). \tag{6}$$

(4) Using standard multiple imputation methodology (Rubin, 1987; Schafer, 1997; Verbeke and Molenberghs, 2000), draw multiple imputations for the unobserved components, given the observed outcomes and the correct pattern-specific density (6). (5) Analyze the multiply-imputed sets of data using the method of choice. This can be another pattern-mixture model, but also a selection model or any other desired model. (6) Inferences can be conducted in the standard multiple imputation way (Rubin, 1987; Schafer, 1997; Verbeke and Molenberghs, 2000).

4.2 Drawing from the Conditional Densities

In the previous section, we have seen how general identifying restrictions (2), with CCMV, NCMV, and ACMV as special cases, lead to the conditional densities for the unobserved components, given the observed ones. This came down to deriving expressions for $\boldsymbol{\omega}$, such as in (5) for ACMV. This endeavor corresponds to parts 2 and 3 of the strategy outline. To carry out item 4, we need to draw imputations from these conditional densities.

Let us proceed by studying the special case of three measurements first. To this end, we consider an identification scheme and we start off by avoiding the specification of a parametric form for these densities. The following steps are required: (1) Estimate the parameters of the identifiable densities: from pattern 3, $f_3(y_1, y_2, y_3)$; from pattern 2, $f_2(y_1, y_2)$;, and from pattern 1 $f_1(y_1)$. Then, for each of the m imputations, we have to execute the following steps. (2) To properly account for the uncertainty with which the parameters are estimated, we need to draw from them as is customarily done in multiple imputation. It will be assumed that in all densities from which we draw, this parameter vector is used. (3) For pattern 2, given an observation in this pattern, with observed values (y_1, y_2), calculate the conditional density $f_3(y_3|y_1, y_2)$ and draw from it. (4) For pattern 1, we now have to distinguish three substeps.

1. There is now only one ω involved: for pattern 1, in order to determine $f_1(y_2|y_1)$, as a combination of $f_2(y_2|y_1)$ and $f_3(y_2|y_1)$. Every ω in the unit interval is valid. Specific cases are: for NCMV, $\omega = 1$; for CCMV, $\omega = 0$; for ACMV, ω is calculated from (5). Note that, given y_1, this is a constant, depending on α_2 and α_3.

   In order to pick one of the two components f_2 or f_3, we need to generate a random uniform variate, U say, except in the boundary NCMV and CCMV cases. Then continue with (b) and (c).

2. If $U \leq \omega$, calculate $f_2(y_2|y_1)$ and draw from it. Otherwise, do the same based on $f_3(y_2|y_1)$.

3. Given the observed y_1 and given y_2 which has just been drawn, calculate the conditional density $f_3(y_3|y_1, y_2)$ and draw from it.

All steps but the first one have to be repeated M times, to obtain the same number of imputed datasets. Inference then proceeds as outlined Rubin (1987), Schafer (1997) and Verbeke and Molenberghs (2000).

In case the observed densities are assumed to be normal, then the corresponding conditional densities are particularly straightforward.

In several cases, the conditional density is a mixture of normal densities. Then an additional and straightforward draw from the components of the mixture is necessary.

A few comments are in place. Except in cases with only a few time points, the number of ω parameters proliferates quite rapidly. There are several ways to deal with it. First, special but important restrictions such as NCMV, CCMV, and ACMV do not suffer from this problem since each of the ω's involved is then determined by the choice of restriction. Second, one might envisage partial but important sensitivity analysis by setting all ω's be equal to a fixed quantity, which is chosen as, for example, a member of a grid filling the unit interval. Third, one could put prior distributions on the ω's, perhaps governed by simple hyperpriors. The first solution is followed in this paper. The other ones require further exploration.

In addition, determining the conditional distribution of the unobserved outcomes, given the observed ones, is easy in the Gaussian case. For categorical outcomes this is easy as well since it comes down to determining conditional multinomial probabilities which are again multinomial. However, for other distributional forms, this can be quite burdensome. In that case, the conditional distributions will have to be replaced by the corresponding ratio of marginal distributions. While this will change the algebra a bit, the methodology will not undergo fundamental changes.

5. Analysis of the Vorozole Study

To concisely illustrate the methodology described in this chapter, we will apply it to the vorozole study, restricted to those subjects with 1, 2, and 3 follow up measurements, respectively. Thus, 190 subjects are included into the analysis, with subsample sizes 35, 86, and 69, respectively. The corresponding pattern probabilities are $\widehat{\pi} = (0.184, 0.453, 0.363)'$. The asymptotic variance-covariance matrix can be derived without difficulty. We will now apply each of the three strategies. We recognize a full analysis, using all patterns, is both interesting and feasible. However, we believe it is beyond the scope of this paper and it will be reported elsewhere.

The patients in this study drop out mainly because they relapse or die. This in itself poses specific challenges that can be addressed within the pattern-mixture framework much easier than in the selection model framework. Indeed, if one is prepared to make the assumption that a patient who dies is representative of a slice of the population with the same characteristics, and with a certain probability to die, then identifying restrictions (i.e., extrapolation beyond the time of death) is meaningful. In case one does not want to extrapolate beyond the moment of death, one can restrict modeling to the observed data only. An intermediate approach would be to allow for extrapolation beyond relapse and not beyond death. (For the current dataset, the information needed in order to do so is unavailable.) Note that, while this may seem a disadvantage of pattern-mixture models, we believe it is an asset, because this framework not only forces one to think about such issues, it also provides a modeling solution, no matter which point of view is adopted. This contrasts with selection models where extrapolation is always done, be it explicitly by modeling the profile, averaged over all patterns.

To apply the identifying restriction of strategy 1, one first needs to fit a model to the observed data. We will opt for a simple model, with parameters specific to each pattern. Such a model can be seen as belonging to the second modeling strategy.

We include time and time-squared ($time^2$) effects, as well as their interactions with treatment. Further, time by baseline value interaction is included as well. While we agree such a choice may seem controversial, it is consistent with the analysis plan and therefore we have opted to leave this term in. Alternatively, one could either remove this term or model raw scores rather than change scores. All effects interact with time, in order to force profiles to pass through the origin, since we are studying change versus baseline. An unstructured 3×3 covariance matrix is assumed for each pattern.

Parameter estimates are presented in Table 1, in the "initial" column. Of course, not all parameters are estimable. This holds for the variance components, where in patterns 1 and 2, the upper 1×1 block and the upper 2×2 block are identified, respectively. In the first pattern, the effects for time-squared are unidentified. The linear effects are identified by virtue of the absence of an intercept term.

Let us present this and later models graphically. Since there is one binary (treatment arm) and one continuous covariate (baseline level of FLIC score), insight can be obtained by plotting the models for selected values of baseline. Precisely, we chose the average value (Figure 1). Bold line type is used for the range over which data are obtained for a particular pattern and extrapolation is indicated using thinner line type. Note that the extrapolation can have surprising effects, even with these relatively simple models. Thus, while this form of extrapolation is simple, its plausibility can be called into question.

This initial model provides a basis, and its graphical representation extra motivation, to consider identifying restriction models. Using the methodology detailed in Section 4, a GAUSS macro and a SAS macro (available from the authors' web pages), was written to conduct the multiple imputation, to fit the model to the imputed datasets, and to combine the results into a single inference. Results are presented in Table 1, for each of the three types of restrictions (CCMV, NCMV, ACMV). For patterns 1 and 2 there is some variability in the parameter estimates across the three strategies, although this is often consistent with random variation (see the standard errors). Since the data in pattern 3 are complete, there is of course no difference between the initial model parameters and those obtained with each of the identifying restriction techniques.

In all of the plots, the same mean response scale was retained, illustrating that the identifying restriction strategies extrapolate much closer to the observed data mean responses. There are some differences among the identifying restriction methods, but this is not graphically represented here. This conclusion needs to be considered carefully. Since these patients drop out mainly because they relapse or die,

Table 1. Multiple imputation estimates and standard errors (in parentheses) for the CCMV, NCMV, and ACMV restrictions applied to the Vorozole study.

Effect*	Initial	CCMV	NCMV	ACMV
Pattern 1				
Time	3.40 (13.94)	13.21 (15.91)	7.56 (16.45)	4.43 (18.78)
Time×*base*	−0.11 (0.13)	−0.16 (0.16)	−0.14 (0.16)	−0.11 (0.17)
Time×*treat*	0.33 (3.91)	−2.09 (2.19)	−1.20 (1.93)	−0.41 (2.52)
$Time^2$		−0.84 (4.21)	−2.12 (4.24)	−0.70 (4.22)
$Time^2 \times treat$		0.01 (0.04)	0.03 (0.04)	0.02 (0.04)
σ_{11}	131.09 (31.34)	151.91 (42.34)	134.54 (32.85)	137.33 (34.18)
σ_{12}		59.84 (40.46)	119.76 (40.38)	97.86 (38.65)
σ_{22}		201.54 (65.38)	257.07 (86.05)	201.87 (80.02)
σ_{13}		55.12 (58.03)	49.88 (44.16)	61.87 (43.22)
σ_{23}		84.99 (48.54)	99.97 (57.47)	110.42 (87.95)
σ_{33}		245.06 (75.56)	241.99 (79.79)	286.16 (117.90)
Pattern 2				
Time	53.85 (14.12)	29.78 (10.43)	33.74 (11.11)	28.69 (11.37)
Time×*base*	−0.46 (0.12)	−0.29 (0.09)	−0.33 (0.10)	−0.29 (0.10)
Time×*treat*	−0.95 (1.86)	−1.68 (1.21)	−1.56 (2.47)	−2.12 (1.36)
$Time^2$	−18.91 (6.36)	−4.45 (2.87)	−7.00 (3.80)	−4.22 (4.20)
$Time^2 \times treat$	0.15 (0.05)	0.04 (0.02)	0.07 (0.03)	0.05 (0.04)
σ_{11}	170.77 (26.14)	175.59 (27.53)	176.49 (27.65)	177.86 (28.19)
σ_{12}	151.84 (29.19)	147.14 (29.39)	149.05 (29.77)	146.98 (29.63)
σ_{22}	292.32 (44.61)	297.38 (46.04)	299.40 (47.22)	297.39 (46.04)
σ_{13}		57.22 (37.96)	89.10 (34.07)	99.18 (35.07)
σ_{23}		71.58 (36.73)	107.62 (47.59)	166.64 (66.45)
σ_{33}		212.68 (101.31)	264.57 (76.73)	300.78 (77.97)
Pattern 3				
Time	29.91 (9.08)	29.91 (9.08)	29.91 (9.08)	29.91 (9.08)
Time×*base*	−0.26 (0.08)	−0.26 (0.08)	−0.26 (0.08)	−0.26 (0.08)
Time×*treat*	0.82 (0.95)	0.82 (0.95)	0.82 (0.95)	0.82 (0.95)
$Time^2$	−6.42 (2.23)	−6.42 (2.23)	−6.42 (2.23)	−6.42 (2.23)
$Time^2 \times treat$	0.05 (0.02)	0.05 (0.02)	0.05 (0.02)	0.05 (0.02)
σ_{11}	206.73 (35.86)	206.73 (35.86)	206.73 (35.86)	206.73 (35.86)
σ_{12}	96.97 (26.57)	96.97 (26.57)	96.97 (26.57)	96.97 (26.57)
σ_{22}	174.12 (31.10)	174.12 (31.10)	174.12 (31.10)	174.12 (31.10)
σ_{13}	87.38 (30.66)	87.38 (30.66)	87.38 (30.66)	87.38 (30.66)
σ_{23}	91.66 (28.86)	91.66 (28.86)	91.66 (28.86)	91.66 (28.86)
σ_{33}	262.16 (44.70)	262.16 (44.70)	262.16 (44.70)	262.16 (44.70)

* *Time*, *base* and *treat* denote the time effect, the baseline effect and the treatment effect, respectively. $Time^2$ denotes the effect of time squared. Interactions between effects are denoted by '×'.

Figure 1. For the average baseline value of 113.57 in the Vorozole study, strategies 1 (ACMV), 2a, and 2b are shown. The bold portion of the curves runs from baseline until the last obtained measurement, and the extrapolated piece is shown as a thin line. The dashed lines refer to megestrol acetate, and the solid lines refer to Vorozole.

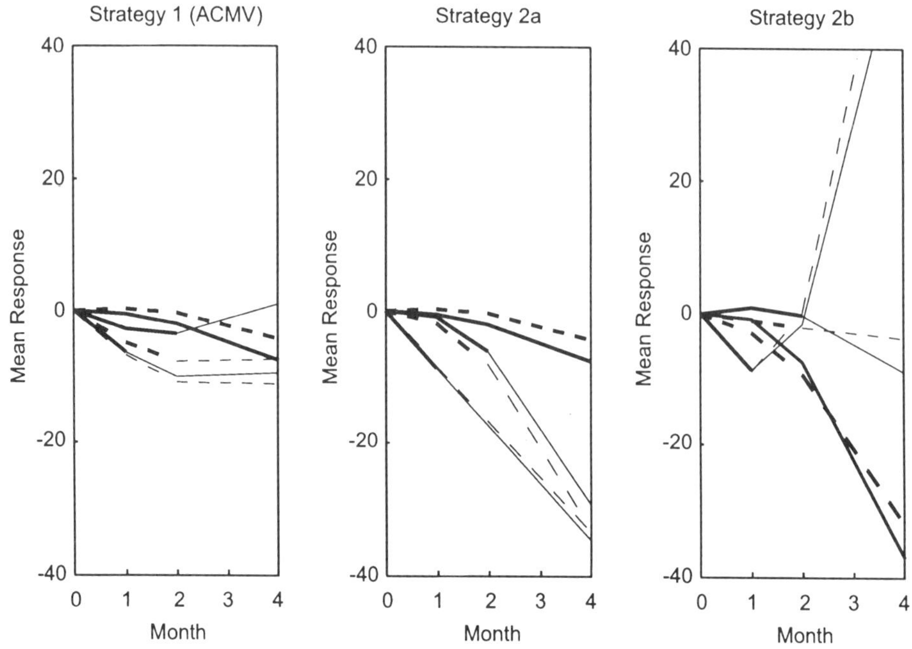

it seems unlikely to expect a rise in quality of life. This consideration is evidence against CCMV, where missing information is always borrowed from the complete group (i.e., the one with the best prognosis). ACMV, which compromises between all strategies may be more realistic, but here NCMV is likely to be better since information is borrowed from the nearest pattern.

Nevertheless, the NCMV prediction looks more plausible since the worst baseline value shows declining profiles, whereas the best one leaves room for improvement. Should one want to explore the effect of assumptions beyond the range of (2), one can allow $\boldsymbol{\omega}_s$ to include components outside of the unit interval. In that situation, one has to ensure that the resulting density is still non-negative over its entire support.

In strategy 2b, *pattern* is included as a covariate. An initial model is considered with the following effects: time, the interaction between time and treatment, baseline value, pattern, and the following interactions: treatment by baseline, treatment by pattern, and baseline bypattern. Further time^2 is included, as well as its interaction with baseline, treatment, and pattern. No interactions beyond the third order are included, and unstructured covariance matrix is common to all three patterns. This implies that the current model is *not* equivalent to a strategy 1 model, where all parameters are pattern-specific. To achieve this goal, every effect would have to be made pattern-dependent. A graphical representation is given in Figure 1. Early dropouts decline immediately, whereas those who stay longer in the study first show a rise and then decline thereafter. However, this is less pronounced for higher baseline values. On the other hand, the extrapolation based on the fitted model is very unrealistic, in the sense that for the early dropout sharp rises are predicted, which is totally implausible.

These findings suggest, again, that a more careful reflection on the extrapolation method is required. This is very well possible in a pattern-mixture context, but then the first strategy, rather than the second and third strategies, has to be used.

To test for a treatment effect, one can follow two strategies. The first focuses on the *marginal* treatment effect (i.e., one calculates the marginal treatment effect from the pattern-specific effects). Delta-method arguments complete the procedure. We obtain p-values 0.801 (CCMV), 0.900 (NCMV), and 0.828 (ACMV). Alternatively, one can consider a 3 degree-of-freedom test, stratified for pattern. The resulting p-values are 0.988 (CCMV), 0.995 (NCMV), and 0.993 (ACMV).

6. Concluding Remarks

In this paper, we have illustrated three distinct strategies to fit pattern-mixture models. In this way, we have brought together several existing practices. Little (1993, 1994) has proposed identifying restrictions, which we here formalized using the connection with MAR and multiple imputation. Strategies 2a and 2b refer to fitting a model per pattern and using pattern as a covariate.

By contrasting these strategies on a single set of data, one obtains a range of conclusions rather than a single one, which provides insight into the sensitivity to the assumptions made. Especially with the identifying restrictions, one has to be very explicit about the assumptions and moreover this approach offers the possibility to consider several forms of restrictions. Special attention should go to the ACMV restrictions, since they are the MAR counterpart within the pattern-mixture context.

In addition, a comparison between the selection and pattern-mixture modeling approaches is useful to obtain additional insight into the data and/or to assess sensitivity.

The identifying restrictions strategy provides further opportunity for sensitivity analysis. Indeed, since CCMV and NCMV are extremes for the $\boldsymbol{\omega}_s$ vector in (2), it is very natural to consider the idea of *ranges* in the allowable space of $\boldsymbol{\omega}_s$. Clearly, any $\boldsymbol{\omega}_s$ which consists of non-negative elements that sum to one is allowable, but also the idea of extrapolation could be useful, where negative components are allowed, given they provide valid conditional densities.

We believe that our approach can play a useful role, as a member of a collection of sensitivity tools. Of course, a sensitivity analysis can be conducted within different frameworks, and there are times where the setting will determine which framework is the more appropriate one (for example Bayesian or frequentist), in conjunction with technical and computational considerations. Draper (1995) has considered ways of dealing with uncertainty in the very natural Bayesian framework and developments in the missing value setting are ongoing. A thorough comparison between the various frameworks will be interesting and worth undertaking in the future.

The SAS and GAUSS macros which have been used to carry out the multiple imputation related tasks are available from the authors' web pages.

ACKNOWLEDGEMENTS

We gratefully acknowledge support from *Fonds Wetenschappelijk Onderzoek-Vlaanderen* Research Project G.0002.98 "Sensitivity Analysis for Incomplete and Coarse Data," and from *Vlaams Instituut voor de Bevordering van het Wetenschappelijk-Technologisch Onderzoek in Industrie.*

REFERENCES

Diggle, P.J., Liang, K.-Y. and Zeger, S.L. (1994). *Analysis of Longitudinal Data.* Oxford: Oxford Science Publications.

Draper, D. (1995). Assessment and propagation of model uncertainty (with discussion). *Journal of the Royal Statistical Society, Series B* **57**, 45–97.

Glynn, R.J., Laird, N.M. and Rubin, D.B (1986). Selection modelling versus mixture modeling with nonignorable nonresponse. In: Wainer, H. (ed.), *Drawing Inferences from Self-Selected Samples.* New York: Springer Verlag, pp 115–142.

Goss, P.E., Winer, E.P., Tannock, I.F., Schwartz, L.H. and Kremer, A.B. (1999). A randomized phase III trial comparing the new potent and selective third-generation aromatase inhibitor vorozole with megestrol acetate in postmenopausal advanced breast cancer patients. *Journal of Clinical Oncology* **17**, 52–63.

Hogan, J.W. and Laird, N.M. (1997). Mixture models for the joint distribution of repeated measures and event times. *Statistics in Medicine* **16**, 239–258.

Kenward, M.G. and Molenberghs, G. (1999). Parametric models for incomplete continuous and categorical longitudinal studies data. *Statistical Methods in Medical Research* **8**, 51–83.

Little, R.J.A. (1993). Pattern-mixture models for multivariate incomplete data. *Journal of the American Statistical Association* **88**, 125–134.

Little, R.J.A. (1994). A class of pattern-mixture models for normal incomplete data. *Biometrika*, **81**, 471–483.

Little, R.J.A. (1995). Modeling the drop-out mechanism in repeated-measures studies. *Journal of the American Statistical Association* **90**, 1112–1121.

Little, R.J.A. and Rubin, D.B. (1987). *Statistical Analysis with Missing Data.* New York: Wiley.

Molenberghs, G., Michiels, B., Kenward, M.G. and Diggle, P.J. (1998). Missing data mechanisms and pattern-mixture models. *Statistica Neerlandica* **52**, 153–161.

Molenberghs, G., Michiels, B. and Lipsitz, S.R. (1999). Selection models and pattern-mixture models for incomplete categorical data with covariates. *Biometrics* **55**, 978–983.

Rubin, D.B. (1976). Inference and missing data. *Biometrika* **63**, 581–592.

Rubin, D.B. (1987). *Multiple Imputation for Nonresponse in Surveys.* New York: Wiley.

Schafer, J.L. (1997). *Analysis of incomplete multivariate data.* London: Chapman and Hall.

Sheiner, L.B., Beal, S.L. and Dunne, A. (1997). Analysis of nonrandomly censored ordered categorical longitudinal data from analgesic trials. *Journal of the American Statistical Association* **92**, 1235–1244.

Schipper, H., Clinch, J. and McMurray, A. (1984). Measuring the quality of life of cancer patients: the Functional-Living Index-Cancer: development and validation. *Journal of Clinical Oncology* **2**, 472–483.

Verbeke, G. and Molenberghs, G. (2000). *Linear Mixed Models for Longitudinal Data.* New York: Springer-Verlag.

Wu, M.C. and Carroll, R.J. (1988). Estimation and comparison of changes in the presence of informative right censoring by modeling the censoring process. *Biometrics* **44**, 175–188.

ANALYSIS OF LONGITUDINAL QUALITY OF LIFE DATA WITH INFORMATIVE DROPOUT

MARGARET C. WU[1], CRAIG B. BORKOWF[2] AND PAUL S. ALBERT[2]

[1]*National Heart, Lung, and Blood Institute,*
[2]*National Cancer Institute*

An important objective of many clinical trials is the estimation and comparison of longitudinal changes in quality-of-life measurements. One difficulty encountered in these trials is that participants may drop out of the study due to worsening disease and miss follow-up evaluations after the time of dropout. When the dropout process depends on the true quality-of-life measurement, it is called informative dropout. If the analysis of the data ignores information about the informative dropout process, the estimates of changes in quality-of-life measurements may be biased. In this chapter we review several approaches for adjusting for informative dropout. We consider the situations where the probability of dropout depends on only the last observed measurement prior to dropout, on only the unobserved measurement at the time of dropout, and on both of these measurements. We illustrate these concepts with an analysis of a clinical trial for the treatment of asthma and provide examples of emphysema and prostate cancer treatment trials in which these approaches are also applicable.

1. Introduction

An important objective of many clinical trials is the estimation and comparison of longitudinal changes in quality-of-life measurements. For instance, in the National Emphysema Treatment Trial (NETT) [1], a multicenter, randomized clinical trial designed to compare medical therapy alone with medical therapy plus lung volume reduction surgery for the treatment of patients with severe bilateral emphysema, important secondary outcomes were the measurement of changes in quality-of-life and respiratory symptoms. Similarly, in the Childhood Asthma Management Program (CAMP) [2], a multicenter, randomized, double-masked clinical trial designed to determine the long-term effects of two treatments for mild to moderate childhood asthma, an important secondary outcome was the change in asthma symptoms measured using patient diaries. Likewise, in a recent randomized clinical trial for advanced prostate cancer, interest focussed on assessing the palliative effect of a new androgen deprivation therapy [3]. The primary endpoints were five quality-of-life measurements of treatment specific symptoms and of physical and emotional functioning, assessed at 1, 3, and 6 months after randomization.

In longitudinal studies, participants are followed at specified time intervals to obtain quality-of-life measurements and other outcomes of interest. However, quality-of-life measurements are often subject to large within-individual random variation

M. Mesbah et al. (eds.), Statistical Methods for Quality of Life Studies, 353–364.

and measurement error. The observed quality-of-life measurements obtained at each follow-up can be viewed as the true response plus a random error term. Consequently, one can use linear random effects models [4] or generalized linear mixed effects models [5] to analyze these measures. In our illustrations, for simplicity, we assume that the longitudinal quality-of-life scores follow linear response curves. Extensions to polynomial response curves or generalized linear response curves are straightforward [6,7].

A complication in such longitudinal studies is that subjects may drop out of a study before the designated termination of the study as a whole. After dropout, all future measurements for a subject, including quality-of-life measurements, are missing. Following the terminology described by Little and Rubin [8] and Diggle et al. [9], when the probability of dropout does not depend on either the observed measurements or the unobserved true response, we say that we have dropout completely at random (DCAR). For example, patients may drop out due to moving away from a study center. If the dropout mechanism relates to the observed quality of life measurements but not the missing value, we say that we have dropout at random (DAR). Conversely, when the probability of dropout depends on the underlying initial value, rate of change, or the true value of the missed quality-of-life measurements, we say that we have informative dropout [10]. For example, subjects may drop out due to sickness and physical limitations caused by worsening of disease. The term ignorable dropout has been used to describe DCAR and DAR mechanisms, while informative dropout is a special type of non-ignorable dropout. The terms ignorable and non-ignorable dropout refer to the fact that likelihood-based estimation is insensitive to ignorable dropout, and may provide biased results when the dropout mechanism is non-ignorable.

In asthma treatment trials, for example, participants may be removed from the study treatment when a prespecified treatment failure occurs. They may then receive a rescue treatment. Measurements following treatment failure status are often excluded from the analysis, so participants experiencing treatment failure can be considered dropouts. The criteria for defining treatment failure often involve the last observed symptom scores, rescue drug usage, and a physician's over-all evaluation. Hence, the dropout process in such trials depends on both the observed and true responses.

It has been shown that in the presence of informative dropout, the usual least squares and maximum likelihood estimation procedures, which do not account for the dropout process, can yield biased estimates of the rate of change in the longitudinal response [4,7,11]. Therefore, generalized linear mixed models (GLMM) for analyzing longitudinal data with informative dropout (or, more generally, missing observations) have been developed that explicitly model the dropout process [10,12–14]. However, such GLMM models currently require specialized software. Alternatively, conditional linear (CL) models can be employed to adjust for informative dropout [6,7,11,14]. CL models condition on certain summary statistics based on the times of observed measurements before dropout and thus make fewer assumptions on the dropout process. Furthermore, CL models can be fit using currently available software for repeated measures analysis, such as PROC MIXED for linear mixed models and PROC NLMIXED for non-linear or generalized linear mixed models in SAS [15]. These programs implement the methods described by Laird and Ware [4], Lindstrom and Bates [16], and Breslow and Clayton [5].

In situations with informative dropout that does not depend on the observed response, the CL model yields nearly unbiased estimates of longitudinal changes [7,17]. However, in situations where the dropout probability depends on the last observed response, the CL model may yield biased estimates [18]. Wu, Albert, and Wu [19] recommend design and analysis strategies to minimize the estimation bias in this situation.

In this chapter we evaluate the use of the CL model to accommodate informative dropout. We consider situations relevant to asthma trials, and evaluate CL models using method-of-moments (MOM) and maximum-likelihood estimation procedures. In Section 2, we review two approaches for accommodating informative dropout, namely modeling the dropout process and the CL model. In Section 3, we evaluate the performance of the CL model under different dropout processes in examples based on asthma clinical trials. Finally, in Section 4 we discuss our main results.

2. Approaches to Account for Informative Dropout and Missing Data

In this chapter we consider the linear mixed model for continuous longitudinal responses. Let $t_1, t_2, \ldots, t_J$ be the planned follow-up times in a study with $t_1 = 0$ corresponding to baseline, $\mathbf{Y}_i = (Y_{i1}, \ldots, Y_{iJ})'$ the complete data vector of continuous quality-of-life measurements for the i-th participant, $\mathbf{X}_i = (X_{i1}, \ldots, X_{iJ})'$ the vector of indicator variables which represent the missing data status (i.e., $X_{ij} = 1$ if present, 0 if missing), and $\mathbf{b}_i = (b_{i1}, b_{i2})'$ the vector of random effects which represent the true individual initial value and the rate of change (slope) over time in the quality-of-life measurements. In general there are two approaches to account for informative missing data, namely modeling the dropout process and the CL model. We review these approaches below.

2.1 Modeling the Dropout Process

The first approach to account for informative missing data is to model the missing data process. This is called the "selection model" approach in the econometrics setting [20]. The joint density of $\mathbf{Y}_i$, $\mathbf{X}_i$, and $\mathbf{b}_i$ is modeled as,

$$f(\mathbf{Y}_i, \mathbf{X}_i, \mathbf{b}_i) = g(\mathbf{Y}_i|\mathbf{b}_i, \mathbf{X}_i) mc(\mathbf{X}_i|\mathbf{b}_i) h(\mathbf{b}_i), \tag{1}$$

where $g(\cdot)$, $mc(\cdot)$, and $h(\cdot)$ are the density functions of $(\mathbf{Y}_i|\mathbf{b}_i)$, $(\mathbf{X}_i|\mathbf{b}_i)$, and $\mathbf{b}_i$, respectively, and $g(\mathbf{Y}_i|\mathbf{b}_i, \mathbf{X}_i) = g(\mathbf{Y}_i|\mathbf{b}_i)$. Parameter estimation for model (1), denoted the "full model," is accomplished by maximum likelihood.

This model is readily interpretable because the dropout process is modeled directly. Furthermore, under the correct dropout model estimation may be more efficient than with the CL model. However, there are two main disadvantages. First, specialized software is required. Second, inferences can be quite sensitive to the choice of the model for missing data [20,21].

2.2 Conditional Linear Model Approach

The second approach is the conditional linear model [7], which is a special case of the pattern mixture model [22,23]. The CL model was developed specifically for longitudinal data with random effects and informative dropout. It consists of a 2-stage linear regression, where sufficient statistics for the dropout process are used as covariates. Under this model the joint density of $\mathbf{Y}_i$, $\mathbf{X}_i$, and $\mathbf{b}_i$ can be expressed as,

$$f(\mathbf{Y}_i, \mathbf{X}_i, \mathbf{b}_i) = g(\mathbf{Y}_i|\mathbf{b}_i)hc(\mathbf{b}_i|\mathbf{X}_i)m(\mathbf{X}_i), \tag{2}$$

where $hc(\cdot)$ and $m(\cdot)$ are density functions of $(\mathbf{b}_i|\mathbf{X}_i)$ and $\mathbf{X}_i$, respectively.

Parameters are estimated by considering the conditional distribution of the responses and random effects given the missing data pattern. Unconditional expected values (e.g., expected rates of change in quality-of-life in each treatment arm) are then obtained by averaging all individual estimates in each treatment arm [6,7,11]. Note that the second factor in the right hand side of (1) is $mc(\mathbf{X}_i|\mathbf{b}_i)$, the prior density of the missing data variable given the random effects, and the second factor in the right hand side of (2) is $hc(\mathbf{b}_i|\mathbf{X}_i)$, the posterior density of the random effects given the missing data variable.

Follmann and Wu [6] proved that if the prior density, $mc(\mathbf{X}_i|\mathbf{b}_i)$ is totally positive of order 2 (see the appendix for the definition) then the posterior expectation of $(\mathbf{b}_i|\mathbf{X}_i)$ is monotone with respect to each element of $\mathbf{X}_i$ irrespective of the distribution of $\mathbf{b}_i$. The exponential family is totally positive of order 2. Furthermore, a linear function is the simplest monotonic function. This result suggests that a second stage linear regression of $\mathbf{b}_i$ on the observed $\mathbf{X}_i$'s (or some monotonic transformation of the $\mathbf{X}_i$'s) can provide a good approximation to the conditional mean $E(\mathbf{b}_i|\mathbf{X}_i)$ for a large class of informative dropout processes.

With this approach for parameter estimation, the 2-stage linear regression can be applied directly using available software for repeated measures with random effects [4,15,16]. There is no need to specify the model for the dropout process.

We now consider which predictor variables to use in the 2-stage regression. Wu and Follmann [17] developed two-dimensional summary measures, $S_i(\mathbf{X}_i)$, of the missing data indicators that are sufficient statistics for the dropout (or missing data) process parameters. These are $S_i(\mathbf{X}_i) = (S_{i1}, S_{i2})'$ with $S_{i1} = T_i$ and $S_{i2} = \sum t_j$, where the sum is over all t_j that are less than T_i, and T_i is the dropout time for the i-th participant. As sufficient statistics, these measures capture all the information of the dropout distribution.

2.3 Linear Response Curve Model

We now consider the CL model for continuous quality-of-life measurements that can be described by linear response curves. Under this model, the 2-stage regression can be specified as:

$$\text{Stage 1: } Y_{ij} = b_{i1} + b_{i2}t_j + \epsilon_{ij}, \tag{3}$$

where $\mathbf{b}_i = (b_{i1}, b_{i2}) \sim N(B_k, \Sigma_b)$ with $B_k = (B_{1k}, B_{2k})'$ for $i \in I_k$ ($k = 1$ or 2 for the 2 treatment groups), and the ϵ_{ij} are independently distributed as $N(0, \sigma_\epsilon^2)$ and are independent of $\mathbf{b}_i$ for $j = 1, 2, \ldots, J$, with

$$\Sigma_b = \begin{vmatrix} \sigma^2_{b_1} & \sigma_{b_1,b_2} \\ \sigma_{b_1,b_2} & \sigma^2_{b_2} \end{vmatrix}.$$

$$\text{Stage 2: } b_{is} = \alpha_{0sk} + \alpha_{1s}S_{i1} + \alpha_{2s}S_{i2} + \epsilon_{is}$$

for $s = 1$ or 2 and $i \in I_k$, where the α's are unknown parameters to be estimated conditioning on the observed S_{i1} and S_{i2} either by the method of moments or the maximum likelihood approach.

The unconditional mean initial value and slope (B_{1k}, B_{2k}) can then be estimated as

$$\hat{B}_{sk} = \hat{\alpha}_{0sk} + \hat{\alpha}_{1s}\bar{S}_{1k} + \hat{\alpha}_{2s}\bar{S}_{2k}$$

where the $\hat{\alpha}$'s are the estimates for the α's, $\bar{S}_{1k} = \sum S_{i1k}/N_k$, and $\bar{S}_{2k} = \sum S_{i2k}/N_k$, the summation is over $i \in I_k$ for $s = 1$ and 2, $k = 1$ and 2, and N_k is the sample size in the k-th treatment arm.

3. Application and Simulation

In this section we investigate the performance of the CL model to adjust for informative dropout under four different types of dropout processes (models for these processes are presented in the Appendix):

(D1) The probability of dropout depends on the underlying rate of change in the true response and this dependence is constant over time. This corresponds to dropout due to worsening disease (see (A1) in the appendix).

(D2) Dropout depends on the underlying true value of the missed response at the time of dropout. This corresponds to dropout caused by death or severe sickness. Under this dropout process the dependence on the underlying rate of change in the response varies over time (see (A2) in the appendix).

(D3) Dropout depends on the last observed response (see (A3) in the appendix).

(D4) Dropout depends on both the last observed response and the true value of the missed response at the time of dropout. This is similar to dropout caused by treatment failure in asthma treatment trials (see (A4) in the appendix).

We now compare the CL approach with other commonly used procedures. We applied each procedure to simulated asthma symptom scores. In CAMP, children aged 5 to 12 were randomly assigned to either placebo, budesonide or nedocromil, and then followed for an average of 4.3 years. The primary outcome was pulmonary function, as measured by forced expiratory volume in the first second (FEV_1) of a spirometry test. An important secondary outcome was asthma symptom score.

Diaries were used to collect daily records of asthma symptoms from all participants. Symptom scores ranged from 0 to 3: 0 = no symptoms, 1 = 1–3 symptoms lasting 2 hours or less, 2 = 4 or more symptoms that interfered with activity, play, school or sleep, and 3 = symptoms lasting more than 2 hours or resulting in staying at home, seeing a doctor or going to a hospital. A baseline symptom score for each participant was determined by averaging the daily symptom scores collected in the 28 days prior to treatment. Follow-up summary scores were similarly computed. All scores were multiplied by 1,000.

As children grow older it is expected that the symptom scores will decrease over time. The linear random effects model with random individual intercepts and slopes can be used to describe the longitudinal symptom scores. The CAMP publication policy dictates that the study data will not be available for our analysis until 3 years after the publication of the primary results. Therefore, our illustrations are based on simulated data. However, the parameter values used in these simulations were obtained from the results of the CAMP study [24]. In our simulations, we assumed a larger treatment effect than that seen in the CAMP study to reduce the necessary sample size. In addition, for simplicity, we considered only two treatment groups (placebo and active treatment).

Thirteen symptom scores were generated for each participant according to equation (3). These correspond to 1 baseline score and 4 follow-up scores per year for 3 years. The baseline mean asthma symptom score was assumed to be 630 in both treatment groups with an expected annual change (decline) of -80 in the placebo group. The standard deviations for the intercept (σ_{b_1}), slope (σ_{b_2}), and the error term (σ_ϵ) were assumed to be 325, 70 and 176, respectively. We further assumed that the intercept and slope random effects were uncorrelated (i.e., $\sigma_{b_1,b_2} = 0$).

Data for this active treatment group were similarly generated assuming that the expected annual change in asthma symptom score was -112. Data for 100 participants were generated for each of the 2 groups. Separate trials were generated for each of the 4 types of dropout processes. The experiments were repeated 400 times for each dropout process.

3.1 Comparison of Statistical Procedures

We compared several estimation procedures. Let UWLE (WLE) denote estimation based on averaging individual slope estimates obtained by unweighted (weighted, using inverse-variance weights) least squares. We let CL2 denote the CL model with 2 sufficient statistics used as covariates and estimation using the method of moments. CL2ML denotes the CL model with the same 2 sufficient statistics used as covariates and estimation using maximum likelihood. The modified CL2 procedure, CL2X, applies the CL2 procedure but excludes the last measurement before dropout. Another modified CL2 procedure, CL2R, applies the CL2 procedure with the last observed response replaced by the measurement made one month earlier. These two procedures were recommended by Wu, Albert and Wu [19] to adjust for informative dropout in situations where dropout is dependent on the last observed response.

CL1 denotes the CL model using one covariate (dropout time) and estimation using the method of moments. Maximum likelihood estimation without any adjustment for informative dropout will be referred to as CL0ML. UWLE corresponds to using all indicators for dropout patterns to adjust for informative dropout [17], while CL0ML and WLE correspond to no adjustment for dropout.

3.2 Results

Each procedure was first evaluated in simulated clinical trials with informative dropout, where the probability of dropout depended on the underlying rate of change in the response (D1) or on the expected true value of the missing response (D2). Table 1 presents the estimated mean annual rate of change (slope) in asthma symptom score obtained from each procedure and the corresponding mean square error (MSE). WLE resulted in biased estimates for the group mean slopes (−91.8 and −88.9 under D1 and D2, respectively, compared to the true mean slope of −80.0 in the placebo group). CL2 provided nearly unbiased estimates without much increase in mean squared error.

Table 1. Estimated slope and mean squared error for each estimation method under two informative dropout mechanisms

Treatment Group and Methods	Dropout Depends on True Rate of Change in Response		Dropout Depends on True Response	
	EST*	MSE*	EST*	MSE*
Placebo				
UWLE	−80.6	420.8	−79.8	451.1
WLE	−91.8	245.9	−88.9	184.1
CL1	−77.2	179.7	−65.7	414.9
CL2	−81.4	225.7	−80.4	244.9
Active Treatment				
UWLE	−110.3	386.0	−110.1	521.1
WLE	−121.4	183.7	−118.7	150.7
CL1	−109.9	136.6	−98.5	353.9
CL2	−112.9	150.0	−111.9	192.9
Difference				
UWLE	−29.7	864.1	−30.3	996.8
WLE	−29.6	205.2	−29.8	209.2
CL1	−32.7	202.1	−32.8	216.5
CL2	−31.5	205.6	−31.5	192.9

*EST = Estimated asthma symptom score slope per year. Expected asthma symptom score slopes are −80.0 per year and −112.0 per year in the placebo and the active treatment groups, respectively. Probit dropout coefficients were 7.0 and 15.3 for the intercept and the slope of the true response, respectively (dropout process D1, see (A1) in the Appendix). The logistic dropout coefficient for true response was 15.2 (dropout process D2, see (A2) in the Appendix). MSE = Mean squared error.

In situations where dropout depends on the true value of the missed response, the CL1 procedure resulted in biased estimates. Although the UWLE procedure gave unbiased estimates, it resulted in much larger mean squared errors than other estimates. Estimates for the between group difference were nearly unbiased for all four procedures evaluated. The biases in the estimated group means tended to cancel each other out in the between group difference.

We next evaluated each procedure in the common situation where dropout depends on the last observed response (D3). Table 2 shows the estimated mean slopes for asthma symptom scores for each of the two treatment groups, the between group difference and the corresponding mean squared errors. In this situation, the CL2, CL2ML, WLE, and UWLE procedures all resulted in biased estimates of the group slope means. There were some minor reductions in estimation bias when the maximum likelihood procedure (CL2ML) was used instead of the method of moments with weighted least squares (CL2). For instance, the estimated mean slope for the placebo group was −52.4 under CL2ML, compared to −47.3 under CL2. Compared to the true mean slope of −80.0, however, the estimates obtained from CL2ML and CL2 were seriously biased. CL2X and CL0ML provided unbiased estimates. For the group slope means, CL0ML mean squared errors were smaller than CL2X. However, for the between group difference, mean squared errors for CL2X smaller than those for CL0ML. Estimates for the between group difference were nearly unbiased for WLE, CL2X, CL2ML and CL0ML. The mean squared errors, however, were larger for CL0ML and CL2ML. Table 3 summarizes performance of each procedure under dropout process D4, where the probability of dropout depends on both the last observed response and the missed true response.

Table 2. Estimated slope and mean squared error for each estimation method under a dropout mechanism that depends on the last observed response[†]

	Placebo		Active Treatment		Difference	
Method	EST*	MSE*	EST*	MSE*	EST*	MSE*
UWLE	−35.1	2512.8	−71.1	2137.6	−36.0	960.4
WLE	−75.8	176.2	−108.5	155.4	−32.7	298.0
CL2	−47.3	1289.9	−82.4	1090.4	−35.1	271.6
CL2ML	−52.4	1273.7	−85.0	1154.9	−32.6	619.5
CL2X	−79.7	446.1	−110.8	379.5	−31.1	295.2
CL0ML	−80.9	267.9	−112.1	212.9	−31.1	477.9

*EST = Estimated asthma symptom score slope per year. Expected asthma symptom score slopes are −80.0 per year and −112.0 per year in the placebo and the active treatment groups, respectively. MSE = Mean squared error.

[†]The dropout process was D3. The logistic dropout coefficient for the observed response at 0.5, 1.5 and 2.5 years of follow-up was 10.1 (see (A3) in the Appendix).

These results indicate that the CL2X, CL2R and CL2ML procedures are nearly unbiased for the group slope means. The UWLE, WLE, CL2, and CL0ML procedures all resulted in biased estimates for the group slope means. In this simulation, the strength of the effect of the observed response on dropout was assumed to be much smaller than the effect of the true response on dropout. (The logistic dropout coefficients in model A4 were 2.1 and 13.1 for the observed last response and the missing true response, respectively.) The fact that CL2ML was unbiased may be due to the difference in magnitude of these two coefficients. We would expect CL2ML to yield biased estimates for other parameter values. Again, estimates for the between

Table 3. Estimated slope and mean squared error for each estimation method under a dropout mechanism that depends on the last observed response and the unobserved true response†

	Placebo		Active Treatment		Difference	
Method	EST*	MSE*	EST*	MSE*	EST*	MSE*
UWLE	−72.9	464.9	−103.7	491.2	−30.8	891.2
WLE	−87.7	177.0	−118.2	146.2	−30.5	218.6
CL2	−75.1	236.1	−106.9	197.5	−31.8	204.1
CL2ML	−79.7	403.8	−111.8	353.4	−32.1	443.8
CL2X	−80.9	430.9	−112.0	333.1	−31.1	290.9
CL0ML	−92.1	357.6	−123.6	350.4	−31.4	402.1
CL2R	−80.6	225.4	−110.5	201.8	−29.9	187.3

*EST = Estimated asthma symptom score slope per year. Expected asthma symptom score slopes are −80.0 per year and −112.0 per year in the placebo and the active treatment groups, respectively. MSE = mean squared error.

†The dropout process was D4. The logistic dropout coefficients were 2.1 for the last observed response obtained at 0.5, 1.5, or 2.5 years of follow-up, and 13.1 for the expected response at 0.75, 1.75, or 2.75 years of follow-up (see (A4) in the Appendix).

group difference were nearly unbiased for all procedures compared. However, the UWLE, CL2ML, CL0ML resulted in much larger mean squared errors.

4. Discussion

In Section 3 we showed that in the presence of informative dropout, the results from the usual estimating procedures (WLE and CL0ML) without accounting for the dropout process can be seriously biased. The conditional linear approach, using the sufficient summary dropout measures as covariates to adjust for informative dropout (CL2), was nearly unbiased. Furthermore, using the dropout time as the only covariate to adjust for dropout (CL1) may give biased results. When applying the conditional linear model, it is important to include both summary measures as predictor variables in the 2-stage regression model.

We also showed that when dropout depends on the observed response but not on the missing response, the usual maximum likelihood estimation without adjustment for dropout (CL0ML) is unbiased. The CL model gives biased estimates of the group means. This is similar to the bias caused by error in the independent variable in the usual regression problem. In this situation, the dropout time depends on the last observed response, which is measured with error. This error is included in both the dropout time (the predictor of the second stage regression) and the last observed measure of the response (the dependent variable). The variance of the error in the last observed response causes the bias. Likewise, our simulations showed that the CL2X procedure, which excludes the last observed response made prior to dropout, can reduce this bias.

When the dropout probability depends on both the observed response and the unobserved true response, all procedures that ignore or adjust for informative dropout give biased estimates. In this case, it is important to use the CL2X procedure. However, the CL2X procedure can be inefficient because fewer measurements are used. Alternatively, the CL2R procedure, which excludes the last observed response and replaces it with an additional measurement, is more efficient.

In the simulations of Section 3, we assumed that the underlying individual rate of change and the initial value were not correlated. This condition was true in the longitudinal ramus height data [25] and data on lung function [10]. In some quality of life measures, the rate of change may be related to the initial value. Nevertheless, we expect that the directions of the results obtained in Section 3 will not be changed by this relationship.

In Sections 2 and 3 we illustrated the application of the conditional linear model to statistical analyses using maximum likelihood and the method of moments procedures. It should be noted that this model can also be applied using the empirical Bayes imputation procedure. Mori et al. [11] illustrated that under the model of Section 2.3, empirical Bayes imputation and the method of moments provided similar estimates for the rate of change in a response variable. More comparisons between these methods and other imputation procedures may be helpful in future research.

In this chapter we restricted our attention to estimation bias and mean squared errors. For variance estimation, we suggest using the bootstrap procedure. Wu et al. [26] illustrated that the bootstrap variance performed well with the CL1 procedure. We expect that it will also work well with the CL2 and CL2X procedures.

REFERENCES

1. National Emphysema Treatment Trial (NETT) Research Group (1999). Rationale and design of the National Emphysema Treatment Trial: a prospective randomized trial of lung volume reduction surgery. *Chest* **116**, 1750–1761.
2. Childhood Asthma Management Program (CAMP) Research Group (1999). The childhood asthma management program (CAMP): design, rationale, and methods. *Controlled Clinical Trials* **20**, 91–120.
3. Moinpour, C.M., Savage, M.J., Troxel, A., Lovato, L.C., Eisenberger, M., Veith, R.W., Higgins, B., Skeel, R., Yee, M., Blumenstein, B.A., Crawford, E.D. and Meyskens, F.L. (1998). Quality of life in advanced prostate cancer: results of a randomized therapeutic trial. *Journal of the National Cancer Institute* **90**, 1537–1544.
4. Laird, N.M. and Ware, J.H. (1982). Random-effects models for longitudinal data. *Biometrics* **38**, 963–974.
5. Breslow, N.E. and Clayton, D.G. (1993). Approximate inference in generalized linear mixed models. *Journal of the American Statistical Association* **88**, 9–25.
6. Follmann, D. and Wu, M. (1995). An approximate generalized linear-model with random effects for informative missing data. *Biometrics* **51**, 151–168.
7. Wu, M.C. and Bailey, K. R. (1989). Estimation and comparison of changes in the presence of informative right censoring: conditional linear models. *Biometrics* **45**, 939–955.

8. Little, R.A. and Rubin, D.B. (1987). *Statistical Analysis with Missing Data.* New York: John Wiley and Sons.
9. Diggle, P.J., Liang, K.Y. and Zeger, S.L. (1994). *Analysis of Longitudinal Data.* Oxford: Oxford University Press.
10. Wu, M.C. and Carroll, R.J. (1988). Estimation and comparison of changes in the presence of informative right censoring by modeling the censoring process. *Biometrics* **44**, 175–188.
11. Mori, M., Woodworth, G.G. and Woolson, R.F. (1992). Application of empirical Bayes inference to estimation of rate of change in the presence of informative right censoring. *Statistics in Medicine* **11**, 621–631.
12. Mori, M., Woolson, R.F. and Woodworth, G.G. (1994). Slope estimation in the presence of informative right censoring: modeling the number of observations as a geometric random variable. *Biometrics* **50**, 39–50.
13. Ten Have, T.R., Kunselman, A.R., Pulstenis, E.P. and Landis, J.R. (1998). Mixed effects logistic regression models for longitudinal binary response data with informative drop-out. *Biometrics* **54**, 367–383.
14. Albert, P.S. and Follmann, D.A. (2000). Modeling repeated count data subject to informative dropout. *Biometrics* **56**, 667–677.
15. SAS Institute, Inc. (1990). *SAS/STAT User's Guide, Version 6, 4th Edition.* Cary, NC: SAS Institute.
16. Lindstrom, M.J. and Bates, D.M. (1990). Nonlinear mixed effects models for repeated measures data. *Biometrics* **46**, 673–687.
17. Wu, M.C. and Follmann, D.A. (1999). Use of summary measures to adjust for informative missingness in repeated measures data with random effects. *Biometrics* **55**, 75–84.
18. Wang-Clow, F., Lange. M., Laird, N.M. and Ware, J.H. (1995). A simulation study of estimators for rates of change in longitudinal studies with attrition. *Statistics in Medicine* **14**, 283–297.
19. Wu, M.C., Albert, P.S. and Wu, B.U. (2001). Adjusting for dropout in clinical trials with repeated measures: design and analysis issues. *Statistics in Medicine*, **20**, 93–108.
20. Goldberger, A.S. (1983). Abnormal selection bias. In: Karlin, S., Amemiya, T. and Goodman, L.A. (eds.). *Studies in Econometrics, Time Series, and Multivariate Statistics.* New York: Academic Press, Inc.
21. Olsen, R.J. (1980). A least-squares correction for selection bias. *Econometrica* **48**, 1815–1820.
22. Hogan, W. and Laird, N.M. (1997). Mixture models for the joint distribution of repeated measures and event times. *Statistics in Medicine* **16**, 239–257.
23. Little, R.J.A. (1993). Pattern mixture models for multivariate incomplete data. *Journal of the American Statistical Association* **88**, 125–134.
24. Childhood Asthma Management Program (CAMP) Research Group (2000). Long-term effects of budesonide or nedocromil in children with asthma. *New England Journal of Medicine* **343**, 1054–1063.
25. Zucker, D.M., Zerbe, G.O. and Wu, M.C. (1995). Inference for the association between coefficients in a multivariate growth curve model. *Biometrics* **51**, 413–424.

26. Wu, M.C., Hunsberger, S. and Zucker, D. (1994). Testing for differences in changes in the presence of informative censoring: parametric and non-parametric methods. *Statistics in Medicine* **13**, 635–646.

APPENDIX

The model used to generate the dropout process in the simulated clinical trials of Section 3 are as:

D1: Probit informative dropout where the probability of dropout depends on the underlying initial value b_{i1}, and the rate of change, b_{i2}, of the true response. That is,

$$P(T_i < t_j | b_i) = \Phi(\theta_{0j} + \theta_1 b_{i1} + \theta_2 b_{i2}). \qquad \text{(A1)}$$

D2: Logistic informative dropout where the probability of dropout depends on the expected true value of the missed response. That is,

$$\text{Logit}\,[P(T_i = t_j | b_i, T_i > t_{j-1})] = \theta_{0j} + \theta_1(b_{i1} + b_{i2}t_j). \qquad \text{(A2)}$$

D3: Logistic informative dropout where the probability of dropout depends on the last observed response but not the underlying missed response. That is,

$$\text{Logit}\,[P(T_i = t_j | T_i > t_{j-1}, Y_{j-1})] = \theta_{0j} + \theta_1 Y_{j-1}. \qquad \text{(A3)}$$

D4: Logistic informative dropout where the probability of dropout depends on both the true value of the underlying missed response and the last observed response. That is,

$$\text{Logit}\,[P(T_i = t_j | T_i > t_{j-1}, Y_{j-1}, b_i)] = \theta_{0j} + \theta_1 Y_{j-1} + \theta_2(b_{i1} + b_{i2}t_j). \qquad \text{(A4)}$$

The parameter values used were $\theta_1 = 7.0$, $\theta_2 = 15.3$ in (A1); $\theta_1 = 15.2$ in (A2); $\theta_1 = 10.1$ in (A3); and $\theta_1 = 2.1$ and $\theta_2 = 13.1$ in (A4).

The total dropout rate assumed for the placebo group was 35% in 3 years and approximately equally distributed in each of the 3 years of follow-up. The same dropout parameter values were used in both treatment groups.

Definition: A function $f(x, a)$ is totally positive of order 2, or TP2, if for all $x < x'$ and $a < a'$, $f(x, a)f(x', a') \geq f(x, a')f(x', a)$.